AYURVEDIC HEALING

A Comprehensive Guide

2006

1

AYURVEDIC HEALING

A COMPREHENSIVE GUIDE
By Dr. David Frawley, O.M.D.

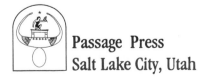

Passage Press
Salt Lake City, Utah

Passage Press is a division of Morson Publishing
Morson Publishing
P.O. Box 21713
Salt Lake City, Utah 84121-0713

**This book is a reference work not intended to treat, diagnose or prescribe.
The information contained herein is no way to be considered as a substitute for consultation with a duly licensed health-care professional.**

All translations from the Sanskrit by David Frawley

Cover design by Kari Jenson & Robben Hixson

Library of Congress Catalog Card Number: 96-72136
ISBN 1-878-423-00-2

CONTENTS

PART II: The Treatment of Disease

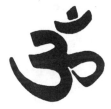

*W*ithin all of us is the archetype of the Divine healer. This Divine healer is the true healer in all beings, not any particular individual or special personality. To heal ourselves or others we must set it in motion within ourselves.

Dhanvantari, an incarnation of the God Vishnu, the immanent Divine consciousness, represents this truth in the tradition of Ayurveda. His statue is found at most Ayurvedic schools and clinics. It is a reminder that however much we know or skillful we become, everything still depends on the grace of the spiritual nature. Hence, this book is dedicated to the Divine healer within you.

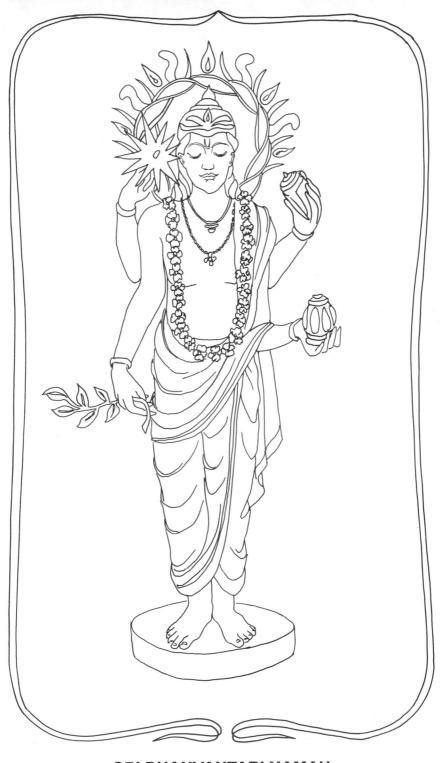

SRI DHANVANTARI NAMAH

FOREWORD

I started reading the manuscript of *Ayurvedic Healing* with a simple curiosity to see how a Western teacher and practitioner of Ayurveda interprets it. I ended my reading with profound admiration of his deep insight and clear grasp of the fundamental principles of this ancient Indian Science of Life.

It was a fascinating experience for me to observe how a Western mind enters with perfect ease into the realms of intuitive knowledge of the East. This book is a splendid attempt to build a bridge of understanding between the Eastern and Western minds and their two often opposite views of life. The author has succeeded in giving a reorientation of our ancient wisdom of India to suit the needs of the modern world. He has rightly pointed out that "Ayurveda today is part of a new movement towards a global medicine that includes the best developments from all lands." The author's effort in this and his other books will certainly help in creating a proper climate for such a synthesis.

Dr. Frawley enjoys some unique advantages as an Ayurvedic spokesmen. He is primarily a Vedic scholar. Ayurveda is part of the Vedas, the oldest record of supreme knowledge and experience of mankind, the essence of which is man's harmony with nature and the individual's oneness with the universe. Ayurveda is to be viewed in such a wider perspective. Dr. Frawley has developed that vision. He is well acquainted with Sanskrit, the language of the original texts of Ayurveda. This has enabled him to reveal the deeper meanings of the terms and concepts mentioned in the texts. Literal translation of the Sanskrit terms into English almost destroys the sense of what was originally meant. Dr. Frawley is faithful to the spirit of the teachings in his translation and adaptation of them.

In addition he is a student of Yoga, the practical science of mind. He has acquired expertise in Vedic Astrology. He has studied and taught Chinese medicine. Naturally, with such a rare combination, he is the most qualified person to introduce Ayurveda to the Western world in light of its contemporary problems and life-style. His attempt symbolizes the world view of health.

The information given in this book covers almost all significant features of the Ayurvedic system and also of Yoga. This includes constitutions of individuals, diet, health care, herbal therapies, specialized methods of relief, cure and revitalization such as: oil massage, Pancha Karma, mantra, meditation, gems and, above all, the spiritual aspects of life. The main emphasis is naturally on diet and herbs with many home remedies.

Many Ayurvedic herbs have been acknowledged by modern researchers for their specific properties. It may be relevant here to quote the latest scientific study on the rejuvenation (Rasayana) concept of Ayurveda by a group of modern pharmacologists in India. They chose five plants for their experimental study. These were ashwagandha (Withania somnifera), shatavari (Asparagus racemosus), haritaki (Terminalia chebula), pippali or long pepper (Piper longum) and guduchi (Tinosporia cordifolia). The study concluded that,

> Based on this experimental evidence we propose that the Rasayanas (rejuvenative substances) of Ayurveda harmonize the functions of the body by modulating the neuroendocrine-immune function. This strengthens the individual's general resistance by stimulating the immune function, a concept similar to 'prohost therapy'. The role of stress and emotion on immunological dysfunction is very well known, so is the role of stress in pathogenesis of many diseases. Therefore, it seems feasible that increased immuno-competence improves the quality of tissues so that they sustain effects of external and internal stress better. *(Ayurveda Revisited,* Dr. Sharadini A. Dahanukar and Dr. Urmila M. Thatte, Bombay, India).

Perhaps Rasayana therapy and Yoga may prove to be the most effective integrated treatment for the health problems in which immune system and emotional problems are involved. Dr. Frawley blazes a new trail in this direction by coordinating such intuitional and scientific wisdoms in his approach.

Lastly, Dr. Frawley has explained the spiritual aspect of life, a vital issue in the ultimate analysis of health and disease. Hindu spirituality believes in individualistic religion and pleads for freedom and spontaneity. This frame of mind transforms human emotions into Divine bliss and restores one's integrity of being, as the *Yoga Sutras* state (I.3.), "then the Seer returns to his own nature."

Ayurveda insists on spiritual and ethical discipline for mental health and normal development of personality. Dr. R.D. Lele, eminent physician and pioneer in Nuclear medicine in India, has appreciated this aspect of Ayurveda in his book *Ayurveda and Modern Medicine.* He states, "The wisdom of Ayurveda lies in incorporating a code of conduct in the Science of Life as a means to ensuring mental health and happiness." Dr. Frawley has dealt with this aspect in all its details.

In conclusion, I must express my happiness as an Indian in welcoming Dr. Frawley to the community of distinguished commentators of Ayurveda and Yoga. He deserves a place of honor in his own right.

Dr. B. L. Vashta
February 1989
Bombay, India

*****

Dr. B. L. Vashta (69) completed his educational course and obtained the qualification of 'Ayurvedic Visharad' (proficiency in Ayurveda) in 1945. He was a professor of Ayurveda for some years, has written many books and is a regular columnist on health in leading Indian magazines. An eminent scholar of Ayurveda, Yoga and Naturopathy, he is also a consultant to major Ayurvedic companies in India. Currently he is advisor of the Institute of Yoga and Ayurveda (Panvel-Bombay, India). He participates in international seminars and conferences and has joined the efforts to spread the knowledge of Ayurveda in India and abroad.

INTRODUCTION

Ayurveda is the knowledge that indicates the appropriate and inappropriate, happy or sorrowful conditions of living, what is auspicious or inauspicious for longevity, as well as the measure of life itself.
—*Charaka Samhita I. 41.*

Ayurveda, which literally means 'the science of life', is the natural healing system of India, its traditional medicine going back to ancient times. It was established by the same great seers and sages who produced India's original systems of Yoga and meditation.

Ayurveda originated as part of 'Vedic Science'. This is an integral spiritual science devised to give a comprehensive understanding of all the universe, which it sees as working according to a single law. Vedic Science includes Yoga, meditation, and astrology, and sets forth Ayurveda as its branch for dealing with the physical body. In this broad and profound background of Vedic Science, Ayurveda includes herbal medicine, dietetics, body work, surgery, psychology and spirituality.

Ayurveda is the healing gift to us from the ancient enlightened Vedic culture. According to astronomical records in ancient Vedic texts, the Vedic system, including Ayurveda, was in practice before 4000 B.C., when the vernal equinox was in the constellations of Orion and Gemini. Recent archeological work in India has discovered Dwaraka, the ancient city of Krishna, under the sea off the coast of Gujarat where Krishna's story described it as submerged. Krishna is said to have lived at the last phase of the Vedic era. The site has been scientifically dated at 1500 B.C. Hence, we know that Ayurveda was already old and predominant in India thousands of years ago.

Ayurveda has gone through several stages of development in its long history. It spread with Vedic and Hindu culture as far east as Indonesia, and to the west it influenced the ancient Greeks, who developed a similar form of medicine. It was used by the Buddhists, who added many new insights to it, and they took it, along with their religion, to many different countries. In this way, Ayurveda became the basis of the healing traditions of Tibet, Sri Lanka, Burma and other Buddhist lands and influenced Chinese medicine. Many great Buddhist sages, like Nagarjuna, perhaps the most important figure in the Mahayana tradition after the Buddha, were Ayurvedic doctors and wrote commentaries on classical Ayurvedic texts. Hence, Ayurveda is a rich tradition, adaptable to many different times, cultures and climates.

Today Ayurveda, in yet another stage of development, is undergoing readaptation to the Western world and modern conditions. This book is part of the new adaptation, yet endeavors to hold to the fundamental and universal principles of this science of life in the process.

Ayurveda is part of a new movement towards a global medicine that includes the best developments in the medicines of all lands. A new naturalistic planetary medicine is emerging, largely through a reexamination of the older Eastern and traditional medicines of native peoples throughout the world. Of all the systems, Ayurveda is probably the best point of synthesis for such a global medicine. It contains the broadest number of healing modalities. It retains much of the language of alchemy, which was a kind of global medical and spiritual tradition in ancient and medieval times. The medicine of India has much in common with both the Chinese and European, and often represents a point of integration between them. We may find that much of the medicine to heal the planet and usher in a new age of world unity is already contained in this, perhaps the oldest of all healing systems.

Ayurvedic Healing is a sequel to my previous book on the Ayurvedic usage of herbs, *The Yoga of Herbs* (coauthored with Dr. Vasant Lad), and is based upon it. *The Yoga of Herbs* presents the background theory of Ayurvedic herbalism and gives a list of accessible herbs for Ayurvedic usage. It defines many common Western herbs in Ayurvedic terms. *Ayurvedic Healing* expands this knowledge and introduces many classical herbal formulas of Ayurveda. It gives special modern Ayurvedic formulas designed specifically for the West and our conditions here. In addition, it provides further Ayurvedic usage and formulas for Western herbs.

It should be noted that this book still presents only a fraction of the useful Ayurvedic herbs and formulas. It presents only those which are available in the West or likely to become so soon. Many others could have been chosen of equal effectiveness.

On this foundation of herbal medicine, *Ayurvedic Healing* is oriented towards the practical treatment of disease and is intended to serve as a basic handbook of Ayurvedic therapy. Many people in response to *The Yoga of Herbs* have requested additional information on specific diseases, and it is partly for them that I have written this book. It adds relevant dietary, life-style and Yogic methods to enhance herbal therapy, including the use of oils, aromas, colors, gems and mantras.

Ayurvedic Healing has two levels; one for the layman and self-care, the other for the natural healer and his practice. The first outlines a general constitutional or life-style treatment for health enhancement and disease prevention. It gives many common or home-remedies for different diseases. It is important to realize that many of our diseases can best be treated by ourselves. Often a few simple therapies done as part of our daily regime can be effective. It is only when our life-style is out of harmony that more severe diseases arise, and more specialized and complicated health care becomes necessary.

The second level provides some of this specialized Ayurvedic medical knowledge and outlines more technical and complicated remedies. These may be better utilized by a health care professional. Also, it should be noted that the accounts of diseases and their treatments are given here only in essence. More specific knowledge and experienced practice may be necessary to deal with severe conditions or acute symptoms.

I have included relevant Western and Chinese remedies for reference purposes. They are not meant to set forth these other systems in detail but to allow a point of connection with the Ayurvedic approach. The Chinese and the Ayurvedic systems have much in common and can often be used to complement or supplement each other. The Ayurvedic system as a global medicine, a version of a universal healing science, encourages such dialogue and synthesis. The United States, like Tibet in ancient times, is being influenced by both of these prime Asian healing systems; we may also arrive at a synthesis of their approaches. Boundaries between healing systems, like political boundaries, are of human invention and do not exist in nature. They belong to the Middle Ages, not to the New Age when a reintegration of human knowledge and culture is necessary.

An Overview of the Disease Process

According to the spiritual tradition of India, diseases have two causes. First, they can arise from physical or biological causes: the imbalance of the biological humors, the elements and prime energies of the physical body. Treatment involves mainly physical or medical methods with a naturalistic basis including herbs, diet, body work and Yogic postures (asanas). In more extreme cases mineral and drug medicines or surgery may be required.

Second, diseases can arise from karmic causes: from the effects of wrong actions we have done in life, meaning from psychological or spiritual causes. These may be wrong occupation, problems in relationship or emotional difficulties, and treatment may require changes in life-style and attitude. Such causes include not living up to our inner purpose or spiritual will in life, what is called in Sanskrit our 'dharma'. Diseases can arise from wrong actions in a previous life, primarily those which brought harm to other beings or misused our power or resources.

Such karmic diseases may require some form of atonement or sacrifice, an 'inner rectification' to reestablish our well being in life. For this Ayurveda uses yoga and a system of divine or spiritual therapy (daiva cikitsa) which includes the use of gems, mantras, prayers, rituals and meditations. These are not medieval superstition but reflect a profound understanding of the deeper levels of the mind and the means of healing the subtler aspects of our being.

According to Ayurveda, the human being consists of three bodies: the physical, astral and causal, or what could be called in Western terms, body, mind and soul. Its system of diagnosis and treatment, though focused on the physical, considers the other two also. Many Ayurvedic methods are ways of correcting disorders in the energy field behind the physical body, as well as the field of consciousness behind it.

Most disease conditions involve both physical and spiritual factors and require treatment on both levels. Ayurveda, traditionally, involves a holistic treatment of the entire human being and our full cosmic nature.

Religion, Spirituality and Healing

The word 'God', for many of us in our culture, often has negative connotations, largely because spiritual truth has been misrepresented by organized and fundamentalist religions. This has been more common in the Western religions of Judaism, Christianity and Islam and their tendency towards exclusivism in their beliefs than in the meditation-oriented teachings of the Orient, which emphasize open-mindedness. Yet a lack of faith in the Divine, which is something like a lack of faith in life or a positive will to live, is found in many diseases. Disease is often a lack of love, including a lack of caring for oneself and one's physical body.

Hence, the first step in healing is often to open up to the Divine or cosmic will and accept the flow of grace. This requires understanding that one's life has a purpose and meaning in the development of the soul and in the spiritual evolution of humanity as a whole. It involves seeking the truth in whatever way is closest to our heart, following the spiritual path truest to our nature. Yet this must include respecting the right of others to follow their own paths. We might call this 'first healing the soul', remembering that the soul, in the Yogic system, is our inner consciousness.

Western medicine has tried to get religion out of medicine. This has been an important and necessary step in the evolution of the mind. Organized religion's dogma, authoritarianism and repressive nature have no place in the realms of knowledge, which require freedom and objectivity for direct perception to occur. Something has been gained by ridding medicine of the outer forms of religion, but something greater has been lost by removing the inner aspect as well.

The essence of healing is integration. Faith, love, devotion, the sense of the unity and sacred nature of humanity and all life are missing in modern medicine. These qualities do not create any dogma, nor do they impose any idea, will or discipline on another. They give the space and the freedom to grow and to see. They create the grace and flow of the cosmic life-force necessary for healing to occur. Without them we are broken and withered inside, and our lives have little meaning. Without them the magic, wonder, beauty and purpose in life are taken away. Most of us today are sick because this spiritual meaning is not present in our lives. We are trapped in the tedium and stimulation of the outer world with practically nothing to nourish our hearts.

Ayurveda cannot accept medicine without religion. From its hallowed ancient perspective, that is like healing without love. This does not mean Ayurveda wishes to impose its religious background on anyone. Along with the regular tools and methods of natural healing, it provides Yogic methods which can be adapted to whatever form (or formlessness) our religious or spiritual life may take. As the Mother of healing, Ayurveda transmits this grace of the Divine Mother.

This is also the beauty of the religious tradition of India. It is not so much an organized religion as a spiritual resource, providing every possible approach to truth so each individual can find what is necessary and meaningful for themselves. It discards nothing, neither does it insist upon anything. It respects the Divine nature and freedom of each individual. Hence its true and original name is the "Sanatana Dharma", the eternal or universal religion, which is the religion of life itself. From this background also came the practice of Ayurveda.

If not a sign of spiritual crisis or change, disease is at the least, a spiritual opportunity. According to the *Upanishads*, the main spiritual teachings of ancient India, disease is the highest form of asceticism (tapas), whereby the truth of life and the truth of one's own self can be revealed. Disease may be a sign of wrong action in life, but it can also be an indication that the soul is directing its energy within. Either way it requires a spiritual reexamination of our lives, particularly if the disease is severe. Hence, self-examination is the first step and fundamental basis of understanding and resolving any disease.

All life is learning and a development of self-knowledge. For disease to become understood it must be viewed in this light. We must, therefore, not just treat disease, but use disease as a tool for understanding ourselves in both our superficial and deeper layers. Once this communion with our inner consciousness is gained, we will find an inner harmony and joy that can overcome all external difficulties. It is on this developing self-awareness that the healing methods and remedial measures suggested herein should be employed.

There is no final Ayurvedic way of looking at or treating a disease. Ayurveda provides energetic guidelines, but these have to be applied on an individual basis. In this book I have presented some diseases in a different way than classical Ayurvedic texts. This has been done according to the need to revise the Ayurvedic view from the past to what is necessary for our conditions today. Other Ayurvedic practitioners may view, or treat, diseases from other angles. This reveals the expansiveness of the Ayurvedic vision, not some inconsistency within it.

I would like to thank Dr. B.L. Vashta for going over this text and for his ongoing assistance in all aspects of my work, and Dr. Subhash Ranade and the Ayurveda Shikshan Mandala in Pune, India for their encouragement, in addition Mr. Anand Puranik for help with my research and studies in India.

May this book contribute to the welfare of all beings. May it stimulate the creative intelligence of all who come into contact with it.

Namaste! Reverence to the Divine Spirit within you!

David Frawley,
Santa Fe, New Mexico
February 1989

PART I

THE PRINCIPLES AND THERAPIES OF THE SCIENCE OF LIFE

Vata, Pitta and Kapha, the group of the three biological humors, in their natural and disturbed states, give life to the body and destroy it.

—Ashtanga Hridaya, I. 6.

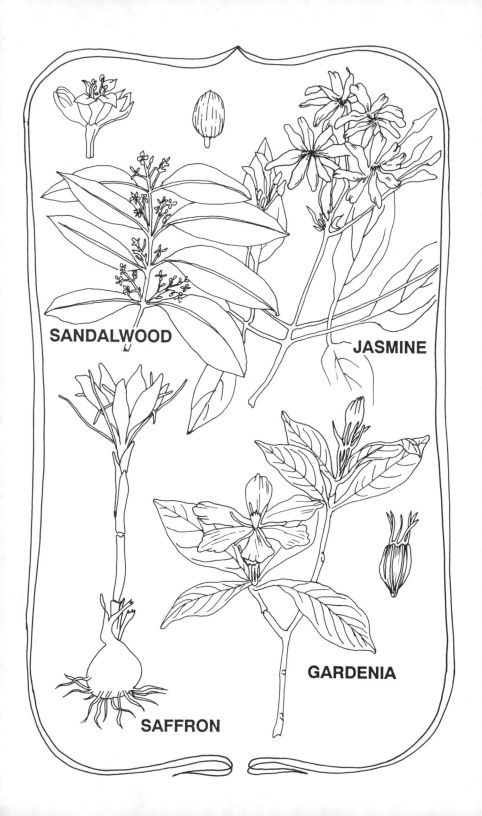

SANDALWOOD

JASMINE

SAFFRON

GARDENIA

1
THE BIOLOGICAL HUMORS
THE DYNAMICS OF THE LIFE-FORCE

The Three Great Cosmic Forces

According to the ancient seers of India, as recorded in the mantras of the *Rig Veda,* the oldest of the scriptures of India, there are three basic forces in existence. First of all, there is a principle of energy that gives force, velocity, direction, animation, motivation. Life is nothing if not a play of forces, continually changing. As modern science confirms, matter is energy and what seems solid is but a static appearance of innumerable, subtle moving forces.

This energy of life was called Prana, meaning the primal breath or life force. All energy follows a movement of inhalation and exhalation like the breath. All material energy is a development of pure energy, which is the power of life itself; energy is life. The ancient seers perceived the energy of the universe as the manifestation of the life-force, ever seeking greater life, awareness, freedom and creative unfoldment.

Hidden in all energy is the working of a conscious will. Energy is will in action in the outer world. Behind will is sentience or consciousness as the power of determination. Hence, this Prana was also called Purusha, the Primal Spirit. Life is being, the consciousness principle. It manifests in nature as the working of intelligence behind the movement of energy. This natural or organic intelligence is conscious and sure in it's plan and method; not conscious by choice or intention but intuitively and spontaneously a movement of pure beauty and harmony. It's glory is manifest in all of nature, from the flowers to the stars.

The second of the triad of forces they perceived as a principle of light, or radiance. Energy is light. Energy, as it moves, undergoes transformation and emits light and heat. There is a natural warmth to all life. And there is a natural light to all energy. There is in all life a principle of reflection, a transparency that manifests as intelligence and consciousness. Hence, in all chemical reactions is concealed the power of light as the ability of consciousness to transform itself. Within the first spark is latent the light of the highest awareness.

The third of these forces was seen as a principle of cohesion. In all manifestation is a common unity. There is an interlinking of forces into a single rhythm. There is an affinity of forces in which all are ultimately linked together in one great harmony. This cohesiveness was seen not only as a chemical property; it also reveals a conscious intent. It manifests the power of love. Love is the real force that holds all things together.

These three are one; life is light, which is love. The energetic principle (life), possesses a radiance (light), which in turn has a bonding power (love). We must ever seek greater life, light and love as this is the nature of the universe itself.

In the Vedas, the spirit of life was symbolized as the great god Indra, the dragon slayer and wielder of the thunderbolt (Sanskrit vajra). The spirit of light was worshipped as Agni, the god of fire, the divinity of vision and of sacrifice. The spirit of love was worshipped as Soma, the nectar of immortality. Hidden in these cryptic mantras is the primal code of all cosmic law, the key to all levels of working of the universal force. Through these mantras we can learn to balance and control the humors they govern. This not only creates health but gives the basis for rejuvenation of the mind and transformation of consciousness. Ayurveda and other branches of Vedic Science, like Yoga, are the development of the prime insights of the Veda in particular directions.

These same three deities, or principles, of life, light and love, are also reflected in ancient European mythology. For example, Zeus, Apollo and Dionysus were worshipped by the Greeks, though here the symbolism is more poetic and less mystical.

These three forces, life, light and love, are symbolized by the three elements of air, fire and water. According to ancient mythology, in the beginning heaven and earth were one. There was no space between them in which living beings could manifest. Then, by the will of the Creator, the gods came into being and separated heaven and earth, drawing apart the two firmaments. In the space between, they set in motion the life-force to allow for creatures to come into being. This life-force became the atmosphere in which the elements of air, fire and water as wind, sun and rain, provided for the development of life.

The Three Biological Humors

According to Ayurveda there are three primary life-forces in the body, or three biological humors. These are called in Sanskrit "Vata," "Pitta" and "Kapha." They correspond primarily to the elements of air, fire and water. As the active or mobile elements, they determine the life processes of growth and decay.

The Ayurvedic term for humor is Dosha, meaning that which darkens, spoils or causes things to decay. When out of balance, the humors are the causative forces in the disease process.

The biological air humor is called Vata, sometimes also translated as wind. In terms of etymology, it means 'that which moves things'. It is the motivating force behind the other two humors, which are considered to be 'lame', incapable of movement without it. It also governs our sensory and mental balance and orientation, and promotes mental adaptability and comprehension.

The biological fire humor is called Pitta, sometimes also translated as bile. Its etymological meaning is 'that which digests things'. It is responsible for all chemical and metabolic transformations in the body. It also governs our mental digestion, our capacity to perceive reality and understand things as they are.

The biological water humor is called Kapha, sometimes also translated as phlegm. Etymologically it means 'that which holds things together'. It provides substance and gives support, and makes up the bulk of our bodily tissues. It also provides our emotional support in life and governs such positive emotional traits as love, compassion, modesty, patience and forgiveness.

Each of these humors exists in a second element which serves as the medium for its manifestation or acts as its container.

Vata, air, is contained in ether, and so it is also said to be composed of ether. It resides in the empty spaces in the body and fills up the subtle channels.

Pitta, fire, exists in the body as water or oil, and so is said to contain an aspect of water. It exists mainly in an acid form, as fire cannot exist directly in the body without destroying it.

Kapha, water, exists in the medium of earth, which contains it, and so it is also said to be composed of earth. Our physical composition is mainly water which is contained within various boundaries of our skin and other tissue linings (earth).

Qualities of the Humors

Each humor has its primary qualities. According to Vagbhatta, one of the great Ayurvedic commentators: "Vata is dry, light, cold, rough, subtle and agitated. Pitta is a little oily, is sharp, hot, light, unpleasant in odor, mobile and liquid. Kapha is wet, cold, heavy, dull, sticky, soft and firm." *(Ashtanga Hridaya I. 11–12).*

Vata (the air humor) is primarily dry, cold and light. Pitta (the fire humor) is primarily hot, moist and light. Kapha (the water humor) is primarily cold, moist and heavy. Each of the humors thus shares one major quality and is opposite in two others.

It is by their attributes that we recognize them. An excess or deficiency of these qualities indicates an excess or deficiency of the humor. This, in turn, brings about various pathological changes in the body.

Actions of the Humors
(Quotes from *Ashtanga Hridaya XI. 1–3*)

Their actions, on both the body and the mind, are described as follows: "The root of the humors, tissues and waste materials of the body is Vata (air). In its natural state it sustains effort, exhalation, inhalation, movement and the discharge of impulses, the equilibrium of the tissues, and the coordination of the senses."

Vata (air) is the most important, or primary, of the three biological humors. It governs the other two and is responsible for all physical processes in general. For this reason, disturbances in Vata tend to have more severe implications than the other two humors, and often affect the mind as well as the entire physical body. Hence, it is the quality of our life, through our care of the life-force, that is the primary factor in both health and disease. "Pitta (fire) governs digestion, heat, visual perception, hunger, thirst, lustre, complexion, understanding, intelligence, courage and softness of the body." Pitta governs all aspects and levels of light and warmth in the body and mind. "Kapha (water) gives stability, lubrication, holding together of the joints and such qualities as patience." Kapha is the material substratum and support of the other two humors and also gives stability to the emotional nature.

Aggravated States of the Humors
(Quotes from *Ashtanga Hridaya XI. 6–8*)

When aggravated the humors give rise to various symptoms and various diseases. "In excess, Vata (air) causes emaciation, debility, liking of warmth, tremors, distention and constipation, as well as insomnia, sensory disorientation, incoherent speech, dizziness, confusion and depression." High Vata (high air) results in the life-force and the mind losing their connection with the body, causing decay and loss of coordination. There is hyperactivity at the expense of the vital fluids and the physical body tends to waste away.

"Pitta (fire) in excess causes yellow color of stool, urine, eyes and skin, as well as hunger, thirst, burning sensation and difficulty sleeping." High Pitta (high fire) results in the accumulation of internal heat or fever, with inflammation and infections. We literally begin to burn ourselves up.

"Kapha (water) causes depression of the digestive fire, nausea, lethargy, heaviness, white color, chills, looseness of the limbs, cough, difficult breathing and excessive sleeping." High Kapha (high water) results in the accumulation of weight and gravity in the body, which inhibits normal function and causes hypoactivity through excess tissue accumulation.

Sites of the Humors

Each humor has its respective site in the body. "Vata (air) is located in the colon, thighs, hips, ears, bones and organ of touch. Its primary site is in the colon. "Pitta (fire) is located in the small intestine, stomach, sweat, sebaceous glands, blood, lymph and the organ of vision. Its primary site is in the small intestine. "Kapha (water) is located in the chest, throat, head, pancreas, sides, stomach, lymph, fat, nose and tongue. Its primary site is the stomach." (*Ashtanga Hridaya XII. 1–3.*)

At these primary sites the humors accumulate, giving rise to the disease process. Treating them at these locations by their respective methods, we can cut the disease process off at the root.

These locations are in terms of their derangements. Vata (air), when deranged, is produced from below, as gas from the colon. Pitta (fire), when deranged, is produced in the middle as bile and acids from the liver and small intestine. Kapha (water), when deranged, is produced above as phlegm in the lungs and stomach.

The Five Forms of Vata (Air)

The five forms of Vata are called, in Sanskrit, "Prana," "Udana," "Samana," "Vyana" and "Apana," for which there are no equivalent terms in English. They are formed by adding various suffixes to the root 'an', which means to breathe or to energize.

Prana (pra-ana) means the forward or primary air or nervous force. Pervading the head and centered in the brain, it moves downward to the chest and throat, governing inhalation and swallowing, as well as sneezing, spitting and belching. It governs the senses, mind, heart and consciousness. It is our portion of the cosmic life energy and directs all the other Vatas in the body. It determines our inspiration or positive spirit in life and connects us with our inner Self. The term 'Prana' is also used in a broader sense to indicate Vata in general, as all Vatas derive from it.

Udana (ud-ana) means the upward moving air or nervous force. Located in the chest and centered in the throat, it governs exhalation and speech. It is also responsible for memory, strength, will and effort.

Udana determines our aspiration in life. At death it rises up from the body and directs us towards various subtle worlds according to the power of our will and the karma that move through it. When fully developed it gives us the power to transcend the outer world, as well as various psychic powers. The practice of Yoga is involved primarily with developing Udana.

Samana (sama-ana) means the equalizing air. It is centered in the small intestine and is the nervous force behind the digestive system.

Vyana (vi-ana) means the diffusive or pervasive air. It is centered in the heart and distributed throughout the entire body. It governs the circulatory system and, through it, the movement of the joints and muscles and the discharge of impulses and secretions.

Apana (apa-ana) means the downward moving air or the air that moves away. It is centered in the colon and governs all downward moving impulses of elimination, urination, menstruation, parturition and sex.

As Udana, the ascending air, carries our life-force upwards and brings about the evolution or liberation of consciousness, Apana, the descending air, carries it down and brings about the devolution or limitation of consciousness. Apana supports and controls all the other forms of Vata, and derangements of it are the basis of most Vata disorders. As a downward moving force, when aggravated it causes decay and disintegration. Hence, the treatment of Apana is the first consideration in the treatment of Vata.

The Five Forms of Pitta (Fire)

The five forms of Pitta are called in Sanskrit "Sadhaka," "Bhrajaka," "Pachaka," "Alochaka" and "Ranjaka." These also have no English equivalents.

Pachaka Pitta is the fire that digests things. It is located in the small intestine and governs the power of digestion. It is the basis and support of the other forms of Pitta, and is the first consideration in the treatment of Pitta, as our primary source of heat is the digestive fire.

Sadhaka Pitta is the fire that determines what is truth or reality. It is located in the brain and the heart and allows us to accomplish the goals of the intellect, intelligence or ego. These include worldly goals of pleasure, wealth and prestige and the spiritual goal of liberation. It governs our mental energy, mental digestion (the digestion of ideas or beliefs) and our power of discrimination. Its development is emphasized in Yoga, particularly the Yoga of Knowledge.

Bhrajaka Pitta is the fire that governs lustre or complexion. It is located in the skin and maintains the complexion and color of skin. When aggravated, for example, it causes skin rashes or discolorations. It governs our digestion of warmth or heat which we experience through the skin.

Alochaka Pitta is the fire that governs visual perception. It is located in the eyes and is responsible for the reception and digestion of light from the external world.

Ranjaka Pitta is the fire that imparts color. It is located in the liver, spleen, stomach and small intestine, and gives color to the blood, bile and stool. It primarily resides in the blood and is involved in most liver disorders.

The Five Forms of Kapha (Water)

The five forms of Kapha are called in Sanskrit "Tarpaka," "Avalambaka," "Kledaka," "Bodhaka" and "Sleshaka."

Tarpaka Kapha is the form of water that gives contentment. It is located in the brain, as the cerebro-spinal fluid, and the heart. It governs emotional calm, stability and happiness, as well as memory. The practice of Yoga also increases the mental form of Kapha as contentment and bliss (Ananda).

Sleshaka Kapha is the form of water that gives lubrication. It is located in the joints as the synovial fluid and is responsible for holding them together.

Kledaka Kapha is the form of water that moistens. It is located in the stomach, as the secretions of the mucous lining. It is responsible for the liquification of food and for the first stage of digestion.

Bodhaka Kapha is the form of water that gives perception. It is located in the mouth and tongue as the saliva that allows us to taste our food. Like Kledaka, it is also part of the first stage of digestion.

Avalambaka Kapha is the form of water that gives support. It is located in the heart and lungs. It is the storehouse of Kapha (phlegm) and upon it depend the actions of the other Kaphas in the body. It is not simply the phlegm produced by the lungs, as that is an excess of Kapha generally. It corresponds to the basic plasma of the body, its primary watery constituent, which is distributed by lung and heart action.

Tissues

According to Ayurveda the human body is composed of seven Dhatus or tissue layers. These form concentric circles from the gross to the subtle. They are: 1. plasma (rasa), sometimes called 'skin', 2. blood (rakta), 3. muscle (mamsa), 4. fat or adipose tissue (medas), 5. bone (asthi), 6. marrow and nerve tissue (majja) and 7. semen or reproductive tissue (shukra).

Kapha (water) is responsible for all the tissues, generally, as it is the basic substance of the body. It is specifically responsible for five: plasma, muscle, fat, marrow and semen. Pitta (fire) creates blood and Vata (air) creates bone.

Diseases of the humors are usually reflected in the tissues they govern. However, any of the humors can enter into any of the tissues and cause various diseases. Diseases are classified not only according to the humors but also according to which tissues the humors have entered.

Bodily Systems (Srotas)

Ayurveda sees the human body as composed of innumerable channels that supply the various tissues of the body. Health is the proper flow through these channels. Disease is improper flow, which may be excessive, deficient, blockage, or flow out of the proper channel altogether. The excess humors move into the channels causing these various wrong flows. The channels are similar to the different physiological systems of Western medicine but also contain subtler energy fields such as the meridian system of Chinese medicine. A complex symptomology of channel system-disorders exists in Ayurveda. Diseases are classified according to the systems they involve. Examination of the channels by various diagnostic measures is one of the main tools for determining the nature and power of disease.

Three channels connect with the outside environment and bring nourishment into the body in the form of breath, food and water.

1. Pranavaha Srotas: the channels that carry Prana, the breath or life-force, primarily the respiratory system (though aspects of the circulatory system are contained in this idea as well). It originates in the heart and the gastrointestinal tract, primarily the colon.

2. Annavaha Srotas: the channels that carry food, the digestive system. Its origins are in the stomach and left side of the body.

3. Ambhuvaha Srotas: the channels that carry water or regulate water metabolism. This does not have an equivalent in Western medicine. (Diabetes, for example, is a disease of this system.) It originates in the palate and the pancreas.

Seven channels supply the seven tissues of the body.

4. Rasavaha Srotas: the channels that carry plasma (rasa). This is similar to the lymphatic system. Its origins are in the heart and blood vessels.

5. Raktavaha Srotas: the channels that carry blood (rakta). This relates to the circulatory system. Its origins are the liver and spleen.

6. Mamsavaha Srotas: the channels that supply muscles (mamsa), or the muscular system. It originates in the ligaments and skin.

7. Medavaha Srotas: the channels that supply fat or adipose tissue (medas), or the adipose system. Its origins are the kidneys and omentum.

8. Asthivaha Srotas: the channels that supply the bones (asthi) or the skeletal system. Its origins are adipose tissue and the hips.

9. Majjavaha Srotas: the channels that supply the marrow and nerve tissue (majja), mainly the nervous system. Its origins are the bones and joints.

10. Shukravaha Srotas: the channels that supply the reproductive tissue (shukra) or the reproductive system. Its origin is the testes or the uterus.

Three additional channels connect to the outside world and allow for the elimination of substances from the body. The waste product of breath is sweat, of food is feces, of water is urine. These three waste materials are called the three Malas and they can also be damaged or obstructed by excess accumulations of the humors.

11. Svedavaha Srotas: the channels that carry sweat (sveda) or the sebaceous system. It originates in adipose tissue and the hair follicles.

12. Purishavaha Srotas: the channels that carry feces (purisha) or the excretory system. It originates in the colon and rectum.

13. Mutravaha Srotas: the channels that carry urine (mutra) or the urinary system. It originates in the bladder and kidneys.

Two special systems exist within the female.

14. Artavavaha Srotas: the channels that carry menstruation.

15. Stanyavaha Srotas: the channels that carry the breast milk, or the system of lactation, treated as the subsystem of the menstrual system.

The mind itself exists as a special system. It connects to the nervous system (majjavaha srotas) and the reproductive system (shukravaha srotas). The movement of energy in all the channels depends upon the stimulus that arises from the mind.

16. Manovaha Srotas: the channels that carry thought or the mental system.

Earlier Western Views of the Humors

Ancient and Medieval Western medicine up to the time of the seventeenth century was based upon a system of biological humors. It had much in common with Ayurvedic medicine and a number of contacts existed, particularly between the Ancient Greeks and Hindus. Apollonius of Tyana, fourth century B.C., a famous Greek sage and hermetic figure, visited India and brought much of its knowledge back with him. He was a highly regarded figure in Western thinking through out the middle ages and later.

In addition, the older pre-Christian healing traditions and folk medicine (like that of the Druids) of our ancient European ancestors, including not only the Greeks and Romans, but also the Kelts, Germans and Slavs, apparently also had something in common with Ayurveda. Their languages were closely related to Sanskrit. Their social structure and spiritual practices were similar to that of Aryan India. Hence, their healing practices, and our knowledge of them is still rather limited, must have been related.

The classical Greek tradition recognized four humors based upon the four elements. First was the Choleric humor that reflected the element of fire. Second was the Sanguine humor that reflected the element of air. Third was the Phlegmatic humor that reflected the element of water. Fourth was the Melancholic humor that reflected the element of earth. These terms for the humors still exist in our language, as well as the ideas of good or bad humor as psychological disease factors.

Each of these four humors, like the three of Ayurveda, was represented by a particular substance in the body. The Choleric humor was represented by yellow bile, the Sanguine humor by blood, the Phlegmatic humor by phlegm and the Melancholic humor by black bile. Each reflected the primary quality of its element. The Choleric humor was hot, the Sanguine dry, the Phlegmatic wet and the Melancholic cold.

We find in this Western system Pitta (bile) and Kapha (phlegm) clearly represented in the Choleric and Phlegmatic types. Both terms in each system mean bile and phlegm.

Vata (air) is most represented by the Melancholic humor. Vata tends towards depression, weak kidneys and the main debilitating and chronic diseases that were placed under the Melancholic humor. High Vata also created darkness or dark exudations (black bile). Astrologically, both were ascribed to a malefically placed Saturn in the chart and its cold, dry and dark influence.

Sanguine often appears as the state of health of balance of the other three humors (though by some is also considered to be Vata). In this way the older natural healing system of Western medicine and Ayurveda are found to be similar in terms of fundamental principles. As usual, each system has its characteristic variations that are not entirely translatable in terms of the other.

In the middle ages and the Renaissance the spice trade brought many Ayurvedic herbs to Europe. The alchemical tradition, popular from Europe to China at that time, was based on Ayurveda, which retains a strong alchemical basis to the present day. Hence we find such great healers of the time, like Hildegard of Bingen (twelfth century German) commonly using Ayurvedic remedies like long pepper (pippali) or galan-gal, almost forgotten later, as well as many gem or mineral remedies Ayurveda is well known for.

The most famous philosopher of Renaissance times and translator of Plato, Marsilio Ficino, mentions many Ayurvedic herbs and Ayurvedic like formulas in his medical works, like *The Book of Life*. These include the herbs of Triphala, (called chebulan, emblica or Triphera and often given in a balsam form), as well as aloe, saffron, cinnamon and cloves, often prepared as in Ayurveda into herbal jellies and taken with gold or silver foil (as is Chyavan prash today). The herbs and preparations of Europe of this era have much more in common with Ayurvedic preparations today than they do with either allopathic medicine or with later Western herbal usages.

Hence studying Ayurveda is not so much learning a foreign and exotic system but discovering our own spiritual and naturalistic healing tradition lost centuries ago. The humors give us the key to this ancient system. They can be used in many ways and are part of the language of a constitutional medicine with branches throughout the world.

2
THE SIX TASTES
THE ENERGETICS OF HEALING SUBSTANCES

Ayurvedic diagnosis of disease is based on the three biological humors; treatment is according to the six tastes. These apply not only to herbs but also to foods and minerals. They are based on the actual taste of the substance when taken in the mouth and reveal an intricate dynamic of herbal properties.

The six tastes are sweet, salty, sour, pungent, bitter and astringent. Each is made up of two of the five elements. Sweet taste, as in sugars and starches, is composed of earth and water; salty, as in table salt or seaweed, of water and fire; sour, fermented food or acid fruit, of earth and fire; pungent, hot spices like cayenne or ginger, of fire and air; bitter, bitter herbs like golden seal or gentian, of air and ether; and astringent, as in herbs containing tannins, like alum or witch hazel, of earth and air.

Heating and Cooling Effects
The six tastes are classified as heating or cooling to different degrees. Hottest generally is pungent, followed by sour and salty. Coldest is bitter, followed by astringent and sweet.

Heavy and Light Properties
They are also classified as heavy and light. Heaviest generally is sweet, followed by salty and astringent. Lightest is bitter, followed by pungent and sour.

Moist and Dry Properties
And they are classified as moist or dry. Wettest generally is sweet, followed by salty and sour. Driest is pungent, followed by bitter and astringent.

Tastes and the Humors
Three tastes increase each of the biological humors and three decrease them. These are general rules. Many combinations and variations exist.

Vata (air) is most increased by bitter taste, which most resembles it, then astringent and pungent. It is most decreased by salty taste, then sour and sweet.

Pitta (fire) is most increased by sour taste, then pungent and salty. It is most decreased by bitter taste, then astringent and sweet.

Kapha (water) is most increased by sweet taste, then salty and sour. It is most decreased by pungent taste, then bitter and astringent.

Actions of the Tastes

Each taste has its specific therapeutic actions. Sweet taste is building and strengthening to all body tissues. It harmonizes the mind and promotes a sense of contentment. It is demulcent (soothing to the mucus membranes), expectorant and mildly laxative. It counters burning sensations.

Salty taste is softening, laxative and sedative. In small amounts it stimulates digestion, in moderate amounts it is purgative, and in very large amounts it causes vomiting.

Sour taste is stimulant, carminative (dispels gas), nourishing and thirst relieving. It increases all tissues but the reproductive.

Pungent taste is stimulant, carminative, and diaphoretic (promotes sweating). It improves metabolism and promotes all organic functions. It promotes heat and digestion and counters cold sensations.

Bitter taste is alterative (blood purifying), cleansing and detoxifying. It reduces all bodily tissues and increases lightness in the mind.

Astringent taste stops bleeding and other excess discharges (such as excess sweating or diarrhea) and promotes healing of the skin and mucus membranes.

Amounts of the Six Tastes Needed

Everyone needs a certain amount of each of the six tastes. The relative proportion differs according to the constitution or humor of the individual. Too much of any taste can become harmful to any constitutional type, as can too little.

Sweet

- Needed in significant amounts for all humors, as food is predominately sweet in taste. More is required for Pitta (fire), moderate for Vata (air), less for Kapha (water).

- Necessary for maintaining tissue growth and development in all three humors.

Salty

- Needed in small amounts for all humors, as it is strong in low concentrations. More is needed for Vata (air), moderate for Pitta (fire), less for Kapha (water).
- Necessary for maintaining mineral balance and holding water.

Sour

- Required in moderation for each humor. More is needed for Vata (air), moderate for Kapha (water), less for Pitta (fire).
- Necessary for maintaining acidity and countering thirst.

Pungent

- Needed in moderation for each humor; more for Kapha (water), moderate for Vata (air), less for Pitta (fire).
- Necessary for maintaining metabolism, improving appetite and digestion.

Bitter

- Needed in small quantities for each humor; more for (Pitta) fire, moderate for Kapha (water), less for Vata (air).
- Necessary for detoxification, but also is depleting.

Astringent

- Needed moderate amounts for each humor, as a secondary food taste; more for Pitta (fire), moderate for Kapha (water), less for Vata (air).
- Necessary for maintaining firmness of tissues.

Comparative Nutritive and Medicinal Values of Tastes

In terms of nutrition, sweet is most important generally for everyone, as it possesses the highest nutritive value. Sour is moderately nutritive but tends to deplete the reproductive secretions. Astringent has some nutritive properties, particularly for the minerals; most green vegetables are regarded as astringent. Salt provides minerals and helps hold water but is not very nutritive in itself. Pungent has slight nutritive properties in various spicy vegetables, like onions, but is generally depleting. Bitter is the least nutritive, or tasty, and is often a sign that vegetables are too old to eat.

In terms of medicinal properties, bitter and astringent are the most commonly used. They treat severe fevers, infections and traumatic injuries that are the most immediate threat to life. Pungent is also very useful for stimulating our defensive reactions and breaking stagnation. These three tastes are the most common in plants, have the most immediate action, and are best for destroying pathogens. Sour, salty and sweet have less medicinal value and are more for long term tonification and slower therapies.

Aggravation of Humors by the Six Tastes
Excess of the Tastes

Each taste in excess causes certain damage, first to the humor it aggravates, then even to the humor it alleviates (if in too large amounts).

For example, too much salt will initially aggravate Kapha (water) by holding more water in the tissues. An excess, however, can even aggravate Vata (air), which it alleviates in normal amounts. This causes thirst, wrinkling of the skin and falling of the hair.

Each taste differs in its power to aggravate humors. Bitter is the most aggravating in small amounts, as it is most depleting; then salty, sour, pungent, astringent and sweet.

The stronger pure forms of each taste are more likely to aggravate the humors. The complex forms are less likely to, as they require assimilation. They do not have so one-sided an action, nor are they as likely to cause autoimmune derangement.

The pure forms of the six tastes are sugar (not only white sugar but any pure sugar), salt, hot spices, alcohol, pure astringents, pure bitters. The first two are those most commonly taken in our culture. They are most responsible for the aggravation of the humors, even those they usually alleviate.

Pure versus Complex Forms of the Six Tastes

Taste	Pure	Complex
1. Sweet	Sugar	Complex carbohydrates
2. Salty	Table salt	Seaweed
3. Pungent	Hot peppers (cayenne)	Mild spices (cardamom, fennel)
4. Sour	Alcohol	Sour food (yogurt, sour fruit)
5. Bitter	Pure bitters (aloe gel)	Mild bitters (golden seal)
6. Astringent	Pure astringents (strong tannins)	Mild astringents (alfalfa, red raspberry)

Pure forms of the six tastes are more likely to aggravate the humors when taken regularly, as in food or with food. Yet they also can possess strong medicinal properties for temporary conditions. Pure forms of the six tastes should be used with care or used therapeutically.

Deficiency of the Tastes

A lack of each taste will also aggravate humors — first those they alleviate, then, if the lack is greater, even those they aggravate. For example, too little sugar will first aggravate Vata (air) and Pitta (fire). But if the deficiency is to the point of malnutrition, it can even weaken a person with Kapha (watery) constitution.

Usually in our culture bitter taste is used too little, then pungent and astringent. The lack of bitter taste causes us to accumulate toxins internally. Hence, most of us can use more of these tastes. We usually have sweet and salty in excess, even if we are Vata (air) types.

Tastes and Organs

Too much sweet damages the spleen (pancreas), too much salty damages the kidneys, too much pungent damages and dries the lungs, too much sour damages the liver, too much bitter damages the heart, too much astringent damages the colon. But too much of any taste, as we have seen, will generally damage the body as a whole. Sweet builds toxins, salty causes looseness, sour causes acidity, pungent causes burning, bitter causes cold and astringent causes contractions.

Tastes and Emotions

The six tastes are also the "flavors" of our various emotions. These can affect us in the same way as diet and herbs, and can increase the therapeutic or disease-causing effects of the tastes that correspond to them.

Sweet	Love, attachment.
Salty	Greed.
Sour	Envy.
Pungent	Hatred.
Bitter	Grief.
Astringent	Fear.

Emotions have the same effect as food or herbs of the same energetic quality. Psychological factors, generally speaking, will outweigh physical factors. Anger can damage the liver as much as alcoholism. So herbs and diet are not enough if the taste of the mind has not changed.

| Hot Emotions | Anger, hatred, envy. |
| Cold Emotions | Fear, grief, sorrow. |

Relationships Between the Six Tastes

These six tastes can be combined for various therapeutic actions. For example, pungent and bitter combine well for their drying and cleansing action (like the Western herbal combination of cayenne and golden seal). Pungent, sour and salty combine well for their mutual action of stimulating digestion. Generally, tastes will further the action which they share in common, while reducing those they do not.

Some tastes tend to balance or complement each other. For example, pungent aids in the digestion of sweet, as in the use of spices with sweets. Sweet helps alleviate the burning sensation of pungent taste, as in taking sugar with cloves. Pungent promotes sweating, while astringent stops it. Bitter counters the craving for sweet.

Six Tastes Pills

In India various herbal formulas are made combining all six tastes. Such pills are given, particularly to children, to insure that adequate amounts of all six tastes are received daily. These pills help educate our sense of taste and harmonize its function.

A simple Ayurvedic version of the six tastes pill is made with equal parts shatavari (sweet), amalaki (sour), rock salt, ginger (pungent), barberry (bitter) and haritaki (astringent). Or we can modify this formula according to the three humors. Vata (air) can take twice the amount proportionally of the sweet, sour and salty herbs, concentrating on the tastes that reduce it. Kapha (water) can take twice the amount of the pungent, bitter and astringent herbs. Pitta can take twice the amount of the sweet, bitter and astringent.

A good Western version can be made with licorice (sweet), hawthorne berries (sour), sea salt, ginger (pungent), barberry (bitter) and red raspberry (astringent).

Dosage is one gram or two 500 mg. tablets every morning.

While not mentioned specifically in the disease treatment section, six tastes pills are useful generally for strengthening digestion and improving absorption, for chronic digestive system disorders and as an intestinal corrective. They are particularly good for those with chronic low appetite and anorexia.

3
CONSTITUTIONAL EXAMINATION
HOW TO DETERMINE
YOUR UNIQUE PSYCHO-PHYSICAL NATURE

Each one of us possesses in our physical makeup all three biological humors. Kapha makes up our flesh and our secretions, the water in our body. Pitta gives us our warmth and capacity to transform substances in the body, our fire. Vata governs our energies and activities, gives us our air. We each replicate the great cosmic forces and through them our own physiology is part of the cosmic dance. However, the proportion of the humors varies according to the individual. One humor will usually predominate and its nature will make its mark upon us in terms of our appearance and disposition.

From the Ayurvedic perspective, the first step in treatment is to ascertain the natural constitution of the individual. This is according to the predominant biological humor as Vata (air), Pitta (fire), or Kapha (water). The predominant humor, in turn, reflects the main energies and qualities within the individual.

Most diseases arise from the excesses brought about by the inborn predominant humor. Generally, all the diseases an individual is prone to can be treated through methods of balancing the constitution.

This constitutional approach is the essence of Ayurveda. It gives Ayurveda broad powers for disease prevention, health maintenance and longevity enhancement, as well as the treatment of disease. Through it, we can prescribe a life plan for ourselves as individuals, for health maintenance and to optimize our human and creative potential. It also allows us to apply Ayurveda along non-medical lines as a form of health education and life-style counseling.

Some individuals are strongly predominant in one humor or another. These we might call pure Vata (pure air), pure Pitta (pure fire) and pure Kapha (pure water) types. Mixed types also exist, when two or more humors stand in relatively equal proportion. Three different dual types exist as Vata-Pitta (air-fire), Vata-Kapha (air-water) and Pitta-Kapha (fire-water). An even type or VPK type is also found, making seven major types in all. It should be noted that mixed types do not necessarily indicate better or worse health. They do serve, however, to complicate treatment.

Efforts to balance one humor may aggravate another. For dual types, therefore, it is often better to try to raise the third humor, the one that is too low. Vata-Pitta (air-fire) types should try to increase Kapha (water). Pitta-Kapha (fire-water) types should try to increase Vata (air). Vata-Kapha (air-water) types should aim at developing Pitta (fire). In this way it will be easier to understand which qualities need to be balanced.

Often we give numbers to denote the proportion of the three humors in the body. Vata 4, Pitta 2, Kapha 1, would show a high-Vata, low-Kapha person. However, there is no fixed way of using numbers to denote the humors and different practitioners may give them different values.

Different degrees of aggravation of the humors can exist as well. There is much difference between high Vata as insomnia and high Vata as paralysis, for example. And the humors can become unbalanced in different ways, relative to their different attributes. High Vata, excess air, can manifest as excess dryness, causing rigidity or reduced motion. It can also manifest one of its other qualities as excess mobility, causing tremors and appearing almost opposite in attributes. The humors give us a simple background for understanding conditions, yet more specific analysis is often necessary regarding the particular qualities that may be out of balance.

Outer circumstances can aggravate the humors not predominant in an individual nature. For example, we live in a very Vata (high air) culture with constant travel, stimulation and communication. Vata disorders are more common here than in other cultures, even in individuals of different predominant humors. Such variations should not be lost sight of when we examine particular constitutions.

What follows is a more detailed examination of constitution than in *The Yoga of Herbs*. The material presented there can be examined as a background.

Note which humor you check the most; this will usually be your predominant humor. Generally speaking, we know ourselves well enough to determine our constitutional natures. Determining those of friends is more difficult. Consulting an Ayurvedic practitioner can be helpful, but even there a difference of opinion sometimes exists. Different people may be more sensitive to one or another humor in your nature depending upon various factors.

Physical Characteristics

The natural constitution is most easily revealed by the fixed attributes of the physical body. These include frame, weight and complexion. Life-long habits and proclivities, and life-long disease tendency are also important.

Though constitution tends to remain the same throughout the life, exceptional factors like a long-term illness can change it.

V is for Vata, the biological air humor, P is for Pitta, fire and K is for Kapha, water.

Frame	V	Tall, thin, short, poorly developed physique.
	P	Medium, moderately developed physique.
	K	Short, stout, big, well developed physique.
Weight	V	Low, prominent bones.
	P	Moderate, good muscles.
	K	Heavy, tends towards obesity.
Complexion	V	Dull, brown, darkish.
	P	Red, ruddy, flushed.
	K	White, pale.
Skin	V	Thin, dry, cold, rough, cracked, prominent veins.
	P	Warm, moist, pink, with moles, freckles, acne.
	K	Thick, white, moist, cold, soft, smooth.
Hair	V	Scanty, coarse, dry, brown, wavy.
	P	Moderate, fine, soft, early grey or bald.
	K	Abundant, oily, thick, wavy, lustrous.
Head	V	Small, unsteady.
	P	Moderate.
	K	Large, steady.
Forehead	V	Small.
	P	With folds.
	K	Large.
Eyebrows	V	Small, thin, unsteady.
	P	Moderate, fine.
	K	Thick, bushy, many hairs.
Eyelashes	V	Small, dry, firm.
	P	Small, thin, fine.
	K	Large, thick, oily, firm.
Eyes	V	Small, dry, thin, brown, dull, unsteady.
	P	Medium, thin, red (inflamed easily), green, piercing.

Eyes	K	Wide, prominent, thick, oily, white, attractive.
Nose	V	Thin, small, dry, crooked.
	P	Medium.
	K	Thick, big, firm, oily.
Lips	V	Thin, small, darkish, dry, unsteady.
	P	Medium, soft, red.
	K	Thick, large, oily, smooth, firm.
Teeth and Gums	V	Thin, dry, small, rough, crooked, receding gums.
	P	Medium, soft, pink, gums bleed easily.
	K	Large, thick, soft pink, oily.
Shoulders	V	Thin, small, flat.
	P	Medium.
	K	Broad, thick, firm, oily.
Chest	V	Thin, small, narrow, poorly developed.
	P	Medium.
	K	Broad, large, well or overly developed.
Arms	V	Thin, small, poorly developed.
	P	Medium.
	K	Large, thick, long, well developed.
Hands	V	Small, thin, dry, cold, rough, fissured, unsteady.
	P	Medium, warm, pink.
	K	Large, thick, oily, cool, firm.
Calves	V	Small, hard.
	P	Loose, soft.
	K	Round, shapely, firm.
Feet	V	Small, thin, dry, rough, fissured, unsteady.
	P	Medium, soft, pink.
	K	Large, thick, hard, firm.
Joints	V	Small, thin, dry, unsteady, cracking.
	P	Medium, soft, loose.
	K	Large, thick, well built.
Nails	V	Small, thin, dry, rough, darkish.
	P	Medium, soft, pink.
	K	Large, thick, smooth, white, firm, oily.
Urine	V	Scanty, difficult, colorless.
	P	Profuse, yellow, red, burning.
	K	Moderate, whitish, milky.

Feces	V	Scanty, dry, hard, difficult or painful, gas, tends towards constipation.
	P	Abundant, loose, tends towards diarrhea, with burning sensation.
	K	Moderate, solid, mucus in stool.
Sweat	V	Scanty, no smell.
Body Odor	P	Profuse, hot, strong smell.
	K	Moderate, cold, pleasant smell.
Appetite	V	Variable, erratic.
	P	Strong, sharp.
	K	Constant, low.
Voice	V	Low, weak, hoarse.
	P	High pitch, sharp.
	K	Pleasant, deep, good tone.
Speech	V	Quick, inconsistent, erratic, talkative.
	P	Moderate, argumentative, convincing.
	K	Slow, definite, not talkative.
Mental	V	Quick, adaptable, indecisive.
Nature	P	Intelligent, penetrating, critical.
	K	Slow, steady, dull.
Memory	V	Poor, notices things easily but easily forgets.
	P	Sharp, clear.
	K	Slow to take notice but will not forget.
Emotional	V	Fearful, anxious, nervous.
Tendencies	P	Angry, irritable, contentious.
	K	Calm, content, attached, sentimental.
Faith	V	Erratic, changeable, rebel.
	P	Determined, fanatic, leader.
	K	Constant, loyal, conservative.
Sleep	V	Light, tends towards insomnia.
	P	Moderate,may wake up but will fall asleep again.
	K	Heavy, difficulty in waking up.
Dreams	V	Flying, moving, restless, nightmares.
	P	Colorful, passionate, conflict.
	K	Romantic, sentimental, few dreams.
Habits	V	Likes moving, travelling, parks, plays, jokes, stories, dancing, artistic activities.
	P	Likes sports, politics, painting, hunting.
	K	Likes water, sailing, flowers, cosmetics, business.

Activity	V	Quick, fast, unsteady, erratic, hyperactive.
	P	Medium, motivated, purposeful, goal seeking.
	K	Slow, steady, stately.
Strength	V	Low, poor endurance, starts and stops quickly.
Exertion	P	Medium, intolerant of heat.
	K	Strong, good endurance, but slow in starting.
Sexual	V	Variable, erratic, deviant, strong desire but low energy, few children.
Nature	P	Moderate, passionate, quarrelsome, dominating.
	K	Low but constant sexual desire, good sexual energy, devoted, many children.
Sensitivity	V	Fear of cold, wind, sensitive to dryness.
	P	Fear of heat, dislike of sun, fire.
	K	Fear of cold, damp, likes wind and sun.
Resistance	V	Poor, variable, weak immune system.
to Disease	P	Medium, prone to infections.
	K	Good, consistent, strong immune system.
Disease	V	Nervous system diseases, pain, arthritis, mental disorders.
Tendency	P	Febrile diseases, infections, inflammatory diseases.
	K	Respiratory system diseases, mucus, edema.
Reaction to	V	Quick, low dosage needed, unexpected side effects or nervous reactions.
Medications	P	Medium, sensitive to aspirin.
	K	Slow, high dosage required, effects slow to manifest.
Pulse	V	Thready, rapid, irregular, weak — like a snake.
	P	Wiry, bounding, moderate — like a frog.
	K	Deep, slow, steady, rolling, slippery — like a swan.

More on Mental Nature

Mental nature usually reflects the biological humors.

Vata (Airy) Mentality

Individuals with Vata (air) physical types, will usually have Vata psychological natures. They will have emotional tendencies towards fear and anxiety. They will be mentally changeable, excitable, indecisive and have good but erratic mental powers. They are good at both grasping and forgetting. They are quick at both attachment and detachment, fast at getting emotional and expressing emotions, as well as forgetting them. Their minds and senses are sensitive, but unsteady. They will not have much courage and tend towards cowardice. Generally they will be of a more solitary nature and not have a lot of friends. However, they are good at forming friendships with people outside their social sphere. They do not make good leaders, but they will not be good followers either. They will not be very materialistic and are not much concerned with accumulating possessions or money. They often spend money quickly and easily.

Pitta (Fiery) Mentality

Those with Pitta (hot) physical natures will also tend towards fiery emotions like irritability and anger. They will be logical, critical, perceptive and intelligent. They are quick to get emotional and have no trouble expressing anger. They are articulate, convincing and often self-righteous. They usually possess strong wills, are dignified and make good leaders. While very helpful and kind to friends and followers, they are cruel and unforgiving to opponents. They are bold, adventurous, daring and reckless. They are inventive, ingenious and often possess good mechanical skills. Their memories are sharp and not sentimental. They are more concerned with the accumulation of power than with material resources but will gather material resources to gain their ends.

Kapha (Watery) Mentality

Those with Kapha (watery) bodies will also tend towards watery emotions, like love and desire, romance and sentimentality. They will be kind, considerate and loyal, but also slow to respond, conservative, shy and obedient. They tend to have many friends and to be very close to their family, community, culture, religion and country, but they can be closed-minded outside their sphere of habitual activity. They travel less and are happier at home. They easily get attached and find it hard to be detached. While they can display affections easily, they are slow to express emotions, particularly anger. Mentally, they are steady with good forethought but need time to consider things properly.

Relationships Between Physical and Psychological Types

There are, of course, exceptions to this correspondence of physical and psychological types. Nature has many different ways of making human beings and every possible variety must be manifested. Moreover, the energetics between the outer and inner aspects of our nature are not always of simple correspondence. A Kapha (heavy) physical type may have a Vata (light) mind, as, for instance, an obese but very talkative school teacher. Hence, we must not treat psychological conditions simply according to the physical humor. The physical body may not reflect the mental nature but may try to balance or compensate for it.

As mental nature is more subtle than physical nature, more variations are possible. As it is more changeable than physical nature, it can more easily take on temporary disturbances different than the physical constitution. Mental disturbances, therefore, are more likely to be different from the physical constitution than are physical diseases. The mind is also very easily disturbed by the disease process and not always in a way that is of the same quality as the disease. Generally, all diseases make us afraid. They bring up the basic fear of death, thereby tending to aggravate Vata (air) or create anxiety in the mind.

When a difference between physical and mental nature exists, we must be careful not to aggravate one in treating the other. Special herbs for the mind may have to be given, considering the state of the mind.

Mental Nature and Astrology

Differences between the physical and mental nature are often revealed through astrology, which gives us a more accurate and detailed picture of the mind than simple Ayurvedic examination. The birth chart itself is a picture of the energies of the mind or astral body. The physical body can also be read from it by isolating certain factors within it. Hence, in treating the mind it is good to consult astrology. It affords a unique overview of the life, personality and the purposes of the soul in the incarnation.

Mental and Spiritual Disposition

In the Vedic system, mental nature is usually judged according to the gunas, the prime attributes of nature (Prakriti) as sattva, rajas and tamas. These indicate the mental traits respectively of clarity, distraction and dullness. The biological humors are given secondary importance in this approach.

These qualities reflect the level of development of the soul. They are not simply intellectual proclivities or emotional types. They show the sensitivity of the mind, its capacity to perceive truth and to act according to it.

The mind itself is called sattva, clarity, as it is the basic clear quality of the mind which allows for perception to occur. Sattva means literally what possesses the same nature as truth or reality (sat). The mind is naturally clear and pure but becomes darkened by negative thoughts and emotions. When pure, it produces enlightenment and self-realization. Sattva is the divine or godly nature. It brings about internalization of the mind, the movement of the consciousness inward and the unification of the head and the heart.

Rajas is distraction or turbulence in the mind that causes us to look outward and seek fulfillment in the external world. It is the mind agitated by desire. Literally, it means stain or smoke. Rajas is disturbed thoughts and imaginings. It includes willfulness, anger, manipulativeness and ego. It involves the seeking of power, stimulation and entertainment. In excess it creates a demonic (asuric) nature.

Tamas is dullness, darkness and inability to perceive. It is the mind clouded by ignorance and fear. It means heaviness and lethargy. Tamas creates sloth, sleep and inattention. It involves lack of mental activity and insensitivity, and domination of the mind by external or subconscious forces. Tamas creates a servile or animal nature.

Usually rajas and tamas go together. Tamas creates the darkening of pure awareness, which allows rajas to project various false imaginations or ego ideas. Rajas, similarly, in excess, depletes our energy through over activity and makes us tamasic, dull and lethargic.

Rajas and tamas are necessary forces in nature. Rajas creates energy, vitality and emotion. Tamas creates stability and allows fixed forms to take shape, thus it underlies our physical body. But these two qualities are out of place in the mind and in the perceptual process. For objective awareness to occur, the mind must be calm. It must be free of distraction or inertia. It must be like a mirror in order for us to see, or like a lake free of ripples to reflect the moon. Part of the purification of the mind is giving rajas and tamas their proper place in the lower aspects of our nature.

The Three Qualities and the Three Humors

There have been a number of attempts to correspond the three humors to these three prime qualities or gunas. Actually any of the three humors can correspond to any of the three gunas. Hence, we have presented the larger picture below.

Disease Tendency of the Three Mental Types

In Ayurveda, the main cause of disease is said to be 'failure of intelligence', prajnaparadha. This is not simply lack of intellectual knowledge or verbal acuity, but a failure of natural wisdom. It is a lack of understanding of the natural harmony of life and how to adapt to it; living out of harmony with nature, the universe and the Divine. This failure of our natural intelligence to operate is caused by external conditioning factors, like fear and desire. It inhibits creative living and traps us in convention or preconception. It manifests as lack of faith in life and in the Divine, a lack of respect for life and becoming uncaring.

Mental disorders specifically are usually caused by failure of intelligence, or vitiation of sattva. This comes from poor education (lack of moral or ethical values in upbringing), causing harm to others, excess stimulation and entertainment, dishonesty, or untruthfulness. Such physical factors as wrong diet, eating too much sugar or meat, and excess sleep can contribute to it.

Sattva is improved by spiritual cultivation, Yogic practices, meditation, spending time in nature, pro-sattva diet, and life regime in harmony with one's constitution. (see chapter on Mental Disorders)

Sattvic types have the greatest freedom from disease. Their nature is harmonious and adaptable. They strive towards balance and have peace of mind which cuts the psychological root of disease. They are considerate of others and take care of themselves. They see all life as a learning experience and try to see the good in all things, including disease.

Rajasic types often have good energy but tend to burn themselves out through excessive activity. Disease symptoms are frequently acute, and recovery is possible with the right remedial measures. They are impatient and inconsistent in dealing with disease and do not wish to take the time or responsibility to get well. They will blame others for their condition.

Tamasic types have more chronic diseases including cancer. Their energy and emotion tend to be stagnant. Their diseases tend to be deep seated, obstinate and difficult to treat. They do not seek proper treatment and usually have poor hygiene. They will accept their disease as fate and will not take advantage of the methods that may cure them.

The Three Mental Types and the Three Humors

One method of balancing the three humors is to move from their tamasic and rajasic sides to their sattvic (spiritual) side. It is usually not possible to transcend one's predominant humor, but one can move to its higher level of functioning. For example, a Kapha (water) type can move from greed, a tamasic emotion, to devotion, a sattvic emotion; this transforms an emotional disease tendency to a power of health and enlightenment. Without sattva we could not perceive anything at all. All of us contain various degrees of these three mental qualities, just as we all have the three humors.

We should examine our mental constitution according to the proportion of the three qualities, sattva, rajas and tamas, we find in ourselves. This will give us a better idea how to improve our minds and balance our disease tendency through Yoga and the cultivation of character.

When we combine the three qualities and the three humors, the following picture of mental development in human beings emerges. Each humor is divided according to the three qualities. We see that no humor is better than the others in terms of the mental nature. The qualities vary, but higher and lower aspects exist in each type.

Seven different mental types can be ascertained for each humor (like the seven different humoral types). These are pure sattva, pure rajas, pure tamas, sattva-rajas, sattva-tamas, rajas-tamas and all three in equal proportion. Totally pure sattva (shuddha sattva) gives enlightenment.

All of us should examine these mental traits and see which most fit our nature. Those which are negative, such as disease-causing habits, we should reduce by the appropriate remedial measures. These include meditation, prayer, mantra, puja or various other forms of self-examination, or surrender to the Divine. Our culture as a whole today is very rajasic. Therefore, some rajasic traits may be more due to circumstances than indicative of our own disposition.

Vata (Airy) Mental Nature

Sattvic (Harmonious) Energetic, adaptable, flexible, quick in comprehension, good in communication, strong sense of human unity, strong healing energy, true enthusiasm, positive spirit, able to initiate things, good capacity for positive change and movement.

Rajasic (Disturbed) Indecisive, unreliable, hyperactive, agitated, restless, disturbed, nervous, anxious, overly talkative, superficial, noisy, disruptive, false enthusiasm.

Tamasic (Darkened) Fearful, servile, dishonest, secretive, depressed, self-destructive, drug addict, prone to sexual perversions, mentally disturbed, suicidal.

Pitta (Fiery) Mental Nature

Sattvic (Harmonious) Intelligent, clear, perceptive, enlightened, discriminating, good will, independent, warm, friendly, courageous, good guide and leader.

Rajasic (Disturbed) Willful, impulsive, ambitious, aggressive, controlling, critical, dominating, manipulating, angry, wrathful, reckless, proud, vain.

Tamasic (Darkened) Hateful, vile, vindictive, destructive, psychopath, criminal, drug dealer, underworld figure.

Kapha (Watery) Mental Nature

Sattvic (Harmonious) Calm, peaceful, content, stable, consistent, loyal, loving, compassionate, forgiving, patient, devoted, receptive, nurturing, supportive, strong faith.

Rajasic (Disturbed) Controlling, attached, greedy, materialistic, sentimental, needing security, seeking comfort and luxury.

Tamasic (Darkened) Dull, gross, lethargic, apathetic, slothful, coarse, slow comprehension, insensitive, a thief.

4
EXAMINATION OF DISEASE
THE PATTERNS OF IMBALANCE

Diseases and the Biological Humors

Diseases reflect the predominant humor which produces them. We can understand the nature of a disease, like that of physical constitution, according to the attributes it presents. We can treat it with the remedies appropriate for the biological humor involved.

Some diseases are more characteristically of one humor than another. The majority of diseases are of a Vata (air) nature, as Vata tends towards disease (decay). Ayurvedic books list more Vata disorders than Pitta and Kapha together: eighty Vata, forty Pitta, and twenty Kapha.

Kapha (water or phlegm) diseases include most respiratory disorders, colds, flus, asthma, bronchitis, swollen glands, edema, benign tumors. The main attributes of Kapha disorders are dampness, excessive tissue growth, and cold.

Pitta (fire or bile) diseases include most febrile and infectious diseases, liver disorders, ulcers, acidity, boils, skin rashes. The main attributes of Pitta disorders are heat, redness, and oiliness.

Vata (air or wind) diseases include most nervous system disorders, insomnia, tremors, epilepsy, paralysis, arthritis. The main attributes of Vata disorders are dryness, cold, impaired or abnormal movement, and wasting away of tissues.

Kapha diseases are characterized primarily by phlegm; Pitta diseases by fever or burning sensation; Vata diseases by pain.

In general, all diseases can be divided into Vata (air), Pitta (fire) or Kapha (water) types according to the attributes of the humor predominant in its qualities. Yet the same disease may be caused by different humors or by combinations of humors. Most common colds are of a Kapha nature with phlegm and congestion as the main symptoms; others may be Pitta in quality with higher fever and more severe sore throat. Though any one disease may be of many types, the treatment for all diseases follows the same main lines and principles, that of the aggravated humor.

This is the method followed in this book. First the general nature of the disease is presented, which may be predominately of one humor. Then the varieties of the disease are distinguished according to all the humors.

The Biological Humors as the Sites of Disease

Most diseases can occur from an imbalance of any of the three humors. For example, arthritis may come about from high Vata, high Pitta or high Kapha. Yet each disease tends to be characterized more by one humor than another, as arthritis being mainly a Vata (air) disorder.

To understand this point better we should realize that the humors, when too high, tend to damage each other. The humors, as the underlying forces of the body, are not only the factors which cause disease but also the sites wherein disease occurs. They relate to the tissues, organs and systems that they rule; so, diseases involving the nervous system show Vata (air) as the site of the disorder. Diseases of this system ruled by Vata will more commonly be Vata. Yet they may be of a Pitta or Kapha nature, as these, when high, can damage Vata.

Usually, a humor will aggravate the factors it rules; that is, it will be the site as well as the causative factor in the disease process. Thus, high Kapha (phlegm) tends to damage the lungs, a Kapha organ. But an excess humor may take, as its disease site, another humor. This often indicates a more severe condition, in which the humor has already damaged its own sites. For example, high Kapha, after damaging the lungs, may then damage the nervous system, as in asthmatic wheezing or epilepsy due to phlegm blocking the subtle channels, thus affecting Vata (air). The humors affect each other, and in more severe diseases, like cancer, all three humors may be out of balance, making treatment extremely complicated.

Ayurvedic textbooks often divide diseases into additional types, but the primary classification is according to the three humors. When a condition is caused by two humors together, the treatment methods for them must be combined. Using this methodology, I have also presented some modern diseases not previously classified in Ayurvedic terms and differentiated them. There is not the space to present all diseases in detail, so some are presented in a more basic form.

Many of the diseases, such as constipation, diarrhea and vomiting, are chosen because they reflect the basic conditions in which the humors become aggravated and show the primary therapies used to treat them.

According to Ayurveda, it is not necessary to know the names or forms of diseases. It is more important to know the attributes of the humors and their states of imbalance behind different diseases. From this standpoint treatment is simpler and more holistic. Once the aggravated humor is ascertained, along with its site of manifestation, an integral regime for reducing it can be implemented. It is the underlying energy of the disease which has to be countered, not merely its face that has to be identified. Ayurveda sees all diseases according to the three humors. Hence, for it, no really new diseases can be found, only variations in the same basic disease-causing factors.

Excess of the Biological Humors
(Quotes from *Ashtanga Hridaya XII. 49–54*)

According to Ayurvedic source books, the classical symptoms of the aggravated or elevated humors are as follows:

"Vata's actions when aggravated are collapse, spasms, piercing pain, numbness, depression, breaking, striking and biting pain, constipation, cracking of the joints, contraction, retention of waste materials in the body, excitability, thirst, trembling, roughness of skin, porosity of tissues, dehydration, agitated movement, stiffness, astringent taste in mouth, dark or reddish brown discoloration." We see in these the drying and disruptive powers of the wind.

"Pitta's actions when aggravated are burning sensation, redness, feeling hot, boils, sweating, pus formation, bleeding, necrosis, exhaustion, fainting, inebriation, pungent and sour taste in the mouth and all discolorations but white and brown." We see in these the burning and fermenting action of fire.

"Kapha when aggravated creates phlegm, hardness of tissues, itching, cold sensation on the skin, heaviness, congestion, obesity, edema, indigestion, excessive sleeping, white color, and sweet and salty tastes in the mouth which take time to notice." These reflect the heaviness and stagnation of water.

Deficiency of the Biological Humors
(Quotes from *Ashtanga Hridaya XI. 14–16*)

The symptoms of the humors when low or deficient are as follows: "Vata when low causes lassitude of the limbs, deficiency of speech and enthusiasm, and confusion of perception, as well as increase in phlegm and the production of toxins (ama)." Vata (air) when low resembles high Kapha (water).

"Pitta when insufficient causes weakness of the digestive fire, cold, and lack of lustre." Pitta (fire) when low resembles both high Vata and high Kapha.

"Kapha when low results in a feeling of emptiness in the stomach, palpitations, and loosening of the joints." Kapha (water) when low resembles high Vata (air).

Disease is thought to be primarily caused by the humors that are too high or aggravated. Low humors are not thought to possess the strength to cause disease.

The following list gives, in a comprehensive way, the disease symptoms common to each of the three humors. These can be added to the factors of constitutional examination for greater clarity. Examination of pulse, tongue and abdomen, as well as questioning the patient, are important.

Symptoms of Aggravated Humors

Vata, the biological air humor, is represented by a **V**, Pitta, the fire humor, by a **P**, Kapha, the water humor, by a **K**.

Color *	**V**	Black, brown, blue black, blue, pink, decrease or absence of normal color.
	P	Red, purple, yellow, green, black, smoky.
	K	White, pale.
Pain	**V**	Most severe; throbbing, biting, churning, beating, tearing, variable, migratory, intermittent.
	P	Medium; burning, steaming.
	K	Least; heavy, dull, constant.
Fever	**V**	Moderate temperature; variable or irregular fever, thirst, anxiety, restlessness.
	P	Highest temperature; burning sensation, thirst, sweating, irritability, delirium.
	K	Low grade fever; dullness, heaviness, constant elevated temperature.
Discharges	**V**	Gas, sound (discharge of gas, cracking of joints, etc.).
	P	Bleeding, pus, bile.
	K	Mucus, salivation.
Mouth	**V**	Astringent taste, dry.
	P	Bitter or pungent taste, increased salivation.
	K	Sweet or salty taste, profuse salivation, mucoid discharges.
Throat	**V**	Dry, rough, pain and constriction of esophagus.
	P	Sore throat, inflammation, burning sensation.
	K	Swelling, dilation, edema.

---

*   As in complexion, discharges, discolorations.

Stomach	V	Decreased secretions, irregular appetite, frequent eructation (belching, hiccup), sense of constriction.
	P	Excessive appetite, sour or pungent eructation, burning sensation, ulcers, cancer.
	K	Slow digestion, sweet or mucoid eructation.
Liver and	V	Dry, rough, scanty secretions, irregular activity.
Gall Bladder	P	Soft, excessive bile production, gall stones, inflammation, abscesses, increased activity.
	K	Enlarged, heavy, firm, scanty bile, decreased activity.
Intestines	V	Dry, peristalsis disorders, distention, gas, constipation.
	P	Profuse secretions, quick peristalsis, inflammation, ulceration, abscesses, tumors, cancer, bleeding, perforation.
	K	Mucus coating, slow peristalsis, obstruction, distention, edema, tumors.
Feces	V	Constipation, painful and difficult bowel movements, dry, small in quantity.
	P	Diarrhea, watery stools, quick or uncontrollable evacuation, burning sensation, increased frequency, moderate amount.
	K	Solid, decreased frequency, large amount, containing mucus, with itching.
Urine	V	Scanty, difficult to discharge, increased frequency or absence of urination, colorless.
	P	Profuse, with burning sensation, increased frequency, yellow, turbid, brown or red in color.
	K	Profuse, decreased frequency, mucoid, white or pale.
Sweat	V	Scanty, irregular.
	P	Profuse, hot.
	K	Moderate, constant.
Mind and	V	Delusion, fear, apathy, sorrow, loss of consciousness, insomnia, desire for hot and hatred of cold things.
Senses	P	Weakness of senses, intoxication, restlessness, violent emotions, delirium, loss of sleep, dizziness, fainting, desire for cold things.
	K	Slow perception, lack of desire, lethargy, stupor, excessive sleeping, desire for hot things.
Onset of	V	Rapid, variable, irregular.
Disease	P	Medium, with fever.
	K	Slow, constant.

Time of	V	Dawn, dusk.
Day when	P	Noon, midnight.
Aggravated	K	Mid-morning, mid-evening.
Season	V	Fall, early winter.
when	P	Summer, late spring.
Aggravated	K	Late winter, early spring.
Exogenous	V	Wind, cold, dryness.
Aggravating	P	Heat, sun, fire, humidity.
Factors	K	Dampness, cold.

THE DISEASE PROCESS

Ojas
The Essential Energy of the Immune System

Ojas is the essential energy of the body. It literally means 'vigor'. It is the subtle essence of the reproductive system and of all the vital secretions. It is the special Ayurvedic concept of a source fluid underlying all our physical capacities. Ojas is not a physical substance. It is the sap of our life energy and exists on a subtle level in the heart chakra. When it is sufficient, there is health. When it is deficient, there is disease. Disease strikes at the locations where it is weak. In modern terms, we could say it is something like the essential energy of the immune system.

Ojas is defined as "the ultimate essence of the reproductive fluids and the heat of the tissues. Located in the heart, it pervades the entire body, giving stability and support. It is moist, of the nature of nectar (Soma), transparent, slightly red and yellow in color. When it is destroyed, one dies; when it is sustained, one lives.

"Ojas is decreased by such factors as anger, hunger, worry, sorrow and overwork. Then one experiences fear and a lack of strength: one constantly worries with disturbed senses. Lacking color, weak in mind, one becomes wasted. Such qualities as patience and faith disappear." Other factors that decrease Ojas include excessive sexual activity and the use of drugs or stimulants, as well as stress, anxiety, devitalized food, unnatural environment and life-style.

It is replenished by special foods like milk and ghee (clarified butter), and by special tonic herbs like ashwagandha (Withania somnifera), shatavari (Asparagus racemosus) and guduchi (Tinospora cordifolia). Meditation practices, mantras such as Om, and sexual moderation are also helpful, as Ojas is essentially sattvic (pure) in nature.

When low, Ojas causes chronic, degenerative diseases, as well as mysterious and hard to treat infectious and nervous disorders. The modern disease AIDS has all the symptoms of a disease of low Ojas. Less severe chronic low-energy conditions are often also related specifically to low Ojas; chronic low grade infections like Epstein-Barr virus or chronic hepatitis. Ojas decreases with age, and the diseases of old age reflect low Ojas, just as low Ojas causes premature aging.

The Three Humors and the Disease Process

According to Ayurveda, the disease process can be summarized in a simple way. The humors undergo increase by aggravating factors (diet, climate, seasons, life-style, emotions, etc.). This causes weakening of the digestive fire, which in turn allows an undigested food mass (called Ama in Sanskrit) to arise. This, with the increased humor, blocks the channels and becomes deposited in any weakened site in the body, from which the disease then manifests.

Ayurveda recognizes six stages in the disease process according to the development and movement of the aggravated humors.

These are called: 1. accumulation (sancaya), 2. aggravation (prakopa), 3. overflow (prasara), 4. relocation (sthana samsraya), 5. manifestation (vyakti), 6. diversification (bheda). The first two refer to the increase of the humors in their respective sites. The other four show their spread to different parts of the body.

Accumulation

The humors begin to increase in their respective locales. Causes include wrong diet, seasonal maladjustments, wrong life style, psychological disturbance, and all the usual factors that increase a particular humor.

Vata (air) accumulates in the colon causing distention, gas, constipation, insomnia, fear, fatigue, dryness and seeking of warmth.

Pitta (fire) accumulates in the small intestine producing burning sensation, fever, hyperacidity, bitter taste in the mouth, yellow coloring of urine and stool, desire for cold things, and anger.

Kapha (water) accumulates in the stomach resulting in lassitude, heaviness, pallor, bloating, indigestion and desire for light food.

Aggravation

The humors continue to increase in their respective sites, bringing about an increase in the symptoms manifested there and, by the pressure of this accumulation, reflected symptoms elsewhere.

Vata (air) causes light-headedness, increased constipation, abdominal pain or spasms, further accumulation of gas with rumbling in the bowels, along with upper abdominal distention.

Pitta (fire) causes increased acidity, acid regurgitation, burning pain in the abdomen, excessive thirst, loss of strength, and difficulty sleeping.

Kapha (water) causes loss of appetite, indigestion, nausea and increased salivation, heaviness in the head and heart, and excess sleeping.

Overflow

The humors have now filled up their respective sites and begin to overflow into the rest of the body. They enter into the plasma and blood, spreading out of the g.i. tract. The humors are no longer localized and can now penetrate into the organs and tissues of the body.

They move in different directions causing various disorders and dysfunctions. The nature and location of these complications depends upon the direction the humors move. (They can move in any direction, up, down, to one side or the other, but will go the way it is easiest for them to travel). They come into close contact with the tissues and waste materials of the body and become mixed with either of them. There will be a worsening of symptoms at their respective sites.

Vata (air) causes dry skin, pain or stiffness of the joints, lower back pain, convulsions, spasm, headache, dry cough, intermittent fever, as well as continued abdominal pain with constipation and painful bowel movements and general fatigue.

Pitta (fire) causes inflammatory skin diseases, conjunctivitis, gingivitis, dizziness, headache, high fever, bilious vomiting, as well as diarrhea with burning sensation.

Kapha (water) causes cough, asthma, swollen glands, low grade fever, vomiting, swelling of the joints, and mucus in the stools.

Relocation

The humors now relocate themselves in other sites in the body where they begin to cause specific diseases. Usually those sites which are weak or vulnerable are the ones taken. For example, in arthritis, they would deposit themselves in the joints and accumulate there. The symptoms now tend to become more fixed, whereas in the overflow state they tend to move around.

Manifestation

The humors manifest specific symptom complexes at these particular sites. We can now identify the disease as asthma, diabetes, arthritis, or whatever it may happen to be.

Diversification

At these particular sites the humors manifest their special characteristics. The disease can be identified according to those attributes of the three humors which it possesses.

For example, Vata (air) type arthritis will evidence severe pain, cold, stiffness, dry skin, and constipation. Pitta (fire) type will show fever, burning sensation, red swelling of the joints and loose stool. Kapha (water) will demonstrate swelling, edema, phlegm and congestion.

The Six Stages and Treatment

The general rule in treatment is that it is always easier to treat the humors while they are still located in their original sites. The stages of accumulation and aggravation, therefore, are easy to cure. The stage of overflow is the transitional stage.

At the relocation phase only the preliminary symptoms of the disease are in evidence and vitality is still strong, so treatment is still simple. The last two stages present a fully developed disease. It has matured and will take time and effort to rectify.

The Three Disease Pathways

Three pathways for diseases are differentiated: outer, inner, and central.

The inner disease pathway (antar marga) consists of the digestive tract. This pathway is called inner because the digestive tract forms a channel through the inside of the body.

Diseases here are easy to treat since it is possible to expel them from the body directly through the digestive tract, which is the main route for eliminating all toxins. They include mainly diseases of the digestive tract.

The outer disease pathway (bahya marga) consists of the plasma (skin) and blood, and the superficial tissues. Diseases here are more difficult to treat because they have already entered into the tissues. They include skin diseases and toxic blood conditions.

The central disease pathway (madhyama marga) consists of the deeper tissues of muscle, fat, bone, bone marrow and nerve tissue, and reproductive tissue. It is called the central disease pathway because it occurs between the outer pathway, the skin, and the inner, the g.i. tract.

The most sensitive points and organs of the body are affected, such as the head, heart, bladder and the joints of the bones.

Diseases here are the most deep-seated and the most difficult to treat. Most severe, chronic and degenerative diseases, from arthritis to cancer, come from this area.

The outer and central disease pathways make up the seven tissues of the body. The first two, skin and blood, are the outer and the next five, muscle, fat, bone, marrow and reproductive fluid, the middle. Hence, diseases are also classified by which tissue the humor resides in.

Movement of the Humors through the Disease Pathways

The factors which cause diseases to move from the digestive tract to the tissues are, "excessive exercise, too much hot or sharp food, wrong life-regime and by being transported by Vata."

They move from the inner tissues back to the digestive tract by "purification of the openings of the channels," particularly by oleation and sweating therapies, as well as by the control of Vata (breath-control, pranayama) and right life-regime.

We see, therefore, that all diseases are produced by an accumulation of the humors. Almost any disease can be caused by any one of the humors, so we have to examine fully all signs and symptoms. The disease process is the same in all diseases. It varies according to humors, stages, direction of movements of the humors, and sites where they become deposited. Ayurveda thus affords us a beautiful, simple, yet comprehensive understanding of the disease process which allows us to treat the disease at the right stage. By understanding this process and following the right regime in life for our constitution, we prevent the humors from accumulating and thus cut off the disease process at its root.

5
AYURVEDIC LIFE-REGIMES
BALANCING THE BIOLOGICAL HUMORS

Om, intelligence remember, remember your labor.
— *Isha Upanishad 14.*

According to Ayurveda, though diseases are of many kinds and pathogens are of many varieties, all are products of disharmonies of the three biological humors, Vata, Pitta and Kapha.

The biological humors are factors of both physical and psychological disease. They indicate wrong humor, emotional disorders or imbalance in the mind. Ayurvedic treatment aims at balancing the humors to neutralize the disease process. It is not, as is the case with Western medicine, so concerned with the classification of disease or the identification of pathogens. These are considered of secondary importance. In merely treating external pathogens, only the symptoms, not the underlying causes, are dealt with. In balancing the humors the root of the disease process is cut off.

Ayurveda and Self-Care
Ayurvedic curative aids are not necessarily complex, nor do they always have to be administered by another. They involve diet, herbs, life-style, Yoga and meditation which we can implement ourselves. The more complex remedies (extensive or strong herbal prescriptions or chemical drugs) and the more specialized methods (such as surgery) usually become necessary only when the disease process has been allowed to continue unchecked for a long time.

The usual rule is: whatever we can do for ourselves to improve our own health will be more effective than what another does for us. When we have failed in our efforts, the doctor, health care professional or clinical facility becomes necessary. Even then, their value is temporary, to bring us back to the point of caring for ourselves. Often small things we do for ourselves, such as giving up wrong foods, will do more for our health in the long run than taking many remedies or consulting many doctors.

There is no substitute for our own right living. It cannot be bought at any price and we cannot expect another to provide it. As long as we are not living in harmony with our nature and constitution we cannot expect ourselves to be really healed by any method. It is the beauty of Ayurveda that it gives each of us the knowledge and means to live in harmony. It provides us with the right regime for our particular type covering all aspects of our nature, physical, psychological and spiritual. But it can only succeed with our own time and effort, devotion and dedication.

One of the failings of modern culture is that it deprives us of the time we need to take care of ourselves and those we love. However, if we really value our well-being we, will take the time. The responsibility is ours, and there is no one to blame but ourselves if we do not make the effort.

Ayurvedic Life-Regimes

What is necessary, therefore, is that we each establish for ourselves our own appropriate life-regime according to our unique constitution. I do not like the word 'routine' because it implies a rigid discipline to be followed mechanically, a rut or a groove to become habituated to. 'Discipline' is also a misleading term for these life practices, because it implies trying to impose some external or ideal pattern upon our resistant nature. It is more a matter of discovering, through sensitivity to ourselves and to life, what is the natural movement of our own being. It is 'Yoga', a coordinating and harnessing of our resources for their maximum energetic effect.

It is necessary that we establish the right rhythm in our lives. This maintains a certain harmony and consistency but remains flexible and responds to the challenges of the moment. The rhythm of our right action in life creates a certain momentum that gives power to our lives and gradually improves all of our faculties.

What is significant is creative living. Creativity is not chaotic. It establishes an order, an absolute order, but one that gives freedom, as through it our energies are longer dispersed through wrong or untimely use. This is the order of intelligence that gives, as Krishnamurti states, "each thing its right place." It mirrors within ourselves the profound beauty and order of nature.

Ayurvedic regimes keep us in harmony with the universe and the cosmic life force. They are the rhythms of creative living, as natural as the breath. They require an effort to establish in the beginning to counter the inertia created by our life out of balance, but they soon create a self-sustaining and expanding force of their own.

These regimes, as presented here, are to help us establish a daily, monthly and yearly program to follow. All serious students of Ayurveda should establish such a program in their own lives. They should write it down. Conditions before implementing the program should be noted, and the results of following it should be kept track of on an ongoing basis. If these regimes are done consistently, there is no limit to how much we can improve our own state of being.

Taking Control of Our Own Karma

What we do every day makes for who we are. Our actions determine the content of our consciousness as well as the energy level of our physical body. An occasional visit to a healer, no matter how famous or expensive, cannot substitute for our own regime or substantially alter its effects. The healing methods we put into practice are of the greatest importance, not what someone does for us. The latter are palliative; the former only can be curative, as they alone indicate a change of nature within us.

What we do every day determines not only who we are in this life but also who we will become in the next. According to the Upanishads, "as is a man's will, so is his action, as is his action, so he becomes." (*Brihadaranyaka Upanishad V. 4.5.*) We must first have the right will or the true resolve to live in harmony. This is called "kratu" in Sanskrit, meaning intelligence in action. Through it we can take control of our own karma and cease to be victims of our own unconscious action.

Moreover, what we do every day is our real religion, for it shows what we truly value in life. From it comes the impressions which we take into our next life. Our wrong habits are not only bad for the health problems they cause us in this life, but they also create a predisposition to such problems in future lives. We may be able to escape their immediate effects, but they will come to us eventually.

Ayurvedic Regimes and the Treatment of Disease

We have seen that diseases and their treatment in Ayurveda are explained according to the biological humors. Kapha (water) constitution individuals tend towards Kapha type or variety of diseases. Pitta (fire) constitutions usually have Pitta diseases. Vata (air) people similarly have a predominance of high Vata symptoms in the diseases they get. Life regimes, therefore, afford us a methodology for preventing, as well as curing, disease.

It is possible, however, to temporarily come down with a disease caused by a humor other than that predominant in one's constitution, so the nature of the disease should be carefully examined. Diseases of a humor different than one's constitution, as a rule, are easier to treat.

A disease can be identified through its underlying humoral imbalance, according to the nature of the symptoms and syndromes it presents. Therefore, through recognizing the underlying humoral imbalance, we can treat a condition even if we do not know technically what it is. For example, if an individual has cough, congestion, profuse white phlegm, excessive salivation and such high Kapha (water) signs, we can implement an anti-Kapha therapy even if we do not know if the condition is bronchitis or another lung disease.

Limitations of Naturalistic Therapies

The main difficulty with this, or any natural form of healing, is that it takes time, as well as effort of our own. It may take a month or more of a natural herbal remedy, particularly in treating a long-standing complaint, to give a noticeable effect. It may take several months of following a constitutional regime to notice major changes. Nor can we expect the mild remedies of natural healing, such as herbs or body work, to succeed if our own life is out of balance, if our diet, work and stress of life-style are antagonistic to them.

Mild natural remedies work on a subtle internal level by correcting and improving the nature of the life-force. This is like the growing of flowers. The natural healer provides the seed but the rest — the water, sunshine and love — must come from us as the seed is planted in the soil of who we are. If that soil is not prepared properly, a natural energy may not be able to take root or to flourish, even if the seed is good.

So, dear friends, if you are serious about natural healing, you must have faith. You must have patience. And you must put *YOURSELF* to work. No one else can heal you any more than anyone else can live life for you. Be respectful of your life and give reverence to the Divine Spirit within you. Be the master of your own destiny.

Life-Regimes and Other Types of Treatment

Ayurvedic life-regimes are simple, non-invasive, non-traumatic and, generally, will not interfere with more specific forms of medical treatment. They can be taken along with other treatment methods including allopathic medicine. They can be used to enhance almost any form of treatment.

Pacifying or Eliminating Excess Humors

Self-care methods given here are mainly for pacifying (shamana) the various humors. For more severe cases, Ayurveda supplements them with stronger elimination methods (shodhana). (see chapters on 'Herbal Therapies'.)

Danger of Excess Treatment

Physical disease is often a result of overfixation upon the physical body and the material world. If we put too much energy into our physical condition we may aggravate the disease process. We must give the body its place and its proper care, but must not let it dominate the other aspects of our lives. We should make the required efforts with faith and patience, devoting the greater part of our energy for the real spiritual and creative issues of our lives.

Many of us today suffer from excess treatment. We have taken too many medications, seen too many different doctors or healers. Our bodies are deranged by too much strain to make them well. Hence, in healing ourselves we should proceed with patience and simplicity. By taking many remedies we may not make things better; even if our condition is not good, we must consider that we may make things worse. Moreover, we must give therapies their time and not switch them too quickly. Nor should we combine many different kinds of treatments at once, particularly those of a strong or forceful nature.

LIFE REGIMES

Sattvic Living

All human beings should follow a sattvic or pure life-style, one that gives peace and clarity of mind. The remedial measures in Ayurveda are generally of a sattvic (harmonious) nature.

Physical purity includes pure diet, with raw or freshly cooked vegetarian food, pure air and water, proper exercise of a calming nature, as well as physical cleanliness. (see 'Sattvic Diet'.)

Purity of mind includes truthfulness, honesty, humility, equanimity, non-violence, friendliness and compassion to all beings. Emotional impurities like anger, hatred, pride, lust and fear are given up; gossip and worry are to be set aside. These are the main bad mental habits which destroy the natural clarity and equipoise of mind.

Purity of life-style includes right livelihood (an occupation that does not bring harm to others), pleasant speech, harmonious or pleasant environment, and avoidance of distraction, noise and all violent or degrading forms of entertainment.

Sattvic life-style includes devotion to the Divine or to truth, compassion, service to humanity, study of spiritual teachings, reverence for spiritual teachers, and the practice of Yoga and meditation.

Purity itself, however, should not become a fault through self-righteousness, hypersensitivity or fanaticism. Good humor and moderation should always be maintained. Natural harmony and adaptability are what is necessary, not the imposition of an artificial standard.

Diet and Herbs

Diet is the most important long-term physical remedial measure. Its effects take time to manifest, often one to six months, but are enduring. As a remedial measure, it is constant, though requiring modification for season, age or specific diseases. Our physical body is composed of food; we cannot expect its condition to change without changing our diet.

Herbs are like subtle foods. They can be taken in small or large doses. Large doses (more than one ounce of herbs per day) should usually not be taken without special study or professional guidance. In small doses herbs are like strong food supplements; and they can and should be taken on a regular basis by almost everyone. They are part of our necessary food articles and provide subtle nutrition. Right nutrition is not only taking our daily bread but also taking our daily herbs.

Oils and Massage

Massage and external application of oils are necessary for most of us on a regular basis. This may be no more than applying a common oil, such as sesame, to the feet or head twice a week. Therapeutic touch communicates to our body and breaks stagnation along its surface. Oil massage nourishes the heart and calms the mind. It gives elasticity to the muscles and ligaments and strengthens the bones.

Essential oils and fragrances are also an important part of life. They open the mind and heart and purify the air and aura. Incense works along the same lines. It aids in purification and helps create an atmosphere receptive to the Divine powers.

Colors and Gems

The right use of colors has a harmonizing effect on the mind and emotions through the senses. Our impressions feed the mind and affect the biological humors.

Gems help balance the aura and harmonize the cosmic influences projected upon us through the stars. They are not merely for ornamentation but offer an additional method of attunement with the subtle energies of life. It is usually helpful to wear or use gem-stones that help balance one's physical and mental nature. This is shown to us through astrology and Ayurveda.

Life-style

Life-style is probably the most important general factor in physical and mental health. Right life-style does not mean suppressing our nature, but bringing out its deeper powers. In Ayurveda, this includes not suppressing our natural urges like eating, sleeping, sex, elimination, urination, sneezing, weeping, coughing, yawning, or farting.

Life-style considerations for everyone involve such physical factors as right amount of rest, sufficient exercise, right exposure to sun, to heat or cold, and a pleasant and natural environment.

The mental factors and ethical attitudes of right life-style are the principles of sattvic living. These are varied according to the constitution. Such factors as right relationship and right attitudes are included here, as well as right livelihood.

Yoga and Meditation

Yoga and meditation relate to the spiritual aspect of life. According to Ayurveda, the soul is the source of life and health. We must therefore live according to the purpose of our soul in order to have peace and well-being. Often disease indicates that we have lost contact with our soul.

Each of us should do some daily Yoga and meditation. This may include Yoga postures, breathing exercises, mantra and visualization, as well as more direct meditation practices aimed at silencing the mind. Without this our life has no real center around which the other practices of right living can be organized.

It should be noted that although Ayurveda includes all these different remedial measures as part of the system of Vedic science, all are not specific to it. Gem therapy is more appropriately part of Vedic astrology. Yoga therapy is a branch of treatment in itself, including a more specific use of asanas, pranayama and mantra. It is important to consult practitioners of these other branches of Vedic Science for more detailed guidance on these subjects; or to access our own direct inner intuition.

Spiritual methods vary more according to differences of cultural and individual temperament than do physical health measures. The mind, as it is not as defined an entity as the physical body, requires greater flexibility in its treatment. These are general guidelines to be adapted with intelligence and consciousness.

Moreover, the biological humors do not comprehend all aspects of our nature, though they have effects on all levels. It is not necessary to stereotype oneself according to one's humor. All that is required is to not neglect the problems which may arise from not compensating for it. The humors are guidelines for tuning into one's nature, but the full attunement is ultimately an individual affair.

Classical Remedial Measures for the Three Humors

According to Ayurvedic source books, "Vata (air) is treated by mild application of oils, mild sweating and purification methods; by sweet, sour, salty and warm food, and by oil massage; by staying indoors, by firm guidance, by anointing the eyes, by wine made from grain or sugar; by warm oil enemas, by moderate cleansing enemas, by comfortable living; by medicines that stimulate the digestive fire, by all kinds of oils, particularly by oil enemas with sesame oil or meat or animal fat broths.

"Pitta (fire) is treated with the ingestion of ghee (clarified butter), by purgation with sweet and cold herbs; by sweet, bitter and astringent foods and herbs; by application of cool, delightful and fragrant essential oils; by the wearing of precious gems around the neck; by frequently anointing the head with camphor, sandalwood and vetivert oils; by relaxing in the moonlight, by beautiful songs, by a cool wind; by unrestrained enjoyment, by friends, by a devoted son; by a beautiful and attractive wife; by ponds with cool water, by houses with large gardens; especially by loving emotions; and by milk and ghee as laxatives.

"Kapha (water) is treated by strong emetic and purgation methods according to the rules; by food that is dry, little in quantity, sharp, hot and pungent, bitter and astringent in taste; by old wine, by sexual enjoyment, by staying up at night; by all kinds of exercise, by mental activity, by dry or strong massage; by smoking of herbs and, generally, by taking pleasure in physical hardship." (*Ashtanga Hridaya XIII. 1–12.*)

We see the Ayurvedic methods traditionally used to balance the humors are complex. They are not our modern "take this pill and come back in a week," but consider all aspects of life.

In addition, we must consider that it is important not only what we do but how we do it. We may take the right remedies, but if we take them with the wrong attitude they cannot be expected to work.

Vata (air) people tend to do things hastily, irregularly or erratically. Pitta (fire) people tend to be fanatical or forceful and may apply things in a rigid or authoritarian manner. Kapha (water) types may be too slow or conservative in what they do. All that we do to balance our constitution should be based on an attitude which also compensates for it.

Below is an outline of the main therapies for each humor. These therapies are described specifically in other chapters.

SYNOPSIS OF TREATMENT
ANTI-VATA THERAPY

Comprehensive Therapy for Reducing Excess Air

All anti-Vata (anti-air) therapies are nurturing, warming, moistening, calming and grounding. They should be done with patience, peace, consistency and regularity.

Diet

A nutritive, strengthening diet is indicated with predominately sweet, sour and salty tastes. Food should be warm, heavy and moist with frequent and regular meals. Spices should be used in cooking to regulate digestion. Cold water or ice should be avoided, as well as stimulating beverages such as coffee, though a small amount of wine or alcohol can be taken with meals.

Herbs

Digestion	Spices and salts should be used: asafoetida, rock salt, garlic, ginger, cumin, fennel, coriander, cardamom, cinnamon, ajwan.
Elimination	Bulk and tonic laxatives are indicated: psyllium and flaxseed, mild laxatives like Triphala, oily purgatives like castor oil.
Energy	Special anti-Vata tonics: garlic, ashwagandha, bala, shatavari, black musali, white musali, kapikacchu, amalaki; other useful available herbs include ginseng, dang gui, lycium berries, marshmallow, comfrey root, solomon's seal, saw palmetto.
Mind	Anti-Vata nervine herbs: calamus, ashwagandha, haritaki, jatamansi, valerian, nutmeg, asafoetida, basil; other useful herbs include zizyphus seeds, biota seeds, camomile.

Oils and Massage

Oil therapy is specific for high Vata with warm, heavy oils like sesame and almond applied moderately on a regular basis. Best sites are the feet, the top of the head, the back and the lower abdomen.

Massage for Vata should be warm, moist, mild, nurturing, relaxing and not inducing pain.

Best essential oils for Vata are warming, calming and clearing like sandalwood, camphor, wintergreen, cinnamon, musk. Most of these are also good for incense.

Colors and Gems

Most colors are good for Vata (which tends towards depression), including yellow, orange and white and a small amount of red. Vata, however, is sensitive and lighter or more pastel shades are preferable to bright or metallic tones. Dark colors, grays, browns and blacks, should be avoided. Green and blue can be used in moderation or with warmer colors.

As gems tend to be heavy and grounding they are often good for Vata. Special gems for the nervous system are indicated, including emerald, jade, peridot set in gold; yellow sapphire, topaz and citrine and other golden stones set in gold. Ruby or garnet can be helpful and improve circulation and energy.

Yoga

Calming and grounding asanas are indicated such as sitting and lying postures, as well as back bends and inverted poses. Calm, deep breathing practices are helpful, such as alternate nostril pranayama or So ham pranayama. Calming and fear-dispelling mantras like Ram, Sham, Hum, Hrim, Shrim are specific.

Meditation

Raja Yoga, integral Yoga is indicated combining knowledge, devotion and psychophysical techniques. Right attitude for meditation involves giving up worry, fear and anxiety, negativity and lack of faith.

Life-style

Most important factors are adequate sleep, not staying up late at night, moderate sun bathing, avoidance of wind and cold, mild exercise, avoidance of overwork or physical hardship, avoidance of excess talking or thinking, moderation in sex, not traveling too much, and avoidance of excess stimulation generally including television, movies and radio.

Purification Practices
Pancha Karma
Enema therapy is indicated as the main anti-Vata treatment in more severe conditions. Nourishing herbs like licorice, ashwagandha or shatavari or oils like sesame are used for tonifying enemas. Vata (air) dispelling herbs like calamus, ginger, fennel and rock salt are good for cleansing enemas.

Nasal therapy is also indicated with the taking of Vata-clearing herbs like calamus, ginger or basil in the form of snuffs, decoctions, medicated oils or ghees.

ANTI-PITTA THERAPY
Comprehensive Therapy for Reducing Excess Fire
All anti-Pitta (anti-fire) therapies should be cooling, calming, moderately cleansing and nurturing. They should be implemented with an attitude of peace, restraint and moderation.

Diet
A balanced strengthening and reducing diet with mainly sweet, bitter and astringent tastes, along with adequate intake of raw food and juices, is indicated. Food should be cool, heavy and dry, even in taste, without excessive spices. Water should be taken cool. Coffee and alcohol should be avoided but tea can be taken.

Herbs

Digestion	Digestive bitters: aloe, gentian, barberry; cooling or mild spices: turmeric, fennel, coriander, cumin, mint.
Elimination	Bitter laxatives: aloe, cascara sagrada, rhubarb and senna; often mild laxatives such as milk, ghee or rose are sufficient, or bulk laxatives such as psyllium.
Energy	Calming and cooling tonics: shatavari, bala, amalaki, saffron, aloe gel, licorice, guduchi; other useful herbs include comfrey root, solomon's seal, marshmallow, dandelion root, burdock root, fo-ti, rehmannia.
Mind	Cooling and calming herbs: gotu kola, bhringaraj, sandalwood, rose, lotus seeds; other useful herbs include skullcap, passion flower, betony, chrysanthemum, hibiscus.

Oils and Massage

Cooling oils such as coconut, sunflower or ghee should be used for massage. Medicated oils, brahmi (gotu kola) or bhringaraj (eclipta), are good. They can be applied to the top of the head, forehead and heart.

Fragrances and flower essences are specific, such as sandalwood, vetivert, henna, rose, lotus, jasmine, gardenia, honeysuckle, iris. They can also be used in the form of incense.

Colors and Gems

The cooling colors white, blue and green are best, but generally any overly strong or very bright colors should be avoided, particularly red. Grays and browns are alright but dark black should be avoided.

Cooling gems are indicated such as moonstone, clear quartz crystal, emerald, jade, peridot, blue sapphire, amethyst set in silver.

Yoga

Cooling and calming asanas are indicated such as most sitting or lying postures, shoulderstand, cooling pranayama — shitali, lunar pranayama, cooling and calming mantras — Om, Sham, Som, Shum, Shim.

Meditation

Yoga of knowledge or self-inquiry is generally appropriate, such as Vedanta, Zen, Vipassana, along with giving up of anger, hostility, argument and overly critical nature.

Life-style

Too much sun and exposure to heat or heaters should be avoided; one should resort to cooling breezes, cool water, moonlight, gardens, flowers, and lakes and practice sweetness of speech, forgiveness and contentment.

Purification Practices
Pancha Karma

Purgation is indicated with strong laxatives — rhubarb, senna and aloe. For self-care, milder laxatives can be used — aloe gel, Triphala or psyllium husks.

ANTI-KAPHA THERAPY
Comprehensive Therapy for Reducing Excess Water

All anti-Kapha (anti-water) therapies are reducing, lightening, stimulating, drying and clearing. They should be applied with force and determination, as well as detachment.

Diet

A primarily reducing diet is used, emphasizing pungent, bitter and astringent tastes. Food should be warm, light and dry, with hot spices. Occasional fasting or skipping a meal is good. Cold or ice water should be avoided. Herbal teas are good and regular tea can be taken as well.

Herbs

Digestion	Hot spices are indicated: cayenne, black pepper, dry ginger, long pepper, mustard, cloves, cinnamon, garlic for improving metabolism; bitters such as aloe, turmeric, barberry and gentian are useful for reducing the need for sugars and fats.
Energy	Pungent or bitter tonics: garlic, long pepper, cinnamon, saffron, ginger, elecampane root, shilajit, guggul, myrrh and aloe gel.
Mind	Stimulants and mind-clearing herbs: calamus, gotu kola, basil, guggul and myrrh; other useful herbs are sage, bayberry, skullcap and betony.

Oils and Massage

Dry or rough massage is good or massage with such light oils as mustard or flaxseed (linseed) oil. Rubbing alcohol or warm herbal oils prepared in alcohol, like wintergreen, camphor, eucalyptus, cinnamon, mustard and cayenne, are good.

Stimulating and cleansing fragrances and incenses, like musk, camphor, cloves, cinnamon, cedar, frankincense and myrrh, should be used.

Colors and Gems

Warm and bright colors should be used, such as yellow, orange, gold and red. White should be avoided along with the white or pale shades of blue and green, also pink. Brown, grey and black can be used in moderation.

Warm gems are indicated: ruby, garnet and cat's eye set in gold. Reducing gems such as blue sapphire, amethyst, lapis, set in gold can also be good but should be combined with the warmer stones.

Yoga

Strong workouts are indicated with less sitting postures, headstands if possible, solar pranayama, bhastrika (breath of fire) and stimulating and clearing mantras like Aim, Hrim, Hum, Om.

Meditation

Yoga of devotion (bhakti Yoga) or service work (karma Yoga), are generally in harmony with the nature. Usually the divine is worshipped as a particular deity or incarnation, like Rama, Krishna or Christ. Renunciation of greed, desire, attachment and sentimentality is indicated for clearing the mind.

Life-Style

Strong and aerobic exercise should be done, with sun bathing, warm breezes, avoidance of cold and damp, following of discipline, physical hardship, staying up at night, avoidance of sleep during the day, mental stimulation, travel, pilgrimage.

Purification Practices
Pancha Karma

Therapeutic vomiting is indicated with such expectorant herbs as calamus, lobelia, licorice, salt. For self-care, expectorant herbs can be taken in lower dosages including bayberry, sage, elecampane and ginger.

BALANCING THE HUMORS IN THE MODERN WORLD

The factors of imbalance implicit in our modern life-style must be considered when implementing these life-regime suggestions. These are aspects of our culture which aggravate the humors. Our dietary emphasis on sugars, ice cream, ice water, soft drinks, carbohydrates, meats and foods fried in oil tends to imbalance Kapha (water). Our competitive social and business practices, our emphasis on personal achievement and success, as well as such habits as smoking and drinking aggravate Pitta (fire). However, the great majority of our practices increase Vata (air).

Vata is aggravated by such modern life-styles as frequent traveling, particularly by airplane. This dissociates us from the ground altogether, literally raising us high into the air. Any form of transportation which removes our direct physical contact with the earth increases Vata, even riding in cars. High speed increases Vata. The faster we drive, the more our Vata, our nervous energy, becomes hyper. Fast forms of sports, excessive running or skiing, for example, also have this effect.

We must consider the physical problems such practices may create over time, particularly for those who work in these fields. Simple therapies should be done to compensate, such as having a foot massage; applying sesame oil to the feet; doing an inverted Yoga posture; or just walking barefoot on the earth.

The mass media as a whole has an influence that strongly aggravates Vata. We are affected not only by its message, which is change and mobility, but also by its nature, the subtle radiations it emits. The physical body has a vital or energy sheath, the basis of Vata (the life-force) as the primary energy of the body. This can be short circuited by excess exposure to waves given off by televisions, computers, etc. We also become habituated to perpetual stimulation. The emphasis on superficial information keeps our minds in a state of want (emptiness that increases Vata) and perpetual distraction. Sitting in front of a computer all day can have an over-stimulating effect; playing computer games even more so.

Rock music, or any other frequent exposure to very loud sounds or a high noise level, disturbs the nervous system and aggravates Vata. Sound is the quality that corresponds to ether (part of Vata, composed of air and ether), so excess or disharmonious sound will increase it.

Most drugs derange Vata, including both medicinal and recreational types, largely through their over-stimulation or disruption of nerve function. Stimulant drugs (uppers), weight reduction pills and most pain-relieving drugs as well as amphetamines and cocaine are strongly disruptive. Marijuana and tobacco, followed by coffee and caffeine-containing soft drinks affect Vata in a milder way. Mind-altering drugs such as L.S.D. or ecstasy aggravate Vata in a potentially severe manner. Artificially-induced, temporarily-heightened sensitization of the nervous system leads to either long term desensitization or hypersensitivity. Symptoms of such Vata derangement include insomnia, constipation, dry skin, weight loss, vertigo or light headedness, loss of memory, loss of sensory acuity or coordination, tremors, palpitations and anxiety.

Eating of junk food or food that has been microwaved aggravates Vata because the life-force in the food has been depleted.

A number of New Age practices are highly Vatogenic (air-increasing). Channeling, forceful meditational practices, excessive imagination, or anything that may disrupt the connection of our life-force with our physical body, can increase Vata.

Excess sexual indulgence aggravates Vata (air) by removing from our body its strongest energy of water (the reproductive fluid) to keep it in check. Homosexual activity tends to aggravate Vata more than heterosexual practices as there is not the balancing influence of the opposite sex to keep Vata (the life-force) in equilibrium.

Our life style of easy divorce, frequent sexual partners in or out of marriage, and broken families takes its toll here. The family or home itself has a Kapha or watery nature that is disrupted by excessive change. Such disturbances derange the Vata or life-force of all of its members, particularly the children who are more impressionable (who have not yet established a life center of their own).

There is no moral judgement in this; it is a question of energetics. Other cultures have their own characteristic imbalances as well. To the degree that we are involved in such activities, we invite imbalance. These factors that imbalance Vata (and sometimes Pitta) are primarily rajasic. They also reduce sattva, harmony of mind. Our primary social values are materialistic; money, pleasure, fame and power. Our primary social behavior is constant action, stimulation, entertainment, seeking, moving from one thing to another. We must consider the spiritual implications of our life styles. Health and harmony of the physical life should be the basis of the development of consciousness. If it is not possible, or not desirable, to change the nature of our activity, we can at least adopt as many of the appropriate remedial measures as possible to compensate for its side-effects.

6

AYURVEDIC DIET

PERSONALIZING YOUR DIETARY REGIME

*I am food, I am the eater of food, I eat the eater of food. I consume the
entire universe. My light is like the Sun.*
— *Taittiriya Upanishad II. 9.6.*

Dietary Therapy

Herbal therapy requires the additional support of the proper diet to be
effective. Diet can enhance, or counter, the effect of herbs. Generally, an
inharmonious diet will either neutralize or greatly limit the effect of the
right herbs.

Herbs and foods follow the same energetics and can be looked at
according to the same principles. Both involve taste, energy, elements and
humors. Herbs provide subtle nutrition; foods provide more gross or
substantial nourishment.

Diet can be an effective treatment in itself. Though dietary results are
slower to manifest, over a period of time they are as certain as that of
herbs. Dietary treatment is usually the safest therapy and can be used by
itself when herbal knowledge may not be adequate for proper prescription.
Diet is the essence of effective self-care.

Wrong diet is the main physical causative factor of disease. Hence,
in correcting the diet, we not only add to the power of healing herbs, we
also eliminate one of the fundamental causes of the condition. In its
constitutional approach, Ayurveda emphasizes correct diet for the individual. This is the main factor in long term treatment of the physical
body, called in Sanskrit, annamaya kosha, the food sheath.

Ayurveda is concerned primarily with the energetics of food as a
means of balancing the biological humors. It is not as concerned with the
specific nutritional requirements, the actual mineral, vitamin and chemical content of food. From its view there is no standard diet for everyone,
nor any minimum daily requirements. Its concern is that the food we take
in, and the manner in which we take it, is in harmony with our nature. As
such, its primary classification of food is according to the humors, the

different food types work on. This affords us a simple yet comprehensive understanding of what is good for us and why.

Diet and the Mind

In Vedantic philosophy the mind (manomaya kosha) is considered to be the essence of food. Uddalaka Aruni, a famous ancient sage, states "The food that is eaten is divided threefold. The gross part becomes excrement. The middle part becomes flesh. The subtle part becomes the mind." *(Chandogya Upanishad VI. 4.1.)* According to the common adage, "we are what we eat." What we eat affects our emotions and can create a predisposition for both psychological and physical disorders. Just as wrong emotions can upset our digestion, so wrong digestion can upset our emotions.

We should consider the spiritual qualities of the food we take in. Does it enhance our mental processes and peace of mind? Or is it disturbing? It is for this reason that meat, however nourishing, is not a good food. It has the energy of death and brings the forces of violence and decay, the negative emotions of fear and hatred along with it. (see also 'Sattvic Diet')

Uddalaka Aruni also tells us, "The water that is drunk is divided threefold. The gross part becomes urine. The middle part becomes blood. The subtle part becomes the life-force (prana)."*(Chandogya Upanishad VI. 4.2.)* Hence, what we drink also nourishes our life-force. Drinking stale water, such as comes out of our taps, or distilled water, and drinking alcohol, coffee or other stimulating beverages, will disturb our life-force and thereby derange our emotions and thoughts.

Ayurvedic Principles of Dietetics

While care should be taken about the nature of food, other factors of food intake should be considered. According to Ayurveda, these include right preparation of food, right combination of foods, right amount of food, right frequency of meals and right times and places for eating. Right emotional or mental state is necessary; good food taken in a bad mood or ill humor can cause disease. Also important is right attitude in the person preparing the food, which should be done with care and good feelings.

Seasons

Diet should be adjustable for climate and seasonal variations, as well as stages of life. Anti-Vata diet should be given emphasis in the fall. Anti-Pitta diet should be followed more in the summer and late spring. Anti-Kapha diet should be followed more in the winter and in early spring.

Individuals whose constitutions are equal in two of the humors, what we call dual types, should vary their diet by season. Vata-Pitta types should follow an anti-Vata diet more in the fall and winter and anti-Pitta in the spring and summer. Vata-Kapha types should follow an anti-Vata diet in the summer and fall and anti-Kapha in the winter and spring. Pitta-Kapha types should follow an anti-Pitta diet in summer and fall and anti-Kapha in winter and spring.

Climate

Anti-Vata diet is more appropriate to cold, dry, windy climates, like the high desert or high plains regions.

Anti-Pitta diet is more suitable for hot climates including the southern United States and the lower desert of the southwest.

Anti-Kapha diet is more appropriate in damp and cold regions like the midwest, most of the east and northeast, and the northwest.

Like dual constitutions, dual climates exist. The hot desert is a Pitta-Vata climate, while the southeast is largely a Pitta-Kapha climate.

Age and Sex

In old age an anti-Vata diet is more appropriate. In middle age an anti-Pitta diet is better. In childhood an anti-Kapha diet should be given more special consideration.

Men should consider a more anti-Pitta diet, women an anti-Kapha diet.

Such general factors, however, should enhance, not replace, the basic diet for balancing one's humor.

Qualities of Food

Food tends to be neutral, neither too hot nor too cold in energy. For this reason the heating or cooling effects of foods are mild. For heating or cooling to manifest, either large quantities or long-term consumption is necessary. Foods can be made hot by cooking and by the addition of spices; colder by taking them cold or raw. Anything very hot, like pepper, or very cold, like bitter herbs, cannot have much food value.

Foods are primarily heavy or light, though most tend to be heavy. It can be made lighter through the use of spices or by consuming less. Foods also are drying or moistening; most often they are moistening. They can be made drier by evaporation or dry-preparing them. They can be made moister by cooking, by the addition of liquids or oils.

DIETS FOR THE THREE HUMORS

For the treatment of most diseases the diet prescribed will be opposite in nature to the biological humor causing the disease. It will generally be the same diet as that for one's constitutional humor; the diseases we get are usually caused by it. These diets should be applied considering the variations mentioned above and according to the proper dietetics. It is not only the types of foods we have to watch, but also our manner of eating.

Nor is it just a simple matter of avoiding the food that is bad for us. We must also improve our digestion through the use of spices, herbs and other regimes. Without these aids even the food that is good for us may not be digestible.

It should be noted that the quality of foods varies according to freshness, preparation and combination, as well as other factors already mentioned. The system presented here is only a general guideline. Some difference of opinion as to food quality may exist among different practitioners (even more so than about the quality of herbs).

KEY TO FOODS LIST

I have classified foods according to Yes and No or what is good or bad for the respective constitution. Under the Yes column, a food marked * is Good to take for the respective constitution, ** is Better, *** is Best. Under the No column, a food marked * is Not Good for the respective constitution, ** is Worse, and *** is Worst. Thus, the best foods for each humor would be marked *** in the Yes column; the Worst Foods would be marked *** in the No column.

A food that is * on the No column, for example, may be taken occasionally, or easily antidoted. Our predominant diet is what matters; we have some latitude within that field, except when we are very ill.

Classification is also according to food categories. Each food type has its general degree of increasing or decreasing the humor. When both the category and the specific food are high for increasing a humor, the effect is greater. Foods not listed can generally be judged by category or by comparing them to related foods.

ANTI-VATA DIET
DIET FOR DECREASING THE BIOLOGICAL AIR HUMOR

General Considerations

Vata (air) types are most likely to suffer from emaciation, malnourishment or wasting away of tissues. Therefore, dietary therapy, improving food quality and quantity, is one of the most important treatments for all Vata disorders. Vata types should generally try to eat more and eat more often.

They require a calming, grounding, nourishing diet. Food should be warm, heavy, moistening and strengthening.

Tastes recommended are sweet, sour and salty. Pungent, bitter and astringent are not advised. Pungent taste, however, can be used as a spice (rather than as food) for regulating appetite unless the individual has extreme enervation or hypersensitivity.

Air types tend to suffer from a variable digestive power. The heavy foods which are good for them may not always be digested properly. Care must be taken that the digestive fire is adequate for the food, or toxins may be produced from the improperly digested food mass.

Dietetics

Meals should be small and frequent but regular. Food should be taken warm or cooked. Fast food, instant food and junk food should be avoided. Not too many different food types should be combined in the same meal. Mild spices and salt can be used.

Meals should not be taken when nervous, anxious or afraid, when excessively thoughtful or worried. Attention should be given to eating. Watching television, reading or other forms of nervous stimulation should be avoided during meals.

Vata types do better if they do not eat alone and if their food is cooked for them. So if you have a Vata friend, one of the best things you can do is to cook a meal for him or her. Vata individuals should learn to cook in order to help balance out their constitutions.

They also have the most irregular and erratic eating habits, and are most in need of a dietary regime. They are likely to forget to eat, not want to cook, or when they cook burn their food. On the other hand, when given a good meal, they may overeat.

Vata people are more likely to suffer from food allergies; some foods that are normally good for them may have to be taken with care. Nightshades (potatoes, tomatoes, eggplant, peppers, chilies) are the most typical in this regard. Yet, often it is not the food that is the problem for Vata people, but their hypersensitivity, which can render anything undigestible. So rather than restricting the diet, it is usually better to take herbs and follow regimes to lower Vata.

Fruit
Yes ✳

Most fruit is all right for Vata as it is pleasant, harmonizing, clearing and increases body fluids. The main exception is dry fruit, which is particularly gas forming (Vatogenic).

However, fruit is generally too light to really lower high Vata (air). It should be taken in moderation, seasonally, and not mixed too much with other foods. Vata types should not become fruitarians (even if they live in Hawaii). Fruit contains a high percentage of the element, ether. It can increase ungroundedness, lack of concentration, lack of will power and some other high Vata traits if it becomes one of the central foods in the diet.

YES		NO	
✳✳	Lemons, limes, grapefruit, prunes (soaked or raw), cherries, grapes, strawberries, raspberries, pineapples, papayas, mango, dates (raw or soaked), figs (raw or soaked)	✳✳✳	Dry fruit
✳	Oranges, bananas, pears, apples (cooked) peaches, plums, apricots, pomegranates, persimmons	✳✳	Melons, cranberies
		✳	Apples (uncooked)

Vegetables
Cooked, Yes ✳: Raw, No ✳

Air types usually cannot live primarily on a vegetable diet as it tends to be too light for them, but they can at least tolerate most vegetables if they are cooked. Preparing them with oils and spices and eating along with whole grains makes them better. Raw vegetables and salads should be taken only moderately or in season with a fair amount of oil dressing.

Cabbage family plants (cabbage, broccoli, cauliflower, brussels sprouts, kale, kohlrabi) tend to cause gas. Mushrooms are diuretic and can be overly drying and aggravate Vata. Raw onions are gas forming but cooked they are one of the best anti-Vata foods. Again, be careful of allergic reactions to nightshades.

Many vegetables in the No category can be made acceptable through application of spices, oils (sesame or ghee), cheese, sour cream, or salt.

YES		NO	
***	Onions (cooked)	**	Onions (raw), mushrooms, cabbage, broccoli, brussels sprouts, lettuce
**	Chilies, sweet potatoes, carrots, beets, cilantro, parsley, radish, avocado, seaweed	*	Cauliflower, alfalfa sprouts, sunflower sprouts, cucumber, celery, asparagus, spinach, chard, eggplant
*	Potatoes, tomatoes, bell peppers, corn (fresh), green beans, peas (fresh), turnips, squash, artichoke, okra, mustard greens, watercress		

Grains
Yes **

Most whole grains are good for Vata, as they are both nourishing and heavy. They can often be digested by Vata types when other foods cannot. Many Vata diseases can be alleviated by a long-term whole grain diet.

Grains which are drying (diuretic) in excess can aggravate Vata, however. Yet, even these are good in some Vata disorders that involve Ama or dampness (as the use of barley to treat arthritis).

Breads are more likely to aggravate Vata because yeast tends to cause gas. Their overall Vata-reducing property is less (yes only to the first degree).

Dried grains such as granola and most chips such as corn chips, also tend to aggravate Vata.

YES		NO	
***	Wheat	**	Granola and dried grains
**	Oats, brown rice, basmati rice, khus khus	*	Corn, buckwheat, millet, rye, barley, quinoa

Beans
No **

Most beans strongly aggravate Vata (cause gas). They are usually drying (diuretic) as well, and promote constipation. Their quality is rajasic, and so they can be over-stimulating. Tofu is one of the better beans for Vata, but more sensitive Vata types still may find it hard to digest.

YES	NO
** Mung	*** Soy, split peas
* Tofu	** Lentils, pinto, peanuts
	* Aduki, lima beans, kidney beans, chick peas

Nuts and Seeds
Yes **

Most nuts and seeds are good for Vata, particularly taken raw or lightly roasted with salt. They are warm, heavy and moist, nourish the lungs, reproductive system and the nerves. But they are also hard to digest and cannot be taken in large quantities at a time. Dry roasted, they are more likely to cause difficulties in digestion (this also goes for peanuts).

YES	NO
*** Almonds, walnuts, peacons, pine nuts	
** Cashews, sesame seeds, filberts, brazil nuts	
* Coconut, sunflower seeds, pumpkin seeds	

Dairy
Yes **

Most dairy is good for Vata as it is heavy, nourishing and moistening. But as it tends to be cooling or heavy, hard to digest, dairy must be taken with proper consideration of the digestive fire. It should be taken warm or with spices; milk should be taken by itself. Fermented dairy products are usually better for Vata as they are already predigested.

YES	NO
*** Buttermilk, ghee	** Ice cream
** Milk, yogurt, kefir, cream, sour cream, butter, cottage cheese	
* Cheese	

Animal Products
Yes *

Meat and fish lower high Vata (air). They can be very effective foods in this respect. Meat can be very grounding. Vata types can most honestly claim to need meat in their diet. They sometimes find that it restores their health when nothing else seems to work (particularly if they have been raised on it).

Even for these conditions, however, chicken and fish are usually enough. Red meat really is seldom required. Eggs are also very good for reducing Vata.

While meat may be helpful short term in high Vata conditions, in general it may not be necessary. It is so tamasic, it has many side effects, including being difficult to digest, increasing Ama and dulling the mind. Because Vata types are the most sensitive, they can also pick up the negative energy of killing from the meat and become disturbed in mind. Even in high Vata conditions, special tonic herbs can be used rather than meat and often with greater effectiveness.

YES		NO	
**	Fish, shell fish, eggs	**	Pork
*	Chicken, turkey	*	Beef, lamb

Oils
Yes **

Most oils are good for Vata. Oil, being moist and warm, is the main substance indicated for lowering high Vata (air), as it possesses the opposite properties. But again, oils can be hard to digest. They may be better applied externally: they can be absorbed more easily through the skin. Most of the vegetable oils tend to be light and are inferior to ghee and sesame oil for lowering Vata.

YES		NO	
***	Sesame, ghee (clarified butter)	*	Safflower, corn, soy, margarine, canola
**	Almond, olive, avocado, butter		
*	Coconut, mustard, peanut		

Sweeteners
Yes *

Most sweeteners or sweet foods are good for Vata. Air types need more sugar than other types for maintaining strength of the tissues and body fluids. Only natural sugars should be used; refined sugar is an artificial food that depletes the life-force. However, pure sweets cause many difficulties in food combining. As Vata types most commonly suffer from gas, they must be particularly careful in how they combine sweets with other foods. Complex carbohydrates tend to be safer and more calming. Although sweet taste is good for Vata, it is not an excuse for indulging in sugars, pastries and candies.

YES	NO
*** Jaggery	** White sugar
** Maple syrup, molasses, raw sugar	
* Honey, fruit sugar	

Spices
Yes **

Most spices are good for Vata, for regulating appetite and dispelling gas. They are particularly useful with heavy or sweet food to allow Vata types to digest them properly. Really hot spices, however, like pepper or mustard, can be overly drying or stimulating and aggravate some high Vata conditions. Yet, particularly in the winter, Vata individuals will find them helpful.

Vata types are most in need of salt, particularly for improving digestion, for which purposes rock salt is best. It should not be taken in excess as salt has the power to aggravate all three humors.

YES	NO
*** Garlic, cardamom, asafoetida, fennel, nutmeg	
** Ginger, cloves, coriander, cumin, cinnamon, basil, fenugreek, rock salt	
* Turmeric, mint, black pepper, cayenne, mustard, horseradish, sea salt	

Beverages

Vata types need to take adequate fluids. Water itself, however, may not be nourishing enough. Dairy is often preferable, or spice or tonic herb teas which can be taken with milk and a natural sweetener. Sour fruit juices are good or water with lemon or lime.

Alcohol, particularly wine or Ayurvedic herbal wines such as draksha, is good in small quantities, 2-4 ounces, with or before meals.

Vitamins and Minerals

Air types do well with oily vitamins like A, D and E. Sour vitamins like Vitamin C are excellent. Minerals are good for them, particularly zinc and calcium, but they can be heavy and hard to digest and are best taken with spices.

ANTI-PITTA DIET
DIET FOR LOWERING THE BIOLOGICAL FIRE HUMOR

General Considerations

Pitta (fire) types require a diet that is cool, slightly dry and a little heavy. They usually possess the best appetites and strongest digestions and can get away with excessive eating or with bad food combinations. The effects of wrong diet may manifest more through toxic blood and infectious diseases than through simple digestive upset. Hence, the correlation between wrong diet and disease is not as easy to make in their case.

Tastes that decrease Pitta are sweet, bitter and astringent. It is increased by sour, salty and pungent. Sharp or strong tastes increase Pitta; mild or bland tastes decrease it. Hence, Pitta types should avoid tasty food.

Dietetics

Pitta types should have their food cool, raw, not heavily spiced and not cooked with a lot of oil. They should avoid fried and overly cooked food, and should be careful not to allow the liver to become clogged by a too rich diet.

Meals should not be taken when angry, irritable or upset. Pitta types should cultivate clarity rather than a critical nature in terms of what they eat. Food should be taken in an attitude of emotional calm and thankfulness. Three regular meals are usually sufficient. Eating late at night should be avoided.

Fruit
Yes **

Most fruit is good for Pitta (fire) as it tends to be cooling, calming, harmonizing and thirst relieving. Even sour fruit can be taken seasonally, and bananas are generally good, except in acute conditions like ulcers or urinary tract infections. Fruit juices are also good.

YES		NO	
***	Apples, pomegranate	**	Grapefruit
**	Pears, pineapple, cranberry, persimmon, melons, prunes, dates, grapes, figs	*	Lemons, limes, bananas, cherries, peaches, apricots, strawberries, papaya
*	Oranges, raspberries, mango, plums		

Vegetables
Yes **

Most vegetables are good for Pitta, particularly if taken raw (though when in debility or low energy, or during the winter, it is still better for Pitta types to take them cooked). They are also good steamed and taken with ghee but should not be fried, particularly deep fried. Nightshades, particularly tomatoes but also sometimes peppers, eggplant and potatoes can aggravate Pitta by their acid content, as can chard and spinach.

YES		NO	
***	Cauliflower, cilantro, alfalfa sprouts, sunflower sprouts, celery	***	Chilies, onions, (raw)
**	Broccoli, cabbage, brussels sprouts, mushrooms, asparagus, lettuce, green beans, peas (fresh), cucumber, okra	**	Tomatoes, avocado
*	Potatoes, parsley, bell peppers, corn (fresh), squash	*	Onions (well cooked), carrots, beets, spinach, chard, sweet potatoes, eggplant, radishes, turnips, watercress, seaweeds

Grains
Yes **

Most whole grains are good for Pitta, as they are strengthening and harmonizing but not overheating. Even those that increase Pitta do so only slightly; They should only be avoided as primary, staple foods in the diet or in acute conditions. Most whole grain breads are also good, as is pasta.

YES	NO
*** Wheat	* Brown rice (short grain), corn, rye, buckwheat
** Basmati rice, oats, barley, granola, quinoa, khus khus	
* Brown rice (long grain), blue corn, millet	

Beans
Yes *

Pitta types, with their good digestive fires, are often better able to digest beans. Even for them, though,beans require spices like cumin so that they do not upset the digestion. Most beans are rather neutral for Pitta. When cooked in lard, as with most refried beans, they aggravate Pitta.

YES	NO
*** Mung, aduki	* Peanuts, lentils
** Tofu, lima	
* Kidney, soy, split peas, chick peas	

Nuts
No *

Nuts are generally oily and warm and hence increase Pitta, all the more so if roasted and salted. However, they are less likely to increase Pitta than meat or fish, particularly when fresh; so they are preferable to these foods when strong nourishing food or protein sources are required.

YES	NO
** Coconut, sunflower	*** Brazil nuts
	** Almonds, cashews, walnuts, filbert, pecans
	* Sesame, pine nuts, pumpkin seeds

Oils
No **

Oils are Pitta (hot) in nature and hence generally avoided by Pitta types. Animal oils are the hottest, then oil from nuts and seeds. Vegetable oils are the least warm in nature. Ghee and butter are best for Pitta as they possess a cooling nature.

YES	NO
*** Ghee	*** Mustard
** Coconut, butter	** Sesame, almond, peanut
* Sunflower, soy, corn	* Olive, canola, safflower, margarine

Dairy
Yes **

Pitta types are usually best able to digest dairy products, particularly milk. They often do well with a milk fast for harmonization of body and mind. Sour dairy products, however, tend to increase Pitta, as they possess enzymes that give them a warm energy. Pitta individuals can better digest ice cream than the other types.

YES	NO
*** Milk, cream	** Buttermilk, yogurt, sour cream, ice cream
** Cheese (unsalted), cottage cheese	* Kefir, cheese (salted)

Animal Products
No **

Meat has a Pitta (fire) increasing nature and provokes anger and aggression. Red meat is most severe in this respect. Pitta types like meat as it makes them feel strong and powerful, but it often brings out their bad side. They usually do not need it and can get by as lacto-vegetarians.

YES	NO
* Chicken or turkey (white meat), egg white	*** Beef, shellfish, lamb
	** Chicken or turkey (red meat), pork, ocean or salt water fish, eggs
	* Fresh water fish

Sweeteners
Yes **

Pitta types can best handle sugar. They often need something sweet to cool and calm them down and harmonize their emotions, but for this same reason can overindulge in it. Honey is alright fresh but becomes hot or Pitta increasing when over six months old.

YES	NO
** Raw sugar, maple sugar, fruit sugar, fresh honey	** White sugar
	* Old honey, molasses, jaggary

Spices
No **

Spicy food is one of the main causes of high Pitta. Nevertheless Pitta types can take some spices, those that are neutral or cool in energy, particularly when eating heavy food.

They should generally avoid salt, but in the summer heat salt can be helpful for maintaining body fluids (along with sour juices).

YES	NO
*** Coriander	*** Cayenne, garlic, black pepper, mustard, horseradish
** Fennel, cilantro	** Ginger, asafoetida, fenugreek, salt
* Cardamom, turmeric, mint, cumin, cinnamon, parsley	* Cloves, basil, nutmeg, rock salt

Beverages

Pitta needs adequate fluid intake. Cool spring water is good. Tea can be taken (black or green), but not coffee. Astringent herb teas are good such as alfalfa, raspberry leaf, hibiscus, dandelion and comfrey, but not too many spice teas. Dairy is good, particularly milk. Pomegranate, pineapple or cranberry fruit juices are good, or vegetable juices such as celery or other green vegetable drinks. Alcohol, beer and wine are to be avoided.

Vitamins and Minerals

Pitta does well with B vitamins. Vitamin K is also good for stopping bleeding. Minerals like calcium and iron are important. Pitta types can usually digest raw vegetables well enough to extract most of what they need. They also can handle large mineral supplements without weakening the digestive fire, which tends to occur with the other humors.

ANTI-KAPHA DIET
DIET FOR DECREASING THE BIOLOGICAL WATER HUMOR

General Considerations

Kapha (water) types do best with a diet that is warm, light and dry. They should avoid food that is cold, heavy and oily. Accumulation of mucus in the system is a sign of taking too much Kapha-promoting foods.

Tastes that increase Kapha are sweet, salty and sour. Those which decrease it are pungent, bitter and astringent. As most food is sweet in taste, Kapha types should take less food. Their main dietary therapy is in eating less and taking more herbs.

Dietetics

Kapha individuals need to eat less in quantity and with less frequency. They should have three meals a day with the main meal at noon, the other two light in nature. They also need to take less time in eating or in preparing food for themselves. They can direct the energy they give to eating towards preparing food for others (like their Vata friends).

It is better for them not to eat in the evening, particularly heavy foods. They should fast seasonally or one day a week. Often it is good for them to avoid breakfast. They should not sleep after eating. Generally, they should eat between 10 a.m. and 6 p.m.

They should be careful not to use food as an emotional support for feeling loved or feeling secure, or as an attachment.

Fruit
No *

Fruit increases water in the system and may cause formation of more mucus. Hence, it is not generally prescribed for Kapha types, particularly when combined with other foods. But it is also light in nature and thus usually does not strongly increase Kapha, which is heavy. Some sour fruit, like lemon and grapefruit, can help reduce fat and dissolve mucus (but not if taken with sugar, though honey is okay). Sweet fruit depresses the digestive fire; that is its main negative action in Kapha types.

YES	NO
** Dry fruit (generally), cranberry, apple	*** Bananas, dates
* Pomegranate, pears	** Persimmons, oranges, pineapple, melons, cherries, plums, figs, grapes, mango, strawberries, raspberries
	* Prunes, papaya, lemon, lime, grapefruit

Vegetables
Yes **

Most vegetables are fine for Kapha, as they tend to be dry and light. Many, such as carrots and celery, are diuretic (reduce water). However, they should be taken warm, preferably steamed and with spices to counteract their generally cold nature, except in warm weather when they can be taken raw. Little oil should be used in their preparation.

YES	NO
*** Chilies, broccoli, cabbage, celery	** Sweet potatoes, cucumber
** Carrots, green beans, peas (fresh), mushrooms, beets, asparagus, lettuce, cilantro, radish, turnips, watercress, mustard greens, alfalfa sprouts, sunflower sprouts, chard	* Tomatoes, squash, corn (fresh), okra, seaweeds

YES	NO
* Potatoes, bell peppers, cauliflower, parsley, spinach, artichoke, eggplant	

Grains
Yes *

Many grains are not good for Kapha, as they tend to be heavy and increase weight. The grains which are good for Kapha are nourishing with diuretic and expectorant (drying) properties. Kapha types do well on a diet of whole grains and steamed vegetables. Breads, however, tend to increase Kapha, as they are more sticky and mucus forming.

YES		NO	
**	Barley, quinoa, dry or popped grains generally	***	Wheat, white rice
*	Corn, millet, buckwheat, rye	**	Brown rice, oats, khus khus
		*	Basmati rice

Beans
Yes **

Most beans are good for Kapha, as they tend to be drying and to increase air. Tofu slightly increases Kapha, but it is still much better than dairy, meat or nuts and is one of the safer protein sources for Kapha.

YES		NO	
***	Aduki	*	Chick peas
**	Soy, lima, lentils		
*	Tofu, mung, kidney, peanut, split peas		

Nuts and Seeds
No **

Most nuts and seeds are not good for Kapha, as they are heavy and mucus forming. They tend to increase congestion. Again, as a protein source, they are preferable to dairy or meat and need not be avoided altogether.

YES	NO
* Sunflower, pumpkin	*** Brazil nuts
	** Almond, cashew, walnut, pecan, filbert, pine nut
	* Sesame, coconut

Oils
No **

Most oils are not good for Kapha, as they are moist and heavy (of the same nature as Kapha). They should be used in small amounts. Animal fats such as lard should be strictly avoided as they are much heavier than vegetable oils. Light oils, especially mustard, are best.

YES	NO
** Mustard, sunflower, safflower, canola	*** Butter
* Corn, soy	** Sesame, almond, olive, avocado
	* Ghee, margarine, peanut

Dairy
No ***

Dairy products, except for buttermilk or goat milk, should generally be avoided by Kapha (water) types. They are especially mucus forming and promote congestion. For Kapha types dairy is often harder to digest than meat and may cause food allergies. Soy milk can be taken as a dairy substitute.

YES	NO
** Buttermilk, soy milk	*** Ice cream, cheese, cream, butter
* Goat milk	** Milk, yogurt, sour cream, cottage cheese
	* Kefir, ghee

Animal Products
No ***

Kapha types generally do not need animal products, as they are less likely to suffer from tissue deficiency. Of meats, fowl is the least aggravating to Kapha. Chicken is better for Kapha than cheese, but any form of meat will tend to increase Kapha in the long run. White or lean meat is better for them; fat should not be eaten.

YES	NO
* Chicken, turkey	******* Pork, beef, lamb
	** Fish, shellfish, eggs

Sweeteners
No ***

Sweet taste is the most highly aggravating for Kapha. Too much of it is their main dietary indiscretion and causes most of their diseases. The exception is honey, which has expectorant properties and a long term drying effect.

YES	NO
* Honey	******* White sugar, brown sugar, maple syrup
	** Molasses, fruit sugar
	* Jaggery

Spices
Yes ***

All spices are good for Kapha including the hot ones. Spicy taste is opposite in properties to Kapha (water), as it is hot and dry. They increase the metabolism to prevent fat and water from accumulating in the tissues.

Salt, however, should be avoided, except in small amounts during the summer or when sweating a lot.

YES	NO
*** Cayenne, black pepper, mustard, horseradish, garlic, ginger, turmeric, cloves, cardamom	******* Sea salt

YES	NO
** Cinnamon, coriander, cumin, basil, cilantro, parsley, asafoetida, fenugreek	** Rock salt
* Nutmeg, fennel, mint.	

Beverages

Kapha types need to take less water and should avoid all ice and cold water. They can take regular tea, herbal teas, spice teas like ginger and cinnamon, astringents like alfalfa, dandelion root or chicory root. Teas can be taken with honey but sugar and milk should not be used frequently. Coffee is alright taken occasionally.

Vitamins and Minerals

Kapha types need less vitamins and minerals and more spices and enzymatic agents than the other types. Usually B vitamins are good for them, but oily vitamins (A, D and E) should not be taken in excess. Heavy mineral supplements can also weaken digestive power further because of their heavy nature.

SATTVIC DIET

"From Sattva is born knowledge, from Rajas greed, from Tamas is confusion, delusion and ignorance." (*Bhagavad Gita XIV. 17.*)

Ayurveda, as a branch of Yoga, is primarily a sattvic (peaceful) form of healing. Sattvic healing methods are natural, gentle, non-violent, non-traumatic, non-invasive, and are done with clarity, love and attention on the part of the healer. Sattvic methods require a rapport between the patient and the healer. They include such methods as herbal medicine, natural dietary therapy, aroma therapy, non-traumatic body work, Yoga therapy.

Rajasic methods are forceful, rough, invasive, traumatic. The healer's motivation is often the seeking of money or other personal goals. Surgery is the most typical rajasic therapy, as are some very strong forms of body work.

Tamasic methods are heavy, dulling, insensitive, inorganic. Drugs, though initially rajasic in their action, are tamasic in the long term. The sterile atmosphere hospitals is tamasic; patients are kept in bed for extended periods of time, without fresh air or exercise, often on a diet with much dead or canned food, watched over by people who have no real caring attitude towards them.

Sattvic or Yogic Diet

Sattvic diet was originally devised for the practice of Yoga and the development of the mind. It is good for those who use their minds a lot, as it improves mental quality and energy. Moreover, it is important in the treatment of mental disorders, as it helps restore harmony and balance. It is good to consider in convalescence from disease or after toxins have been removed. Sattvic diet aids in tonification and rebuilding of a higher quality tissue in the body, particularly for those who wish to improve their state of consciousness. It is often combined with rejuvenation (rasayana) therapies, particularly those for the rejuvenation of the mind (Brahma rasayana) or nervous system.

Sattvic diet consists only of pure foods, light in nature, mildly cooling in energy, that do not disturb the mind. Only foods rich in the life-force or Prana are to be taken. These include organic fresh fruit and vegetables. All foods produced by harming living beings are to be avoided, such as meat and fish. Foods prepared in toxic environments or with an excess of chemical fertilizers or sprays are to be avoided.

Sattvic diet is a generally healthful and balancing diet safe for all three humors, though the diets for the humors can also be modified along sattvic lines. However, as sattvic diet is for improving the mind, it may not be nourishing enough for those who have to do physical labor. It sensitizes the mind and gives greater sense of sympathy and compassion. This may not be helpful for those who are hypersensitive and easily disturbed by noise and stress. As such it may not be grounding enough for Vata (high air) conditions.

Classification of food here follows the three Gunas or qualities of primal nature, Prakriti, as discussed in the section on mental constitution. Sattva is pure, light, clear, calming, harmonizing, opens the mind and promotes wakefulness. Rajas is cloudy, agitated, turbulent, energizing and disturbs the emotions. Tamas is dark, heavy, dulling and promotes lethargy. It closes the mind.

Sattvic Diet and the Six Tastes

Of the six tastes, only sweet is considered generally sattvic, as it is pleasant, harmonizing and nourishing and reflects the energy of love. Pungent, sour and salty are rajasic, as they are stimulating. Bitter and astringent are tamasic, as their long term affect is to cause rigidity.

Pungent taste irritates the nerves by its dispersing property. Sour and salty aggravate the emotions through heating the blood. Bitter and astringent have a constricting affect. This classification of the six tastes is general.

Too much sweet becomes tamasic or dulling. This is particularly true of old or artificially prepared sweets. Some bitter herbs, like gotu kola, are sattvic as bitter taste can help open the mind. Some spices, like ginger, with sweet fragrances are sattvic. Excessive eating is tamasic, light eating is sattvic. Sattvic diet is bland and even in taste, not going to any extremes.

Fruit

Fruit is sattvic (pure) in nature. It is sweet, light and promotes contentment. It has large amounts of the element ether, which controls and balances all the other elements. All fruit is generally good for a Yogic diet or improving the mind. It harmonizes the stomach, relieves thirst, calms the heart and improves perception. It both cleanses and nourishes body fluids. It is preferable to take it fresh and in season.

Some yogis, however, avoid heavy, sweet fruit, such as bananas, as they are mucus forming and may clog the channels.

Vegetables

Most vegetables are good for a sattvic diet, though not as much as fruit. Mushrooms are thought to be tamasic, as they are allied with decay. (It is interesting to note, however, that the Chinese Buddhists include many mushrooms as good for a diet promoting meditation).

Pungent vegetables — garlic, onions, radishes and chilies — are rajasic and tamasic and tend to overstimulate the sexual nerves. Excess of cabbage family plants — cabbage, broccoli, brussels sprouts and mustard, and cauliflower to a lesser extent — are rajasic or gas forming. Potatoes and sweet potatoes can be a little heavy or mucus forming in excess.

Otherwise fresh or steamed vegetables or vegetable juices are generally good. Celery is particularly good for the brain.

Grains

Grains, much like fruit, are generally sattvic in nature, especially rice (basmati or long grain brown rice). Wheat and oats are also good. Grains are better in the winter season, or when more physical strength is required, and are usually the main staple food in a sattvic diet. Whole grains are preferable but breads are also sattvic.

Beans

Beans are usually rajasic in nature. They are irritating, gas-forming and heavy. As such, they are generally not recommended in a Yogic diet.

Exceptions are mung beans, aduki beans and tofu. Equal parts split mung beans and basmati rice (kicharee) is the basic Yogic staple diet and the main simple food for purification or for convalescence in Ayurveda.

Nuts

Seeds and nuts are sattvic in nature. They should be taken fresh or lightly roasted, not heavily roasted and salted, which renders them tamasic. Almonds, pine nuts and walnuts are particularly good. As nuts are a little heavy, they should not be taken in large quantities at a time. Nuts and seeds go rancid (become tamasic) easily.

Dairy

Dairy products are sattvic in nature; pasteurized, etc., however, they can become tamasic. Milk is produced by the love of the cow for its calf. Milk fast, or buttermilk fast, is an important part of a Yogic diet. Dairy is good in convalescence, particularly from conditions of bleeding or blood loss, or wasting diseases. Yogurt is also good but is a little heavy and should not be taken in excess, as it can clog the channels. Most cheese is very heavy and so not recommended on a regular basis.

Oils

Most oils are heavy and not recommended in large amounts. Ghee, clarified butter, is sattvic, promotes intelligence and perception and can be freely used. It can be added to rice or vegetables. Sesame oil is sattvic, as is coconut. Olive oil is also good but not with garlic (which makes it rajasic).

Sweeteners

Sweet taste in moderation is sattvic, but refined sugars are tamasic. Yogic diet takes raw sugars in small amounts, including honey (not heated) and raw sugar, particularly jaggery. Honey when heated is said to become toxic (tamasic). It is said that sweet feeds Shakti (the power of awareness).

Spices

Most spices are rajasic, but a number of exceptions exist. Sattvic spices include ginger, cinnamon, cardamom, fennel and coriander, as well as turmeric. They help balance the effect of too much fruit, dairy or other dampness-forming foods.

Some yogis also use black pepper or long pepper to help dry mucus and keep the channels open. Here rajas is used to counter tamas, thus producing sattva indirectly. Such strategic variations should be kept in mind.

Salt is to be avoided except in the summer or in hot climates. Then it is best combined with lime.

Beverages

Pure spring water can be taken or sattvic herb teas or milk. Coffee and other stimulants should be avoided. Green or black tea, however, is sometimes taken and is thought to improve mental functioning.

Dietetics

Meals should be simple and infrequent. The main meal is usually taken around noon, with no heavy food after sunset. Sattvic meals require preparation with love and awareness. These enhance the sattvic (spiritual) and life-supporting properties of any food that is prepared.

Herbs

Many good herbs for the brain are useful here. Gotu kola (brahmi) gives clarity, calm and coolness to the mind. Calamus is particularly good for clearing the channels, promoting perception and improving speech. Other useful herbs are the Triphala formula, particularly amalaki, aloe gel, jatamansi, ashwagandha, shatavari, saffron, rose, lotus, bhringaraj.

Good Western and Chinese herbs for the mind include skullcap, sage, mint, zizyphus, biota seeds.

Most tonic herbs such as ashwagandha, shatavari, ginseng, astragalus or comfrey root are Sattvic and can be an important energy supplement to a Sattvic diet. Chyavan prash, Brahma rasayan and such Ayurvedic jellies are very sattvic.

Essential Oils and Incense

Most essential oils are sattvic in nature, including most incense. Best are sandalwood, saffron, camphor, vetivert, frankincense, lotus, rose.

Rajasic and Tamasic Diets

Rajasic and tamasic foods are not generally recommended, as they disturb or dull the mind and produce diseases. We should understand them in order to avoid them.

Rajasic foods aggravate Vata and Pitta (air and fire), tamasic foods increase Kapha (water) and Ama (toxins). Rajasic foods cause hyperactivity, restlessness, irritability, insomnia, increase toxins in the blood, cause bleeding and may promote hypertension. Tamasic foods cause hypoactivity, lethargy, apathy, excess sleep, accumulate phlegm and waste materials.

Rajasic food includes most overly tasty food. It is excessively spicy, salty and sour: chilies, garlic, onions, wines, pickles, excess salt, mayonnaise, sour cream, vinegar. Meat is also rajasic (irritating), particularly red meat, though that has tamasic properties as well. Food too hot in temperature is rajasic. Most fried food or roasted and salted food is rajasic. Rajasic food is usually taken with stimulating (rajasic) beverages like coffee or alcohol.

Tamasic food is food which is stale, old, recooked, rancid, artificial, greasy or heavy. It includes all 'dead' food, all meat and fish, particularly pork and animal organ parts. Most canned food comes here also. Pasteurized milk or other pasteurized dairy products become tamasic (pasteurization is a kind of cooking, so pasteurized milk is recooked food). Excess intake of fats, oils, sugars and pastries is tamasic. White sugar and white flour have a long term tamasic effect (though short term white sugar is rajasic). Food that is too cold is also tamasic.

Sattvic Diet with Diets for the Humors

Diets for the humors can be modified according to these three qualities.

Sattvic Vata Diet
Spiritual Anti-air Diet

Vata constitutions tend towards rajas. Their diet, therefore, includes articles which are sattvic or tamasic. For sattvic Vata diet, these tamasic items should be eliminated: garlic and onions, eggs, meat and fish. Rajasic spices, which are sometimes used for Vata, cayenne, black pepper, mustard, asafoetida, should also be used with discretion. Salt should not be used in excess.

Tamasic herbs, sedatives such as nutmeg and valerian, should not be used regularly. Still, when suffering disease, rajasic or tamasic herbs can be used, but no animal remedies unless one's life is threatened by the disease.

Sattvic Pitta Diet
Spiritual Anti-fire Diet

Pitta types also tend towards rajas, but not as much as Vata. They can more easily follow a sattvic diet. Regular anti-Pitta diet is predominately sattvic. Exceptions are beans (other than mung, aduki and tofu), turnips and radishes and animal products, which should not be taken. Excess of sugar and overeating are also contrary to this approach.

Rajasic and tamasic herbs, those pungent, bitter or strongly astringent in taste, should be used with discretion.

Sattvic Kapha Diet
Spiritual Anti-water Diet

Kapha people tend towards tamas, as they develop more heaviness, inertia, congestion and stagnation. Generally, many rajasic foods and spices are recommended for them. Sattvic Kapha diet is, therefore, more restrictive. Primarily, it requires, in addition to the regular Kapha diet, reducing hot spices, avoiding beans (except mung, aduki and tofu), and avoiding all meat and animal products. Sattvic spices should be used, and whole grains for strength.

AYURVEDIC THERAPIES
THE METHODS OF REINTEGRATION

Tonification and Reduction

There are many different therapies applied in Ayurveda. They can all be defined under two groups, tonification and reduction (also called supplementation and elimination). Reduction, langhana, literally means "to lighten;" supplementation, brimhana, means "to make heavy."

Reduction therapies decrease excesses in the body and are indicated for overweight, accumulation of toxins, and aggravated humors. They aim at elimination of factors that may cause disease. Tonification methods nourish deficiencies in the body and are indicated for underweight, debility, or tissue weakness. They work at building up inadequate energy or lack of substance in the body that may bring disease about.

Reduction is indicated in the acute stage of disease, when the attack is strong. In Ayurveda, reducing methods are also employed to eliminate deep-seated toxins, as part of a disease prevention, internal cleansing program.

Tonification is indicated in chronic disease, in convalescence or after reduction methods have been used. The usual rule is first to reduce and then to tonify. If we tonify first we may feed toxins or excess humors in the body and make conditions worse. In this regard, almost all of us can benefit from some reduction methods, if only to purify our systems to make use of tonics. However, there are some conditions where an individual is too weak for any reduction methods, and tonification must be given first. The two methods may be combined to some degree, particularly for milder and long term therapy.

Chinese and Ayurvedic Views Compared

This twofold division of therapies is similar in Chinese Medicine. In Chinese Medicine, reduction is used for external pathogenic factors; such as heat, cold, wind, damp or dryness. Therapeutic methods, such as promoting sweating, elimination or urination, are employed to remove these factors and the diseases they cause. In Ayurveda, reduction is twofold, of toxins from indigestion (ama) or of the excess humors. The methods employed are similar; but in Ayurveda disease is mainly looked at as a consequence of internal factors.

In Chinese Medicine, tonification is of yin, yang, chi or blood, the primary constituents of the body. In Ayurveda, tonification is of the tissues damaged by disease and the underlying humors, the same basic idea.

Attitudes for Reduction and Tonification

Reduction therapy is called 'discontenting' (asantarpana), as it includes practices of discipline, hard living and giving things up. It makes us doubt ourselves more and question who we are and what we are doing in life.

Tonification is called 'gladdening' (santarpana) therapy as it consists of methods to give us greater nourishment, care, relaxation, ease and enjoyment in life. Tonification therapy aims at making us feel better about ourselves in life. It encourages faith, love and positive attitude.

Indications

Reduction is indicated primarily for Kapha (water) and tonification for Vata (air). This is because the main attribute of Kapha is heaviness, and that of Vata lightness. Pitta (fire) usually requires a mixed therapy, some reduction and some tonification. Aspects of reduction have been dealt with under anti-Kapha regime and diet. Aspects of tonification have been dealt with under anti-Vata regime and diet. Here they are presented more specifically.

The reduction methods for Kapha, then, are strong; fasting or vomiting therapy. For Vata they are mild; enema therapy or nutritive diet. For Pitta they are moderate; purgation.

Tonification methods for Vata, conversely, are strong, with powerful tonic herbs such as ashwagandha or ginseng. Tonification for Kapha is mild, with herbs for supplementation that are not too heavy; like elecampane or long pepper. Tonification for Pitta is moderate with cooling tonics such as shatavari or aloe gel.

REDUCTION THERAPY

Reduction therapy in Ayurveda has two parts, called palliation and purification. Palliation, Shamana, means literally calming or pacifying. It is largely for reducing Ama, the undigested food mass, and calming the humors so they can be dispelled from the body through purification therapy. The humor may be mixed with toxic accumulations, which irritate it and make its symptoms more complex. This mass must first be separated from the humor to enable us to work on it directly.

Palliation Therapy

Palliation is said to have seven parts, "herbs for burning up toxins, herbs for stimulating the digestion, fasting from food, fasting from water, exercise, sunbathing and exposure to wind." (*Ashtanga Hridaya XIV. 7.*) These methods all serve to strengthen the digestive fire, Agni, and destroy toxins. They cleanse the digestive tract and allow the toxins in the deeper tissues to drain into it, so they can be eliminated.

For in-depth analysis of palliation therapy, see chapter: 'Detoxification Therapies and Diet'.

Purification Therapy

Purification, Shodhana, is a special form of therapy for elimination of the disease-causing humors. It does not signify any application of reduction methods, nor can it be done without the proper preparation. The beauty and power of Ayurvedic elimination therapy is its system for guiding the toxins to their sites for elimination. Merely to flush out various organs or systems is not effective if the toxins have not been directed to these sites.

Purification therapy is indicated when the aggravated humors are in the g.i. tract. If they are lodged in the tissues or mixed with the tissues, waste materials of the body or with Ama, the undigested food mass, they cannot be directly eliminated. Palliation methods must first be applied.

Ayurvedic Purification Therapy
Pancha Karma

Purification therapy is said to consist of five parts, "cleansing enemas, cleansing nasal medication, purgation, emesis, and blood-letting." (*Ashtanga Hridaya XIV. 5.*) These are more commonly known as 'Pancha Karma', the five cleansing actions - medicated enemas, nasal medications, therapeutic purgation, therapeutic vomiting, and therapeutic release of toxic blood. They are considered to be the most radical way to cleanse the body and thereby eliminate, once and for all, the disease-causing humors.

These methods can be applied in acute diseases, for instance the use of vomiting therapy to treat asthmatic attacks. Or the patient can be prepared to take them for internal cleansing, such as the use of vomiting therapy for high Kapha constitution as in obesity. The patient should have some strength to undergo Pancha Karma, as the methods can be strongly reducing.

Some of these methods can be used as part of other therapies. Enemas with tonic herbs, for example, are part of tonification therapy.

It is not the purpose of this book to explain the practice of Pancha Karma in detail. Much of it is a clinical practice that can only be done in a limited way without the proper equipment and facilities. Ayurvedic nurses are trained to administer the therapy, including measuring the eliminated substance. However, I will at least outline the main approaches of this important line of treatment. It is a phenomena not yet well understood in this country, and a number of misconceptions about it have already become prevalent. The first thing to understand is that it is a system of several therapies and can be applied in different ways. Its methods are varied according to the individual, specific disease, season, culture and so on. Many of its methods can be used in a more general way or as part of self-care.

Preliminary Practices (Purva Karma)
Preparation

Palliation therapy, consisting of preliminary detoxification and Ama-reducing methods according to one's humor, should usually be followed for a period prior to Pancha Karma. One week would be considered a short time for this, one month an average time, six months a long time. In acute conditions, however, shorter term palliation therapy can be done.

Oleation and Sweating Methods

Application of oils, Snehana, also called 'oleation therapy' is an important therapeutic method in Ayurveda, with oils used both externally and internally. Steam therapy or therapeutic sweating, Svedana, is another important method. They are significant parts of Pancha Karma but in addition are useful in themselves for treating various conditions and for health maintenance. They are the main preliminary practices of Pancha Karma.

After adequate detoxification, a period of daily oil application and sweating therapy should be done for at least one week for health maintenance and three weeks for treatment of severe diseases. Warm sesame oil is applied all over the body in large amounts. Special medicated oils (like Narayan or Mahanarayan oil) can be applied in smaller amounts to specific disease sites. The skill in massage is not the issue here. Body work is an important art in itself. Oleation therapy is concerned with the application of oil, not with body massage. Oils are taken internally at the same time, most commonly ghee (clarified butter).

Sweating is done shortly thereafter in a sweat box or with the steam of diaphoretic herbs (camphor, eucalyptus, mint, bayberry) or with tonics (Dashamula and bala) for weaker types. Herbs can be decocted in a pressure cooker, to which a hose is attached at the top (called nadi sveda). The medicated steam is applied to specific sites in the body, such as swollen joints in arthritis.

Some are of the impression that oil and sweating therapies, Snehana and Svedana, are Pancha Karma, that they are two of its five methods. It should be noted that oil and sweating therapies are not the whole of Pancha Karma or even the primary part, but only the main preliminary practice. They do, however, take more time than the primary practices. Much of Pancha Karma therapy is in preparing the toxins for elimination, mainly through oil and sweating therapies. The actual elimination methods can be done quickly once the preparation is made. If one stops with these preliminary practices, one has not actually done Pancha Karma.

Oil application and sweating therapy are designed to help bring the aggravated humors into the digestive tract for elimination. They soften and liquify them to direct them from the external disease pathway, the plasma and blood, to the internal, the g.i. tract. If one stops there, one has merely brought the aggravated humors back to their site of accumulation, which will cause distress and disease. If they are not eliminated, they will be reabsorbed and go back to the tissues where they were lodged.

If Vata (air) is brought out through these methods but not eliminated through the primary therapeutic measures of Pancha Karma, such as enema treatment, it will cause variable appetite, gas, distention, constipation and insomnia. If Pitta (fire) is brought out and not eliminated it will cause irritability, fever and hyperacidity. If Kapha (water) is brought out, it will cause loss of appetite, tiredness and congestion.

Heavy application of oils, also, will depress the digestive fire and cause such digestive disorders as loss of appetite or constipation. Hence, it should not be done excessively, or it should be balanced out by taking ginger, or other spicy herbs, to improve the digestive fire.

Many of the same effects of short-period intense oil massage can be gained by mild daily application of oils over a long period of time. Saunas, warm baths or showers or diaphoretic teas, such as cinnamon and ginger, can be used for sweating therapy. Even so, the five major cleansing actions, like enemas or purgation, should be done occasionally to make sure the humors are not accumulating. Also, herbs and spices to protect the digestive fire should be used whenever many oils are taken in.

Primary Practices (Pradhana Karma)
Therapeutic Vomiting (Vamana)

Artificially induced vomiting should be approached with care. If we strain ourselves to vomit, we can damage our nerve reflexes; therefore, it is usually contraindicated for Vata constitution. It is possible to learn to do it for ourselves with a little patience and practice. It can even be done on a regular basis to cleanse the stomach and can be used sometimes as part of palliation therapy.

Strong teas of licorice, salt, calamus, camomile or lobelia are used. A mild carminative tea like mint or fennel should be taken first in amounts of one pint. One should then apply a finger down the throat. Once the vomiting reflex arises, one should follow it out all the way. It is easier to empty the stomach through one or two strong reflexes than through a series of weak ones. It is also less likely to produce side effects. It is important to empty the stomach thoroughly.

Vomiting is contraindicated for the weak, emaciated, anorexic, young, old, convalescent, or those suffering from dry cough. It is mainly for those with congestion of phlegm in the lungs and stomach, those usually of Kapha (water) constitution. The best season is spring, particularly late spring when the weather has warmed up. It should not be done during stormy or rainy weather. It gives better results if done around the time of the full moon. Best time is morning after sunrise.

Much of the effect of short-term emetic therapy can be gained through the long-term use of expectorant herbs, like ginger and calamus; formulas such as Trikatu; and through following the anti-Kapha diet.

Purgation

Purgation, Virechana, is the simplest of the Pancha Karma methods and it is easy to see its effect. A strong purgative is given — rhubarb, senna, aloe or castor oil. Four parts rhubarb root can be mixed with one part each fennel, ginger and licorice and taken 2–5 gms. before sleep with honey or warm water. Or two teaspoons of castor oil can be taken in warm milk with ginger. Triphala, a mild Ayurvedic purgative, is only strong enough if taken in large doses, usually 10–30 gms.

Purgation is used to eliminate high Pitta (fire) from its site in the small intestine. Note that purgation is not so much for treating the large intestine. This is because purgatives cleanse both the small and large intestine. This cleansing of the small intestine can weaken the digestive fire, and so it is not always advisable in Vata types.

Purgation therapy can be used whenever we need to cleanse the intestines. It can treat constipation, old fevers, acute diarrhea, dysentery, food poisoning or any of the diseases of excess bile and toxic blood.

Purgative herbs are usually given in the evening, so that five to eight bowel movements occur the next day, flushing out the intestines. Late spring and summer are the best seasons.

Purgation therapy is contraindicated for the very young, the very old, the weak, debilitated, emaciated, pregnant or those suffering from chronic diarrhea.

Cleansing Enemas

Enemas (basti) are a mild therapy and can be used for many conditions. There are many different kinds of enemas, some of which are useful for tonification, others for reduction. Cleansing enemas (Niruha basti) are used in Pancha Karma to dispel high Vata (air) from its site in the large intestine. They are made with decoctions of anti-Vata herbs. Strictly speaking, tonifying or building enemas are not Pancha Karma but they are often given after the cleansing enemas as part of the follow up practices and rejuvenation.

A typical cleansing enema can be made with such herbs as calamus, fennel and ginger, along with 1–2 tsps. rock salt and up to 1/2 cup of sesame oil per quart of normal decoction. Without the addition of the oil or demulcent herbs like licorice, cleansing enemas can be too drying and depleting.

Nasal Application of Herbs

Ayurveda lists a whole variety of herbal preparations, including decoctions, oils, ghee, and the smoking of herbs for direct action on the nasal passage. This is called Nasya, literally, 'what relates to the nose', in Sanskrit. For the purification action of Pancha Karma, cleansing herbs are given through the nose, either as snuffs, decoctions or oils. Good herbs include calamus, bayberry, sage, basil, gotu kola.

Calamus, bayberry, sage or ginger powder can be snuffed to clear the sinuses. Calamus or gotu kola oil or ghee can be applied in drops to cleanse or nourish the brain. Cloves, calamus and bayberry can be smoked to cleanse the nasal passages.

Nasya is useful for many Vata (air) and Kapha (water) disorders. It allows for direct action on Prana and the brain. It has strong decongestion action and allows a more specific application of expectorant herbs. It is helpful in some Pitta (fire) disorders, as well as any diseases of the head and nasal passages.

Massage of oil to the head and face, along with inhalation of steam, is useful to help dislodge the toxins and make the nasal treatment more effective. This is a more local form of oil and steam therapy, which is the preliminary treatment for Nasya.

Therapeutic Release of Toxic Blood

In proper application of blood-releasing therapy, toxic blood is taken out of various sites in the body, usually along the back. The blood should be dark in color. Once it becomes bright red, the treatment should stop. The amount taken out is generally from two to eight ounces.

Some people recommend the donating of blood instead. While this does aid in new blood formation, it may not always be the toxic blood that is eliminated.

This therapeutic bleeding therapy is not used as much in Pancha Karma as it once was, but it is still common in all systems of Oriental medicines.

Follow-up Practices (Uttara Karma)

Pancha Karma treatment has several follow up practices. It is not an isolated therapy that can be done once and forgotten, but must be integrated into one's life-regime. First, it may be necessary to repeat the whole process of Pancha Karma. More than one session may be needed to cleanse deep-seated toxins, particularly if shortened (week long sessions or less) versions of Pancha Karma are followed. It may be repeated after one to three months. Often it is good to do it every year.

Second, after Pancha Karma, we should return to a diet and life-style in harmony with our constitution, or establish one if we have not done so already. Pancha Karma is meant to allow us to more effectively implement our life regimes, not to substitute for them. If we follow Pancha Karma with a return to bad habits, we may make our condition worse by suppressing the healing energy of our body that we have just developed.

Most important, if the treatment has been successful, we should be ready for a higher form of tonification therapy. Having eliminated the disease-causing humors, we can now rebuild our damaged tissues on a new level of purity and strength.

Rejuvenation

Rejuvenation (Rasayana) is a special form of tonification therapy. It properly follows deep cleansing like Pancha Karma, and the elimination of the excess humors from the body, because real renewal is only possible once the factors of decay have been taken away. Hence, though many of its methods are the same, it is different from general tonification therapy which can be given in any debilitated condition, even before or without Pancha Karma.

Rejuvenation diet is the same as tonification diet. The herbal treatment is largely the same as well. Emphasis is on substances to increase

Ojas (primary vitality) and improve Sattva (mental clarity). For this reason some of the heavier substances for tonic therapy, such as meat, are not taken.

When rejuvenation of the mind (Brahma rasayan) is the aim, sattvic and tonification diets have to be combined. Special herbs for the mind, gotu kola, calamus and ghee (or the Brahma rasayan herbal jelly), must be used, and asana, pranayama and mantra Yogic methods followed, preferably in a retreat situation for a period of at least one month.

DETOXIFICATION THERAPIES AND DIET
Levels of Detoxification

Ayurveda delineates two levels of detoxification treatment. The first is what could be called 'preliminary detoxification', involving normalizing digestion (and with it, elimination), indicated as 'palliation therapy'. The second, and deeper, level is removing the excess humors from the body, what has been described as 'purification therapy'.

Palliation therapy is easier to do and does not require the preparation of Pancha Karma and the stronger purification therapy methods. It can be employed as part of a mild detoxification approach for those not needing to or not able to undergo the deeper cleansing therapies. Done occasionally or over a period of time, its methods can be as effective as the deeper cleansing practices.

Western and Chinese medicine do not discriminate between these two levels of cleansing. They may combine a method of deeper cleansing, like purgatives, with a preliminary detoxification method, like spices to improve digestion; what they usually do is more like this first level of Ayurvedic cleansing. They do not have a system for distinguishing the humors from other, more superficial, toxins that may need to be eliminated. In making this division, Ayurveda brings clarity into detoxification programs and helps guard against side effects of excess or wrongly administered detoxification therapies.

Preliminary Detoxification

The first stage of most healing processes usually involves a preliminary detoxification program. Most individuals suffer from an accumulation of toxins, undigested food particles or waste materials (Ama in Sanskrit). These not only tend to cause disease, but also block the assimilation of nutrients. Without first clearing this accumulation, the right herbs and foods cannot be absorbed properly. Most diseases are Ama-caused or Ama-related, including chronic diseases like allergies, arthritis and cancer.

Preliminary detoxification approach, like the deeper cleansing therapies of Pancha Karma, is best done in warm months, late spring and summer but has more latitude, as its methods are not as strong. Late spring, May in most regions, is the natural season for detoxification.

Almost everyone can benefit from mild detoxification in the spring season, such as eating fresh greens, raw foods and cooling herbs to cleanse the blood. With the rising of heat and promotion of growth externally, internal toxins, which have been accumulated through the winter season, begin to surface. It is important to eliminate them at this time so they do not cause diseases through the summer season.

Ama Conditions
By-Products of Wrong Digestion

Ama conditions, the accumulation of undigested food or waste materials, differ according to the humors. Ama conditions are called Sama (in Sanskrit 'sa' means 'with', hence, 'sama' means 'with ama'). There are Kapha Ama conditions, called 'Sama Kapha' (toxic water), wherein toxins combine with the predominant Kapha (water) humor. Similarly, we can have Sama Pitta (toxic fire) and Sama Vata (toxic air) conditions. (see 'Detoxification, the Management of Ama' in the *Yoga of Herbs*)

Sama Kapha is revealed by indigestion and congestion along with difficult expectoration of thick phlegm.

Sama Pitta shows indigestion, hyperacidity and diarrhea, along with fever or toxic blood conditions.

Sama Vata occurs with indigestion along with abdominal distention, gas and constipation.

An anti-Ama approach can be applied to any of the humors or combined with any of the therapies for them.

Ama is evidenced by tongue coating, bad breath and foul body odor along with poor digestion and feelings of heaviness and dullness. Anti-Ama therapies should be considered until these clear. In this process of detoxification, as toxins are released, headache or other side effects may arise.

Herbs for Detoxification

Of the six tastes, sweet, salty and sour increase Ama. They not only increase body tissues but also feed toxins. Astringent is neutral. Though it can help dry up Ama, it can hold it in the body by its contracting action. Pungent and bitter tastes are effective against Ama. Bitter taste reduces it, and pungent taste destroys it.

The main herbal method of treating Ama is to burn it up with herbs to increase the digestive fire. Ama is opposite in properties to the digestive fire, Agni, and serves to block its functioning. Hence, herbs that stimulate Agni, or are fiery in nature, are used.

Best are the hot spices: cayenne, black pepper, dry ginger, long pepper, asafoetida and mustard. Other helpful warm spices include cardamom, cumin, coriander, basil and fennel.

The best formulas are Trikatu and Asafoetida 8. When these are not available, a compound can be made with equal parts cayenne, black pepper and dry ginger and taken in dosages of 500 mg. to 1 gm. of the powder in capsules or with honey two to three times a day.

These herbs are generally safe for Sama Kapha and Sama Vata conditions. In Sama Pitta conditions they are helpful, but care must be taken that they do not aggravate Pitta by their hot nature, in which case they should be combined with bitters.

Herbal bitters help scrape Ama (toxic accumulations) out of the tissues and relieve fever or infection due to it. They are good where there is fermentation, heat, or inflammation and are particularly good for cleansing Ama from the blood. They are most effective in Sama Pitta and Sama Kapha conditions and are sometimes useful in small amounts in Sama Vata conditions when the condition is long standing. They are good for any Ama condition that has come about through eating too much sweet or fatty food.

Best are pure bitters like golden seal, gentian, barberry and quassia. Chinese pure bitters are coptis, scute, phellodendron, gentian, and gardenia. Ayurvedic pure bitters include katuka, neem, and aloe. The 'Swedish Bitters' formula is also good.

Ayurvedic formulas include Tikta and Mahasudarshan powder. When these are not available, gentian, barberry and turmeric can be combined in equal parts and taken in dosages of 500 mg. to 1 gm. of the powder in capsules or with honey two to three times a day.

Fasting

Fasting is an important part of any detoxification approach but requires some strength on the part of the patient, particularly when fasting more than a few days. Often it is a good step in starting a detoxification diet; 3–5 days for Vata (air), 5–7 days for Pitta (fire), one to two weeks for Kapha (water).

Vegetable juice fast can be done, but fruit juice fast may not be advisable, as sweet taste can increase Ama. Lemon juice, however, is good, particularly mixed with ginger juice.

Fasting is often combined with taking herbs to improve the digestive fire: pungent herbs, as above, (formulas like Trikatu) or spice teas like ginger, cinnamon, cardamom, and fennel, or Bitters, as above, like aloe gel, can be helpful.

Fasting is an important initial treatment for many diseases as it dispels toxins and enkindles the digestive fire. When appetite returns, however, it is important not to continue the fast, as long-term fasting can suppress the digestive fire. Signs of proper fasting include clear tongue coating, pleasant body odor, normalization of appetite and digestion, feelings of clearness, lightness and lack of tiredness.

Purgatives, Colonics and Enemas

Cleansing the bowels is another route of detoxification that can be combined with fasting or detoxification diet. In Ayurveda, purgatives and enemas, as already described, are mainly part of deeper cleansing approaches (Pancha Karma), and have stronger effects as part of this process. However, they are sometimes used in a more simple way or to help cleanse Ama out of the system.

Purgation can be helpful where there is constipation or irregular bowel movements. If the stool sinks rather than floats, it indicates Ama. Purgation is particularly useful for accumulated masses of undigested food in the colon. These can be found by palpation. They will be hard, irregular and usually not painful to touch. Purgation is also useful for food poisoning or toxic digestion conditions. It should not be employed where there is chronic loose stool, diarrhea, debility or emaciation, even when tongue coating or other Ama signs exist.

As colonics are the strongest and most direct way to cleanse the colon, they can be helpful in detoxification. In this regard Kapha (water) can usually take more, Pitta (fire) moderately, and Vata (air), the least.

Colonics are not advisable for the weak, emaciated, debilitated, anorexic, tired, or those suffering from nervous system disorders or fear and anxiety. However, one or two cleansing colonics may be good for the majority of people.

A colonic should be followed up with herbs to promote digestion, as it very strongly reduces the digestive fire.

Although colonics can often be helpful in cleaning out deep-seated accumulations in the colon, Ayurveda prefers the primary methods of emesis, purgation and enemas for a more direct and effective purification of the humors.

Purgative herbs have the same effects as colonics. They will cleanse the small and the large intestine, though their cleansing action is not as thorough as colonics. It is often helpful to take purgatives the first day of a fast. Additional purges may be taken every three days to a week during the fast, particularly if strong evidence of Ama exists.

Demulcent and bulk laxatives, such as psyllium and flaxseed, are not advisable in many detoxification conditions, as they can further clog or congest the system. Bitter purgatives, rhubarb and aloe are helpful, along with such hot spices as ginger to protect the digestive fire and help burn up Ama.

Enemas are also cleansing to the colon. They are often better (particularly for Vata) than colonics, as their action is not so drastic. The cleansing enemas of Pancha Karma can be useful here also.

Triphala

Triphala, a combination of three tropical myrobalan fruits, is one of the best medicines coming out of India. It is the safest and most strengthening of the purgative herbs. The same results (as with the stronger methods) can be achieved by taking the formula Triphala in moderate dosages over longer periods of time, along with a generally anti-Ama diet. Enough Triphala, usually 3–10 gms., should be taken before sleep to ensure a normal evacuation upon rising. It can be taken as tablets or infused in warm water with a little honey (it does taste bad and its taste is difficult to mask). Dosage can be adjusted based upon personal experience and can gradually be reduced over the period of time.

Triphala not only gradually cleanses the bowels of all toxins, but also improves the digestive fire. So it does not have the side effects of other purgatives. In addition, it has a strengthening and nutritive effect upon the deeper tissues.

It is often good to take Triphala along with digestive spices such as Trikatu. This gives a balanced approach for cleansing both the stomach and colon and makes for a good metabolic regulator. It is useful not only in Ama conditions, but also as part of a regular diet for preventing Ama from building up.

Aloe Gel

When Triphala is not available aloe gel can be used. (Be sure to get the undiluted gel; it is often diluted with water as a juice). Aloe gel is often better for Sama Pitta (toxic fire) or Sama Kapha (toxic water). It also can cleanse the colon over a long period of time without overly reducing the digestive fire. Take two to three teaspoons two or three times a day, preferably with a little spice — ginger, black pepper or turmeric.

Along with anti-Ama diet or with regular diet to reduce the biological humor, aloe gel is an effective method of maintaining cleansing of the tissues and the digestive tract without any debilitating side effects.

****

According to Ayurveda, certain foods that are likely to not be digested properly cause a build-up of toxins and waste materials (Ama) in the system. These are foods that are heavy, greasy, stale or old, including: cheese, pork, lard, white sugar and white flour products. Yogurt is often included here, as it tends to clog the channels.

Ama-forming foods are mainly Kapha (watery) in nature, so that an anti-Ama diet is like an anti-Kapha diet. It is similar to the regular Western health food, mucus-free, live and raw food diet. Such a diet is used in Ayurveda, but it is not given to everyone; it is only part of a preliminary cleansing treatment.

Detoxifying or Anti-Ama Diet
Fruit

For detoxification most fruit should be taken only in small amounts. Sweet fruits and fruit juices should be avoided, especially bananas, pears, persimmons, grape or cherry juice. Some sour fruit juices, lemon, lime or grapefruit and astringent fruit like cranberry or pomegranate can be helpful.

Vegetables

Most vegetables are good detoxifiers; they are best raw but steamed is also good. Sprouts — alfalfa, sunflower, buckwheat, wheat, rice and barley — are first choice, as they contain special enzymes that help digest Ama. Vegetable juices such as celery, parsley, cilantro and spinach are good, but carrot is often too sweet, particularly by itself. The heavier root vegetables, like potatoes and sweet potatoes, should be taken with more care. Mushrooms should be used with caution.

Grains

Most whole grains are good, but breads and pastries should be avoided, particularly those with white flour. Sweet and heavy grains, wheat and oats, should be taken sparingly. Wheat can cause allergies in people with high Ama. Kicharee — equal parts long grain rice and split mung beans — is an excellent food for detoxification. Barley is also good.

Beans

Most beans should be avoided as they cause gas, which tends to produce Ama. Mung beans, however, are good for most Ama (toxic) conditions, particularly for Sama Pitta (toxic fire).

Nuts and Seeds

Most nuts, particularly when roasted or salted, are heavy and mucus-forming. They should be generally avoided in Ama conditions. Sunflower, pumpkin, sesame and other seeds are better but not to be taken in large amounts.

Dairy

Dairy is highly Amagenic (ama-increasing), particularly when pasteurized. Milk is very mucus-forming, as is yogurt, cheese and butter even more so. Generally, dairy should be avoided, though buttermilk (not salted) can be taken. It is better to take acidophilus in pill form than to eat yogurt.

Animal Products

Animal products strongly feed toxins. Animal fats, lard and red meat particularly, should be avoided. Pork is the worst. Fish, including shellfish, can also be very mucus increasing, especially when it is not fresh. Chicken and turkey are the safest meats to take, specifically the white meat. But it is better to avoid animal products altogether, including eggs.

Oils

Oils should be avoided as they are mucus forming. Ghee — clarified butter — can be taken in small amounts. Dry oils such as mustard or flaxseed can be used.

Sweeteners

Sweeteners should be avoided; honey is the safest, but it should not be heated or cooked with. White sugar is the most Amagenic (toxin forming) of all foods, and brown sugar is not much better.

Spices

All spices are generally good for Ama conditions, including hot spices as indicated under herbs.

Salt increases Ama and should be used sparingly, preferably rock salt, which is lighter and easier to digest than sea salt.

Beverages

Cold drinks should be avoided, especially those with ice. Cool spring water or distilled water is good. Herbal teas are excellent. Hot spice teas like ginger, cinnamon and cardamom are best.

Coffee should be avoided, but a little black tea is all right.

Dietetics

The anti-ama is the most restrictive of the diets. Food combinations should be kept simple with only a few different kinds per meal. Do not drink too much with meals. Food should be taken raw or cooked fresh. Reheated, canned or old food should not be taken. There should be several hours between meals and usually three meals a day should be taken. No food should be taken before 10 in the morning or after sunset. The main meal should be at noon. Meals should be light and easy to digest. All overeating should be avoided.

Cautionary Note

As this is a fairly reducing diet, it should be implemented carefully. Vata (air) people, generally, should not follow this diet more than two weeks; Pitta (fire) one month; Kapha (water) can follow it for longer periods. It can be modified according to the diets for the three humors, particularly when taken over a longer period.

It should not be given to those who are overly weak, emaciated, devitalized, the very old or very young, nor should it be continued if the individual becomes debilitated. Signs of excess detoxifying diet include insomnia, palpitations, low energy, fainting, absence of menstruation, and long term loss of appetite. The Western raw food diet, which is similar, also has such side effects when given in excess. Though it is a helpful tool, it has its limits.

TONIFICATION THERAPY

Tonification, or supplementation therapy, is indicated for the elderly, for pregnant women, for women who have just given birth, for children, for the debilitated, emaciated, convalescent, in anemia, malnutrition and in states of nervous exhaustion. It is the primary therapy for Vata (air) types and Vata conditions.

The main season for tonification therapy is the fall, when the dryness and lightness of Vata (air) prevails. Yet it can be initiated any time when severe debility exists. Most of us require a certain degree of tonification or oleation (oil) therapy in the late fall. The therapy helps give us the weight and strength to endure the vicissitudes of winter. It is particularly useful in cold climates or when we will be doing outdoor work and exercise in the cold.

Tonification is contraindicated in Ama conditions (where an undigested food mass exists), for the obese, during colds or flus, congestive disorders, fevers or infectious diseases. It should be applied with care when allergies exist. As tonic foods and herbs are hard to digest, the state of the digestive fire must always be considered.

Means of Tonification

Tonification is described as nourishing the body with "meat, milk, raw sugar, ghee and honey, with oil enemas; by sleeping and resting freely; by oil massage; by baths and by comfortable life-style." (*Ashtanga Hridaya XIV. 9–10.*) The main method is dietary: rich, nutritive food, along with strong, tonic herbs, mild massage, rest and relaxation. Oleation therapy includes external, as well as internal, use of oils.

Work, both physical and mental, should be reduced as much as possible. One should go to bed early and sleep as much as desired. Sexual activity should be reduced; sexual abstinence, according to the *Yoga Sutras,* the classical work on Yoga, is the best means of gaining energy. Breath control and breathing exercises such as Pranayama or the Chinese Qi Gong, also build energy in a primary way. Stimulation, including most of our mass media entertainment, should be reduced.

It is preferable to take a vacation in nature, like a mountain cabin, or at least stay in a comfortable and peaceful place for a period of time. It may not be possible for us to do all of these; but tonification therapy can still be effective if we persist in several major tonification actions over time.

Tonification is simpler than elimination therapy. Many different methods and routes of elimination exist, like purgation, vomiting or sweating; tonification involves one primary method, increased nutrition. It is not just a matter of eating more. Ayurveda uses ways to increase nutrition through the skin, the nose and the colon. These allow a broader tonification therapy and show the comprehensive nature of the Ayurvedic approach.

External Application of Oils

In Pancha Karma (Purification Therapy), oils are applied externally to help liquify toxins, so they can be eliminated more easily. In tonification therapy, oils are applied to nourish the body through the skin. The effects of such nutrients extend to the bones and nerve tissue, a direct penetration into the deeper tissues.

Because external application of oils bypasses the digestive tract, many oils can be used which would be difficult to digest. Good oils include sesame, almond, olive, coconut, and avocado, and various special medicated sesame oils. As mentioned previously, care must be taken as external oils tend to depress the digestive fire and the other fires of the body (like Bhrajaka Pitta which imparts lustre to the skin).

Internal Use of Oils

Oils are the main substance for tonification internally as well. We can add such oils to our diet as ghee, butter, sesame oil or various animal fats and meat broths.

Tonifying Enemas

Oils can be taken internally in the form of enemas. Generally, it is safe for Vata (air) types to take 1/2 cup of warm sesame oil in the rectum in the evening (and preferably hold it until morning) as part of tonification therapy.

Tonic herbs can be taken this way also. Ashwagandha, shatavari or licorice can be made into decoctions and taken rectally. Milk decoctions or meat and bone soups can be used.

Tonifying Nasal Medications

Tonic substances can also be taken in through the nose. Ghee, sesame oil or herbs to nourish the brain, such as gotu kola, calamus or licorice, are the best choice.

Foods for Tonification Therapy

Tonification diet is similar to an anti-Vata (anti-air) diet; it can be adjusted according to the humors. This diet can be used for finding meat substitutes. It can be followed to increase vigor for doing harder work, even for those who are otherwise healthy.

Dairy Products

Dairy is the best form of animal food as it does not involve injury to the animal. It is an effective meat substitute and an important food for debility or convalescence. Milk fast and buttermilk fast are often good initially.

Milk is the best general dairy food for restoring vigor and vitality. It strengthens the lungs, stomach and reproductive system and increases Ojas. Ghee is the best food for restoring vitality, nourishing the nerves and improving Ojas. It also strengthens the digestive fire. Buttermilk, though not the most building, is the easiest to take and improves absorption. Hence, it is often taken first.

Good dairy products for oleation therapy include, in general order of preference: ghee, butter, cream, milk, buttermilk, yogurt, sour cream, cottage cheese, cream cheese, cheese.

Oils

Oils are the essence of oleation (tonification) therapy. They are important meat substitutes as well. Helpful oils include, in general order of strength: ghee, butter, sesame, almond, olive, avocado.

Nuts and Seeds

Nuts and seeds strengthen the nerves and the reproductive system and improve vitality. They are excellent meat substitutes. Nut butters are also good. Good nuts for oleation therapy include: almonds, walnuts, pine nuts, cashews, coconut, black sesame seeds, lotus seeds.

Grains

Whole grains have good strengthening properties. They are mild and easy to digest in convalescence but are not as directly strengthening as dairy or nuts. Strongest are wheat, oats and brown rice. Whole grain breads can also be helpful. Wheat gluten itself is very good. Kicharee — equal parts basmati rice and split mung beans — is one of the best basic foods for tonification or reduction methods. It often can be digested when nothing else can.

Beans

Beans are good sources of protein and thereby work as meat substitutes. As they increase Vata, however, they are better meat substitutes for Kapha and Pitta. A few are especially good foods for convalescence or for improving vitality, such as: black gram, chick peas, mung, tofu.

Strengthening Fruit and Vegetables

Most fruit and vegetables are too light or mild to provide strengthening properties. There are, however, some exceptions: sugars in fruit are strengthening, improve vigor and help rebuild all tissues; some mushrooms are considered good meat substitutes and generally to be Chi or energy tonics by Chinese Buddhists.

Strengthening fruit includes dates, raisins, figs and jujubes, also pomegranate and black grape juices.

Strengthening vegetables are predominately starchy, and include okra, potatoes, sweet potatoes, yams and Jerusalem artichokes. Onions, particularly when well cooked in ghee, are one of the most strengthening foods.

Strengthening Spices
Curries

Spices can have the very yang, warming, strengthening effect of meat, particularly when combined with oils such as ghee. The combination of spices and oils in curries is the basis of Indian cooking, which normally does not use meat. Even though most spices are not tonifying, they are still important for maintaining the digestive fire.

The best strengthening spices are garlic, ginger, cinnamon and long pepper, which give vigor.

Black pepper, cardamom, cloves, fennel, cumin, cayenne and asafoetida are also useful, particularly cooked in oils such as ghee and taken along with other tonic foods.

Raw Sugar

Raw sugars give strength and help build all body tissues, but care should be taken with food combination. Ayurveda considers jaggery, crude raw sugar, to be the best, as it is the richest in minerals and the easiest to digest. Other helpful sugars include: honey, raw sugar, maple syrup, rock candy, molasses, malt sugar, lactose, fructose.

Salt

Adequate salt intake is part of tonification diet, particularly rock salt.

Tonic and Rejuvenative Herbs

There is a whole class of tonic herbs in Ayurvedic and Chinese medicine (see also *Yoga of Herbs,* 'Tonics'), as well as several Western herbs of similar properties. These are the prime tonic and rejuvenative substances to take.

Ayurvedic herbs are ashwagandha, shatavari, aloe gel, amalaki, bala, kapikacchu, shilajit, black musali, white musali, vidari khanda, and vamsha rocana.

Formulas include Chyavan prash, Ashwagandha compound, Shatavari compound, Dhatupaushtic powder and Triphala.

Chinese herbs are ginseng, astragalus, fo ti, rehmannia, lycium, schizandra, dioscorea, dang gui and cuscuta.

Chinese formulas include Four Gentlemen, Four Materials, Women's Precious Pill, Major Ten, Rehmannia 6, Rehmannia 8.

Western herbs are licorice, comfrey root, marshmallow, slippery elm, solomon's seal, saw palmetto, spikenard.

TONIC HERBAL PREPARATIONS
Milk Decoctions

Powerful tonic drinks can be prepared by cooking powdered tonic herbs like ashwagandha, shatavari, comfrey root or ginseng in raw milk. To enhance the tonic effect, one or two teaspoons of ghee, or a little raw sugar (honey and ghee should not be used in equal proportions, as this is thought to be toxic) can be added per cup before drinking. A small amount of a spice like ginger should be added as well.

HERBAL JELLIES

Ayurveda has a whole class of medicated jellies, prepared with such ingredients as tonic herbs, ghee, honey, raw sugar and various spices. They work best as part of tonification therapy.

Chyavan Prash

This is the most famous Ayurvedic jelly. Its prime ingredient is the tropical fruit amla or amalaki. Amla is the highest natural source of vitamin C. It retains the vitamin C content because it is bound up with the tannins in the fruit. Amla is a powerful tonic and builds the blood and reproductive fluids and nourishes the heart, lungs and kidneys.

Brahma Rasayan

This herbal jelly is prepared with gotu kola (brahmi). It is excellent for tonifying the mind and nerves and building the prana (life-force).

HERBAL WINES

Ayurvedic herbal wines have warming and tonifying properties that make them into strengthening foods. They help build tissues and also improve agni. Many of them are prepared with tonic herbs, such as ashwagandha, whose properties they enhance.

Draksha

This is the main basic herbal wine prepared with raisins and spices. It is not only good for maintaining the strength of the digestive fire, but also helps restore vitality.

Other good herbal wines include Ashwagandha wine, Aloe wine and Bala wine.

MEDICATED OILS

Most medicated oils are for external application. They are essential for the external part of tonification therapy. Many are made with tonic herbs such as ashwagandha, shatavari and bala and can help rejuvenate the body through absorption via the skin.

MEDICATED GHEES

Tonic herbs prepared in ghee gain enhanced strengthening properties. Ghee builds Ojas, sexual vitality, gives strength to the nerves and the mind, and helps increase fat and muscle in the body, without being overly heavy. Most easy to make is licorice ghee. For the mind, calamus ghee is best. Ashwagandha ghee is very good also. Almost any tonic herb can be made as a ghee.

Please note the section on Classical Ayurvedic formulas for more information on these preparations.

8
BALANCING
ENERGY

The physical body is a manifestation of our life-force; imbalances in the life-force produce disease. The biological humors are merely three different statuses or orientations of the life-force. Hence, the basis for balancing energy is improving the quality of our life through our life-regimes.

Low Energy

Behind most disease states — particularly those which are chronic, degenerative or hard to treat — is a state of low energy. Most modern methods of treating disease, such as antibiotics, reduce vitality further. Modern life style, in general, disrupts our connection with the life-force of nature and the soul and makes us prone to low energy.

There are several sources of energy. First, there is our congenital vitality. This depends upon karmic factors and is given at birth. Hence, it is difficult to change.

Second, there is the energy we draw in from outside sources. These are primarily two, food and breath. Wrong diet decreases our true energy input from food and is a causative factor in most diseases; thus the general importance of dietary therapy. Wrong breathing, including shallow or hurried respiration, is another important factor; thus the importance of Pranayama or breath control.

Third, there are factors which produce energy via the mind. Meditation, silence or peace of mind increase energy. Distraction of mind, primarily gossip, worry and any excess thinking dissipate mental energy.

Deep sleep is also important for renewing the mind. This is our natural, or given, form of meditation. When this does not occur, our energy is not able to renew itself. The same factors which distract the mind (which vitiate sattva) disrupt deep sleep.

Everything we do in life is a form of reception and transmission of energy. This includes not only eating, breathing and thinking, but all sensory activities, in which we are gathering impressions that feed the mind. When these are wholesome, as with impressions from nature, the mind is given positive energy and creativity. When these are un-wholesome, as artificial stimulation of the senses or an unnatural living environment, the mind develops negative energy and becomes destruc-tive.

Another important way to gather energy is through abstinence from sexual activity, particularly abstinence allied with meditation. This brings our congenital source of energy to its maximum and, in time, can take us beyond congenital energy limitations. On the other hand, excessive or wrong sexual activity is perhaps the main causative factor in low energy, as it reduces our central energy store (Ojas) even further.

Once our primary energy or Ojas is reduced below its threshold, it becomes very difficult to replenish. This results in chronic disease. Therefore, it is most important that we do not allow our energy to fall below its critical level. Factors, besides sexual dissipation, which reduce energy include drugs and other negative life actions, such as harming others.

The Power of the Soul

Our most important source of energy is our own soul (Jivatman), which is the source of Prana, the life-force, and Ojas. If we are not in contact with that internal source of energy, we are entirely dependent upon external sources of energy, which are always limited and always possess a certain entropy or tendency towards decay. Connecting with our internal source of inspiration, discovering our spiritual aspiration in life, and following our true dharma or right vocation are ways of attuning ourselves to our soul.

To Increase Energy

Increasing energy requires, first of all, removing those factors which reduce it: all negative life-energy areas including negative attitudes and emotions, as well as locations or situations that are draining or devitaliz-ing. We must establish right diet, right breathing, adequate restful sleep (deep sleep) and moderate use of sexual energy. Important also are right thinking and not dissipating mental energy, which depend upon the proper intake of impressions from the external world.

If our energy is chronically low, we must be either dissipating it or not renewing it properly. There is really nothing mysterious about low energy, though it often consists of a combination of subtle factors that cannot be treated simplistically or mechanically.

For renewing energy, tonic and supplementation therapy is important. Substances to increase Ojas — like milk, ghee, ashwagandha, bala — are important. Chyavan prash or Ashwagandha compound or the Energy Tonic (no. 2) are helpful. For mental energy, energizing mantras are important such as Om, Ram and Hum. Gems for chronic low energy are ruby, garnet, red coral and other warming stones, which revive and circulate energy, set in gold. Also useful are blue sapphire or amethyst to ward off negative energy, and diamond, zircon, yellow sapphire or yellow topaz to increase internal energy.

Blocked Energy

There are two states of low energy which are often related. The first is when the energy is simply low or insufficient. The second is when it is blocked. When energy is blocked it appears low, but it is simply not flowing properly. This is more common in the young, whose congenital energy source is not yet exhausted by time. Symptoms of blocked energy involve feelings of suppression, tension, being pent up, with occasional outbursts. Blocked energy leads to deficient energy in the long run. Many complicated cases of combined deficient and blocked energy exist and are hard to treat.

In its uncomplicated form, blocked energy is treated differently than deficient energy. Activity is required to move the energy, such as purification therapy including Pancha Karma. For diet: spices to promote digestion and the digestive fire. For herbs: those which move or clear the energy pathways (generally spicy digestive, circulatory and nervine stimulants), like calamus or turmeric. Many aromatic oils have important clearing energy such as camphor or myrrh. Physical exercise and creative mental activity are required.

Often it is necessary to make some move to break stagnation in our life style. This may require change of job, residence or relationship, or otherwise breaking up our pattern of inertia.

Excess Energy

Other diseases arise from excess energy. This is an excess of an inferior quality or negative energy that comes from external sources like too much meat, alcohol and spices. It also comes on a psychic level from controlling, dominating or influencing others. Most infectious, congestive and acute diseases originate in excess energy. It is a condition of too strong ego. Excess energy is treated by reducing therapy, including the stronger forms of Pancha Karma.

Hyperactivity

Hyperactivity is usually a sign of dissipation. It leads to low energy, and is often a sign that the energy level is getting low. When it reaches a certain level, it no longer has the power to consolidate itself. This results in hyperactivity, which in turn results in exhaustion. It requires a combination of mildly tonifying and sedating (reducing) therapies.

Some individuals are karmically or congenitally hyperactive. While they may get away with this when young, it often causes low vitality or chronic diseases when older. Hyperactivity is often a form of distraction and indicates that there is something in life we are trying to avoid.

The Aura

Most disease involves disruption in the vital energy field, or the aura. The aura reveals any energy imbalances we may have. It is the field of our positive vitality, the light emitted by our essential vitality (Ojas). The aura wards off disease and maintains the organic integrity not only of the body but of the mind.

The condition of the aura can be read through the complexion of the skin, the lustre of the eyes, and, to some extent, the pulse. It is revealed by the energy and integrity of the character and by the degree of creativity an individual may possess. By Yogic power or the power of concentration, it can be intuited or perceived. Astrology gives us a key to it, as it is created by the colors of our planetary rays.

Pranayama, gems, mantra and meditation have the most power to improve the aura. The aura is the total effect of our daily thought and action, so right life-regime in general improves it.

Dark gems, such as blue sapphire or amethyst, seal off or protect the aura; warm gems, ruby, garnet or red coral, energize it; nurturing gems, pearl, diamond, yellow sapphire, feed it.

Mantras like Om expand the aura, those like Ram protect it. Those like Hum ward off any negative energy that may disrupt it. Peace and silence of mind both energize and consolidate it.

To renew our aura we need to create our own sacred space. This may be a meditation room, an altar or any other defined sacred area wherein we do a daily practice or ritual, a daily sacred activity connecting us to the cosmic Being or inner Self. Such action must be outside ordinary motivations of personal achievement or acquisition.

Most allopathic practices, like the use of medical drugs, machines, or staying in hospitals, weaken the aura. Excess stimulation or dissipation of any kind damages it. This includes too much activity, excessive sex, over use of the senses, and such factors as radiation, environmental pollution or overexposure to mass media influences.

The aura is weakened whenever we give our minds over to an external influence, as the aura on an inner level is a function of the power of our consciousness. External influences are of an astral or psychological nature, as well as physical. Giving up our minds to the power of another personality weakens the aura. Many forms of channeling or mediumship, wherein we allow other entities to inhabit or work through us, can also have this effect.

Balancing Energy and Spiritual Development

We cannot, through our own human and egotistic efforts, find what is truth or the eternal. Our very efforts are products of time and fragmentation, a movement of desire. Yet hidden within Nature (Prakriti) is a Power of spiritual development (Shakti), an energy of Divine grace.

We can, however, harmonize our Prakriti, our organic nature as psycho-physical entities, mind-body complexes. This allows that hidden Power or Shakti to come forth. We cannot make this Power come forth, but once our nature is balanced, in it will come the spontaneous manifestation of that grace. Then the Power, or Shakti, will lead the way, giving us the energy and capacity for spiritual growth and change. Nature is a vehicle, a vessel for the Yoga Shakti or the power of conscious evolution. But the Shakti cannot function if the vessel is broken, if the vehicle is not coordinated.

Ayurvedic and Yogic life-regimes are given to harmonize our natures, to allow the Divine grace a field to work in. Hence, though they work with outward aspects of our nature like posture and diet, if these are not in order, we cannot expect the inner depths of our being to come forth. Therefore, we should not neglect these life-regimes in our deeper creative or meditational activities.

PART II

TREATMENT OF DISEASE

In the following section diseases are listed according to the bodily systems. All diseases of any particular system can be treated generally according to the principles for treating that system as a whole. For example, most diseases of the nervous system, such as epilepsy or paralysis, can be treated according to the principles and formulas for treating the nerves.As diseases of the same system are often related, much of the material under one disease in that system may be relevant for treating the others. The diseases chosen here are common and typical. Some are given more extensive analysis but the others could be approached in the same manner. It is not possible to list all diseases, nor to repeat all the information for treating a particular system under all of its different disorders.

In examining any particular disease, please note the information provided on that system as a whole. These suggestions should be integrated with the life-regime principles of Part I. For more detail on formulas and therapeutic treatments, as well as for additional formulas, Part III can be consulted. The goal is to provide a comprehensive yet simple method for treating disease through understanding the underlying humoral imbalance.

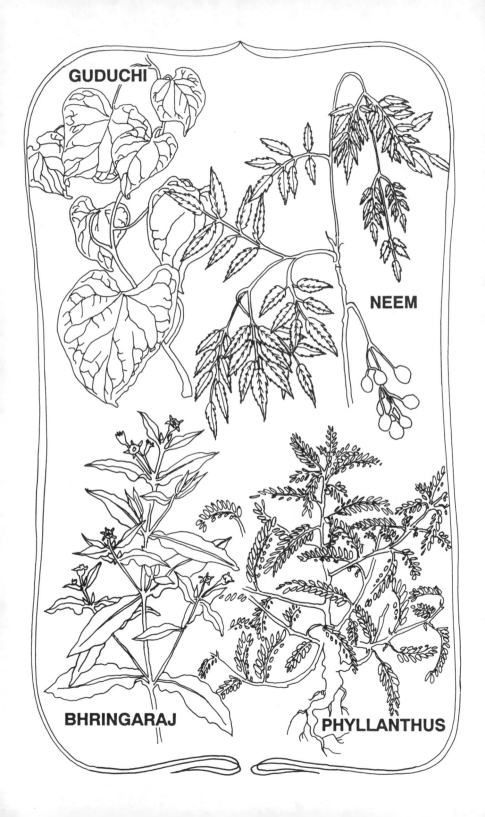

GUDUCHĪ

NEEM

BHRINGARAJ

PHYLLANTHUS

1
DIGESTIVE SYSTEM
DISORDERS

A being the size of the thumb dwells in the middle of our nature like a flame without smoke. He is the Lord of what has been and what will be. He is yesterday and he is tomorrow. — *Katha Upanishad, 2.12–13.*

The Digestive Fire

There is a god, that is to say, a cosmic power, which dwells within us, who determines how we function on a physical level. Without propitiating that deity, we must suffer from disease. That god is our own digestive fire, called "Agni" in Ayurveda (which literally means "the transforming will or force" and exists on higher levels also as the power of discernment). It is important not only that we feed ourselves and nourish our body properly; the digestive fire must also be fed and cared for to give it the power to adequately extract our nourishment.

Most diseases arise from poor or wrong functioning of the digestive system. The digestive fire, Agni, is central to health. It is not only responsible for absorbing nutrients in food, but also destroys any pathogens and renders the food acceptable to our systems. Undigested food becomes like a pathogen in the body, breeding toxins and upsetting the autoimmune system.

When Agni is normal, there is good digestion, circulation, and complexion; pleasant breath and body odor; adequate energy and strong resistance to disease. When Agni is abnormal there is poor digestion, poor circulation, bad complexion; offensive body odor, intestinal gas, constipation; low energy and poor resistance to disease. Hence, treating the digestive system — regulating Agni — is considered a radical (root) treatment for most diseases.

States of the Digestive Fire

Agni has four states in Ayurveda; high, low, variable and balanced. Agni is usually high in Pitta (fire) types, with excessive appetite. Circulation is strong, but toxins in the blood and bleeding are more common. The stool will tend to be loose with some diarrhea. Resistance to disease is generally good, but when they do occur, diseases are apt to be sudden and severe (like febrile disorders or heart attacks).

Agni is usually low in Kapha (water) types, with poor appetite, low metabolism and tendency to gain weight even without excess food consumption. There will be excess mucus and congestion. Circulation is poor and colds and flu are more common, but diseases are not often severe.

Agni tends to be variable in Vata (air) types with periods of strong appetite, even extreme hunger, alternating with loss of appetite and forgetting to eat. Gas, distention and constipation are usually signs of variable Agni. Circulation is also variable, as is resistance to disease. More debilitating diseases and long term derangement of the nervous system are more likely.

Signs of balanced Agni are a normal and regular appetite that is constant and easily satisfied with natural, not strongly spiced, foods. Bowel movements will be regular and there will be little production of gas or bloating. Sensory acuity and mental clarity will also usually be strong.

Herbs for the Digestive Fire

Agni is increased by pungent, sour and salty tastes and decreased by those which are sweet, astringent and bitter, though bitter taste in small amounts before meals can also increase Agni. Spices are usually the best thing for increasing Agni. The digestive fire has the same nature as spicy taste. It is hot, dry, light and fragrant. Hence, the right intake of spices can be a major aid in the treatment of most diseases.

When one's Agni is high, spices should generally be avoided, but digestive bitters — aloe, barberry and gentian — can be taken (typically such formulas in Ayurveda as Tikta or Mahasudarshan churna). These lower the digestive fire without increasing toxins.

When Agni is low, hot spices can be taken — cayenne, ginger, black pepper (typically the Trikatu formula) — but all spices are good.

When Agni is variable, spices and salts should be taken — asafoetida, ginger, cumin, rock salt (typically the Asafoetida 8 formula).

When Agni is normal, mild sattvic (harmonizing) spices — cardamom, turmeric, coriander and fennel — can be taken to maintain balance.

As a general formula for maintaining the digestive fire, particularly in low or variable states, Ayurvedic formula no. 1, the Digestive Tonic (an improved form of Trikatu) can be taken, 2–3 tablets 1/2 hour before meal. Vata (air) types can take with warm water, Kapha (water) with honey, Pitta (fire) with cool water or aloe gel as a vehicle.

Agni can also be increased by exercise, including Yoga postures (asana), by deep breathing (pranayama), meditation, by fasting or light eating and by sleeping less. Staring at a ghee lamp is also helpful.

It is decreased by most damp, heavy, oily and sweet foods with the exception of ghee (clarified butter), which in small amounts increases it. Sedentary life-style, excessive sleep or too much sex are additional factors which weaken the digestive fire.

Stages of Digestion

According to Ayurveda, digestion occurs in three stages. The first stage is dominated by Kapha (water) in the mouth and stomach. It includes the saliva and the alkaline secretions of the stomach lining. Here the water and earth elements are extracted from the food. Kapha types have an excess of these secretions with consequent nausea, bringing up of mucus, profuse salivation and poor appetite. Excess eating of sweet and salty foods will increase these secretions and also cause these symptoms.

The second stage is dominated by Pitta (fire), with the secretion of acids in the small intestine. Here the fire element is extracted from the food. Pitta types suffer from hyperacidity and burning sensation in the stomach. Excess eating of sour and pungent substances increases these secretions.

The third stage is dominated by Vata (air) in the large intestine with the formation of the stool. Here the air and ether elements are extracted from the food. Vata types suffer from gas and constipation. Excess eating of light, dry, bitter, astringent or pungent substances increases these symptoms.

The Six Tastes and the Digestive Process

The six tastes mirror the digestive process in this order: sweet, sour, salty, pungent, bitter and astringent. Sweet taste is digested first, particularly that of sugars. Therefore, sweets should be eaten first. If eaten after other foods, sweets will stop the digestive process, allowing an undigested food mass to form and to ferment. Salty taste is digested second and turns into sweet taste in the stomach.

Sour taste is digested when the food enters into the small intestine. Pungent taste is digested when the food enters into the large intestine. Hence, it is good to have some sour or pungent spice, chutneys or yogurt, in the middle of the meal.

Bitter and astringent tastes are digested last. They serve to close off the digestive process and help produce the stool. After meals it is good to have astringent teas such as regular black tea, or herb teas, alfalfa, raspberry leaf or strawberry leaf. If bitter and astringent tastes are eaten first (except bitter herbs in small amounts before meals) they will reduce the appetite and weaken the digestive process, reducing assimilation of nutrients.

By this logic salads are better at the end of a meal; and desserts (if they are not too heavy or too large in quantity, which naturally will depress the digestive process whenever and however they are taken) are better taken at the start of meals. Thus, another important dietetic factor to consider is the order in which we eat our foods. Proper order may allow us to digest foods and food combinations which we otherwise could not.

Indigestion

Improper digestion results in the accumulation of an undigested food mass (ama). Ama formation is indicated when the stools are poorly formed, breath is unpleasant, appetite is abnormal and a coating appears on the tongue. This undigested mass stagnates and ferments and eventually, entering the blood stream, and moves to different parts of the body causing various diseases.

For Kapha (water) types this undigested mass accumulates along with phlegm in the stomach, and moves from there into the lungs and the rest of the body causing Kapha disorders.

For Pitta (fire) it accumulates along with acid in the small intestine, moves into the liver and the blood and the rest of the body causing various Pitta disorders.

For Vata (air) it accumulates with gas in the large intestine and moves from there into the blood and into the nerve tissue causing various Vata disorders.

Treatment of Ama
(The byproduct of indigestion)

Most herbs to improve digestion, as does anything that improves Agni, also counter Ama. Spices are best for destroying Ama or inhibiting its formation, particularly the very hot spices such as cayenne. Bitters are useful for reducing Ama in the tissues and can help destroy it, particularly pure bitters like golden seal. The drying and detoxifying action of strong pungent and bitter herbs together is often good for eliminating deep-seated toxins.

Astringent taste restrains Ama but can hold it in the body. Sweet is the strongest taste for increasing it. Salty and sour also cause it to ferment further. (see section on 'Preliminary Detoxification and Anti-Ama Diet')

The Need for Regular Examination of the Digestive System

Even a person who has no immediate disease problem should examine the state of the digestion, including tongue, breath, appetite and elimination, making sure that toxins are not forming. It is easiest to stop the disease process at its origin in the digestive tract. Once it moves into the tissues, it becomes more difficult. Thus, in treating all disease and for disease prevention, we must consider first the digestive system.

The Digestive System and Medications

We must always consider the strength of digestion for whatever herb is given. Any herb not properly digested will, like undigested food, tend to turn into a poison. The same is true of minerals and vitamins. For this reason many of the formulas for treating the digestive system are useful adjuncts for insuring the assimilation of other herbal formulas.

DISEASES OF THE LARGE INTESTINE

Our pattern of elimination shows us the final product of our digestion. The colon is the last and most significant area of digestion, wherein nutrients are absorbed to feed the bones, brain and nervous system. Proper management of the colon is the foundation for treating the digestive system. For this reason, diseases of the large intestine often come first in the Ayurvedic listing of digestive system disorders.

Diarrhea shows a lack of absorption of proper nutrients. Constipation shows retention of waste materials in the body. These are the two main disorders of the colon, and such other colon diseases as colitis or diverticulitis, can be treated through them. Other diseases also based upon them, and treatable through them, include most Vata (air) disorders and many Pitta (fire) disorders. Both constipation and diarrhea are due to an excess or accumulation of Apana Vayu, the downward moving air. Constipation is an excess of its dry attribute, whereas diarrhea is an excess of its mobile attribute.

A stool which is poorly formed, has a strong unpleasant odor, or sinks quickly in water, indicates indigestion and the formation of Ama (toxins). It is as important to be aware of our pattern of elimination as of the state of our appetite.

Colon disorders relate to the first or root chakra. They often are based on fear, the need for security and support, lack of groundedness and other first chakra emotional disharmonies. In their treatment we must also take care of our emotional root in life.

Many spices are good for strengthening absorption in the colon. These include ginger, cayenne, black pepper, and especially, asafoetida, basil and nutmeg. In taking spices for our digestive fire, we should consider those for the colon as well. The prime Ayurvedic formula for colon digestion is Asafoetida 8.

Diarrhea and Dysentery

Diarrhea is a condition of frequent, loose or watery stools. If it becomes severe, dehydration can occur along with collapse of energy and potential threat to life.

Diarrhea may be due to exogenous factors such as heavy meals or difficult to digest foods. Such are foods which are too oily, too watery, too dry, too hard, too hot or too cold. Wrong food combinations, such as milk with meat or fish; or eating another meal before the previous meal is digested; irregularity in eating habits; or eating unaccustomed foods, may be additional causes. Impure food and water, food poisoning, parasites, changes in seasons, stomach flu or emotional disturbances — panic or grief — can also bring it about.

Differentiation

Diarrhea is most commonly a Pitta (fire) condition, as Pitta tends to accumulate dampness and has the mildest tone of the colon. Yet it may also be due to high Vata (air), high Kapha (water), high Ama (toxins) or psychological factors.

Pitta diarrhea is usually yellow, foul smelling, and may be mixed with pus or blood. It tends to be hot and there may be a burning sensation at the rectum. There may be thirst, dryness and possibly fever. This is what is usually seen in most acute cases of bacterial dysentery.

Vata diarrhea involves pain, cramping, tenesmus, passing of gas and frequent motions without much stool being passed. Diarrhea and constipation may alternate, or a period of constipation or lack of bowel movements may precede the diarrhea.

Kapha diarrhea is whitish in color, viscous and contains phlegm. There is a feeling of heaviness, torpor and lassitude. Motions are not frequent but tend to have more quantity.

In Chinese medicine, diarrhea is classified as either excess or deficient. Excess type is usually owing to the accumulation of damp-heat in the stomach and large intestine. It is very similar to the Pitta-type in Ayurveda and is often acute. Deficient type may be owing to chi (energy) or yang deficiency. Its treatment has similarities to the Vata and Kapha kinds but does not directly correspond.

General Treatment

In the beginning astringents (stool-binding herbs such as alum, oak bark or raspberry) should not be used, as they can cause the toxins to be held in the body. There should be fasting with herbs to burn up toxins (spices and bitters). An initial purgative — castor oil or rhubarb — should be taken to flush the colon of toxins. Many anti-parasitical herbs may be helpful — wormwood, mugwort, pomegranate, vidanga.

Foods for improving absorption in the small intestine should be taken first; buttermilk is good, along with a bland whole grain diet, mung gruel or kicharee. An anti-Ama or detoxifying approach is best. Good spices for diarrhea include ginger, long pepper, saffron, coriander and cardamom. The best common spice for stopping diarrhea is nutmeg.

Ayurvedic formula no. 9, Herbal Absorption is excellent, as well as Nutmeg compound.

A good general Western herbal formula is equal parts nutmeg, raspberry leaf, mullein leaf and marshmallow.

Should severe or watery diarrhea persist for more than a few days, the use of astringents to bind the stool will be required, as well as the administration of tonic herbs — ashwagandha or ginseng — to restore collapsed vitality.

Pitta (Fire) Diarrhea

An anti-Pitta diet is required; hot spices should be avoided, particularly chilies, even garlic. Do not take any form of alcohol. Oily, greasy and fried foods will also make the condition worse. No oil massage should be given. The abdomen should be kept cool.

Herbal therapy involves first the use of bitter herbs, then secondarily, astringents. Typical herbal bitters are good, such as barberry or golden seal. Or an initial bitter purgativer — hubarb root or senna leaves.

Ayurvedic herbs include bilva, kutaj, katuka, gentian, chiretta, cyperus, aloe and barberry. Formulas include Bilva compound, Cyperus wine and Kutaj wine.

Chinese bitters for diarrhea are coptis, scute and phellodendron. Other specific anti-dysentery herbs include purslane and anemone. Formulas for diarrhea include Coptis and Scute combination.

Useful Western herbs include bitters — golden seal, barberry, gentian and wormwood — and astringents — raspberry leaf, alum root and potentilla. For blood in the stool astringent and demulcent herbs such as raspberry leaf, mullein leaf, marshmallow are indicated. The general anti-diarrhea formula (listed above) can be given with barberry or golden seal for added fire-clearing action.

Vata (Air) Type

Anti-Vata diet is indicated and carminative spices — ginger, cardamom, fennel, asafoetida. Buttermilk is specific, particularly with nutmeg. Castor oil can be given first to cleanse the colon.

Other important Ayurvedic herbs are haritaki (in small doses), kutaj and pomegranate rind. Ayurvedic formulas include Nutmeg compound, Asafoetida 8 and Cardamom compound. The Herbal Absorption formula is also useful, or the general anti-diarrhea formula can be used with fresh ginger.

Kapha (Water) Type

Kapha diarrhea involves mucus in the stool. Treatment consists of an anti-Kapha diet. Dairy, fats, oils, sweets, pastries and breads should be avoided. Hot spices work well including cayenne, dry ginger and black pepper and most herbs to increase the digestive fire.

Other useful herbs include expectorant and digestive stimulants such as calamus, bayberry, basil and sage. The Ayurvedic formula Trikatu or Clove combination can be taken.

Amoebic Dysentery

Amoebic dysentery is commonly picked up in travelling, particularly through third world countries where sanitation is not very good. The specific Ayurvedic compound for it is Vatsaka compound. Kutaj is the main Ayurvedic herb and its formulas.

Eating of garlic can be a preventative. Wormwood is very good (one ounce infused in a pint of water and taken daily for 3–7 days). The common summer weed purslane, particularly taken fresh, is good eaten or infused, one ounce three to four times a day.

Amoebic dysentery easily becomes a chronic condition and may cause emaciation or wasting away of tissues. Then tonics like ashwagandha or ginseng are necessary.

Bacillary Dysentery

Bacillary dysentery treatment is much like that for Pitta diarrhea; it is initially an infectious disorder, and much that is said there is relevant here. The specific Ayurvedic compound is Kutaj wine or jelly. Kutaj tablet is also good. Many bitters such as chiretta, katuka, barberry, neem, golden seal, wormwood, rhubarb and coptis have antibacterial and anti-inflammatory action on the digestive tract and are used in this condition. One ounce of these herbs can be infused in a pint of water and taken daily.

If it becomes chronic, spices are required as well — ginger and garlic, or restorative tonics like ashwagandha or ginseng.

Infantile Diarrhea

Infantile diarrhea and griping is usually caused by an inability to digest mother's milk or cow's milk. It is mainly a Kapha (water) or Ama (toxic) condition.

Spices to help digest milk should be given like fennel, dill, cardamom and calamus. These can be taken by the mother or by the infant in small, pinchful dosages. Dill water, sold at most Indian markets, is very good. Nutmeg is also good for stopping the condition, particularly taken with a banana. More care is needed, however, as babies easily suffer from dehydration.

Constipation

Almost everyone suffers from the accumulation of toxins in the colon, evidenced by a coating at the back of the tongue. According to Ayurveda, normal and healthy colon function is indicated by lack of tongue coating (except for a normal thin white coating). One should have an easy bowel movement the first thing in the morning. The stool should float (if it sinks it indicates Ama, poor digestion and the accumulation of toxins).

Toxins in the colon and constipation, however, cannot always be simply treated with purgatives or colonics. These can weaken the tone of the colon and breed dependency. Their action on the system is strong and often traumatic; it can unbalance other organ functioning and, particularly, aggravate Vata, the biological air humor. Symptoms of excessive use of colonics and purgatives include lack of appetite, excessive weight loss, insomnia, diarrhea or continued constipation, palpitations, anxiety and vertigo or feeling faint.

The main cause of constipation on a physical level is dietary — eating food that is difficult to digest. It may also occur as the complication of a fever or infectious disease. Other factors include sleeping late in the morning, or not heeding the urge to go. Our American life-style of getting up quickly and rushing off to work tends to block the natural urge towards elimination. Sex in the morning causes apana, the downward moving air, to be weakened and can aggravate the condition. Coffee or tea in the morning may promote constipation, as they tend to be diuretic (drying).

Mental factors include insomnia, nervousness, stress, worry, grief and fear, as well as any excess stimulation of the nervous system (too much television). Medical factors such as being bedridden or taking too many drugs or medications (particularly diuretics) can come into play.

General Treatment

According to Ayurveda, the digestion must improved with the right use of spices; the Agni or digestive fire must be normalized. Laxatives that tonify the colon or improve colon function are safer and often preferable to short-term quick purgatives.

Strong purgatives such as senna and rhubarb are better for acute conditions. Castor oil is also good for more severe constipation and is not as drying to the colon as these bitter purgatives. Acute constipation is evidenced by fever, thick tongue coating, severe bloating, gas or abdominal pain. It usually indicates Ama, toxemia or some kind of food poisoning (which may be caused by bad food combinations). Hence, fasting or light diet should also be followed. Care should be taken, however, if the pain is in the lower right abdomen. This can indicate appendicitis, in which case purgatives, though sometimes helpful, can be quite dangerous.

For chronic constipation diet should be addressed first, with adequate intake of oily or bulk foods. These include dairy, nuts, whole grains, bran, raw fruit and raw vegetables. Many fruit juices are good — prune, grape, cherry, but not so much apple or cranberry, which can cause constipation. More oils or fats may be needed in the diet. Sesame oil is excellent, as is olive oil.

Triphala

Specific for chronic constipation or toxins in the colon is the famous Ayurvedic compound, 'Triphala' or the 'Three Fruits', consisting of the fruit of three tropical trees, called 'myrobalan plums', haritaki, amalaki, bibhitaki. It is good for constipation in any of the three humors, though not always effective in acute conditions. It is an excellent general colon cleanser as well as a tonic and rejuvenative (rasayana) for the colon. Moreover, it nourishes the nervous system and helps improve the appetite. As a metabolic regulator, it will reduce fat in overweight conditions, while building the blood, muscles and nerves in underweight conditions. Dosage is 5–15 gms. once a day in warm water before sleep.

Aloe gel, 1–2 tsps. 3 times a day, is another good general treatment for most types of constipation. It possesses both cleansing and lubricating action, though it is not as tonifying to the colon as Triphala.

The Colon Tonic (no. 5) is an improved form of Triphala, with a higher dosage of the main laxative in the formula, haritaki. It has broad spectrum usage, with honey for Kapha (water) types, with cool water or ghee for Pitta (fire) and with warm water for Vata (air).

In terms of life-style, it is important to arise at dawn (Vata time and colon time) and to empty the bowels. Often a glass of warm water or herbal tea will help stimulate peristalsis. Yoga postures or a mild massage of the lower abdomen are helpful.

Squatting, rather than sitting on the toilet, is a more natural position for elimination and helps relieve blockages or spasms in the intestines that may inhibit normal evacuation.

A good breakfast, particularly of oily or laxative foods, such as oatmeal with milk or ghee, may bring about normal evacuation if it has not occurred by that point. Or taking prune or grape juices may do the job. Cold food, like cold cereals, may block normal elimination.

Types of Constipation

Ayurveda recognizes three states of the colon; mild, medium and hard, according to our constitutional condition, as Pitta (fire), Kapha (water) or Vata (air).

Those with mild state of the colon tend to loose or oily stool. If they become constipated, any mild laxative, such as warm milk, will usually be sufficient. Constipation will not often become chronic. This is more characteristic of Pitta constitution as Pitta tends towards oiliness.

Medium state of the colon characterizes Kapha. Stronger laxatives may be needed or more long-term usage.

Hard or difficult state of the colon characterizes Vata. Strong laxatives may be necessary short-term, and constipation is often chronic and difficult to remedy.

Hence, constipation is usually a Vata (air) disorder, particularly as a long-standing condition or in the elderly. It may also be due to high Pitta (heat which dries out the stool) or high Kapha (mucus congestion clogging the colon). Not uncommonly, it is an Ama condition. Ama, undigested food, accumulates in the small intestine and is retained in the large intestine owing to blockage of the downward moving air (apana).

Chinese View

In Chinese medicine, acute constipation is thought to be due to fever and high fire. It is similar to Pitta constipation in Ayurveda and like it treated with bitter purgatives.

Chronic constipation is considered mainly due to deficiency of body fluids with progressive dryness in the colon. It is treated with bulk and lubricating laxatives, such as cannabis seeds, and is like the Vata type.

Vata (Air) Constipation

As the main site for Vata is the large intestine, high Vata is characterized by dryness in the colon, the accumulation of intestinal gas, with abdominal distention and constipation. The tongue usually has an accumulation of brownish fur at the back. There may be bad breath or the passing of gas, along with pain, tenesmus and anxiety. Headache may occur.

Causes are wrong diet with too much dry or light food, taking of drugs (most drugs have a diuretic or drying effect that aggravates Vata), smoking, excessive thinking, worrying, fear and anxiety, overstimulation of the nervous system, and old age. Constipation can cause, or be involved in, many Vata (wind) disorders including arthritis, neurosis, epilepsy and paralysis. Therefore, treating constipation can be a root treatment for many nervous system disorders.

Treatment

An anti-Vata diet should be followed with proper spices for balancing digestion. Oily food — dairy or nuts — should be taken. Adequate oils — sesame oil, olive oil or ghee — should be included to insure lubrication of the colon. Adequate bulk should be taken as well, such as whole grains (oats is best) or bran. Warm milk with a teaspoon of ghee can be taken before sleep for mild conditions. Beans, dry grains, cabbage family plants, mushrooms and other light or drying food should be avoided.

Spices to balance digestion — asafoetida, ginger, cardamom or fennel — should be taken with food to alleviate gas and promote the downward movement of Vata (apana).

Sesame oil or other anti-Vata oils can be applied externally, but not if there is severe bloating or distention (usually an Ama condition) as they can aggravate the condition. Sesame oil will lubricate the lungs via the skin and the large intestine via the lungs.

Typical Ayurvedic formulas include Triphala, 5–15 gms. taken in warm water before sleep. For stronger laxative action the amount of Haritaki can be doubled or Triphala fried in castor oil can be used. For more obstinate constipation, particularly with disturbance of the nervous system, 1–3 tsps. of castor oil can be taken before sleep.

Laxative salts (epsom salt) can be useful. Lavanbhaskar powder is a good Ayurvedic formula using various salts, as it increases Agni and promotes elimination. Asafoetida 8 is helpful for generally regulating peristalsis and it has mild laxative action.

Many bulk laxatives such as psyllium (the husks are preferable) and flaxseed, used both in Western herbalism and in Ayurveda, can be used in milder conditions of Vata constipation. Psyllium husk powder, 1–2 tsps. in warm water before sleep, is the best and seldom causes griping. Aloe gel is also useful as a lubricating laxative for Vata. It may be a little cold for many Vata types, so a small amount of ginger juice or powder should be added to it. Bulk laxatives, such as oils are heavy and should be balanced by spices (asafoetida or ginger), so they do not cause congestion.

In severe Vata constipation, however, tonic or lubricating laxatives may not be strong enough. Stronger laxatives such as rhubarb or senna may have to be used temporarily. But these bitter laxatives will aggravate Vata in the long run by their cold and drying action. They should be combined with gas dispelling spices (ginger or fennel) to prevent griping. A stronger oily laxative, castor oil 2–3 tsps. before sleep, is better.

Typical Chinese formulas include Cannabis Seed combination as a bulk laxative and Major or Minor Rhubarb temporarily for more severe constipation.

Western herbalism uses most of the laxatives already mentioned — rhubarb, epsom salt, psyllium and castor oil.

Enema Therapy*

Enema therapy (basti) is helpful for acute or chronic constipation. First, a cleansing enema is given, particularly when foul smelling gas occurs. Use Vata reducing herbs — Triphala, fennel, cardamom, or calamus — along with a smaller amount of a demulcent — licorice or sesame oil.

Then an oil enema should follow with 1/2 cup sesame oil in 1/2 cup warm water, held for a minimum of 20 minutes.

Tonic herbs can also be taken as nutritive enemas including ashwagandha, bala and shatavari, especially when constipation is accompanied by general debility or old age debility. They can be taken in oil, like sesame oil, or as milk decoctions.

Caution

The presence of the stool in the colon upholds the earth element in the body, which is necessary for keeping the air element from rising too high. Excess elimination therapy can cause anxiety, insomnia, palpitations, fainting, heart pain and other symptoms of high Vata. Again, one should proceed gently with Vata.

---

*   See also section on Enema Therapy in 'Detoxification'

Pitta (Fire) Type

Pitta constipation often occurs during the course or towards the end of a febrile disease. In Ayurveda, purgatives are contraindicated in new fevers but prescribed in old fevers. They are often given after the fever is gone to clear out residual heat and toxins.

In Chinese medicine, purgatives are often given during high fevers, as another method of draining the fever, but care is taken that the fever is 'ripe'. Indications of a ripe, or firm, fever are constipation, distention, gas and strong abdominal pain.

Pitta constipation involves irritability, anger, thirst, sweating with body odor, and burning sensation. It is characterized by a red tongue with yellow coating. The breath will be unpleasant. The face may be flushed or red. There may be headache, or insomnia with violent dreams.

Causes are those which increase Pitta, including too much spicy, sour or salty food, too much meat or greasy food. In constipation the hot attribute of Pitta is aggravated. Hence, hot spices, overexposure to the sun or heat, inadequate intake of fluids, etc. will be strong aggravating factors.

Pitta type constipation often involves liver dysfunction with congestion or obstruction of the bile. It is not simply a colon problem, as it usually is with Vata. Detoxification of the liver is often necessary. (See section on 'Liver Disorders'.)

Treatment

Anti-Pitta diet should be implemented, avoiding too many oils, fats or sweets, which can overtax the liver. Release of anger and letting go of stress and anger may be necessary if constipation is due to emotional causes. Often warm milk and ghee or licorice tea will be enough to stimulate evacuation. In India a rose confection is used for this purpose. Only when accompanied with high fever and thirst will constipation be severe in Pitta constitutions.

Most bitter laxatives can be used safely when this condition is acute. They also help cleanse the liver. Otherwise, bulk laxatives may be sufficient. Aloe gel combines both properties and can be taken, 1–2 tbs. before sleep. Taken on a regular basis, 1–2 tsps. 2–3 times a day, it will usually prevent constipation in Pitta individuals. In severe cases aloe powder can be taken, 1–2 gms. before sleep, to which a little coriander or fennel can be added to stop griping.

Ayurvedic herbs include aloe, amalaki, rose, psyllium. Formulas include Triphala (taken with ghee or aloe juice) and Aloe herbal wine.

Chinese herbal formulas include Major or Minor Rhubarb decoction, according to whether the condition is strong or moderate.

Typical Western herbs include rhubarb, senna leaf (strong action) and barberry, yellow dock, cascara sagrada (mild action).

For most chronic or mild conditions 1–2 tsps. of psyllium husk powder in warm water before sleep is sufficient.

Purgation Therapy (see also section on Purgation Therapy)

Purgation therapy (virechana) is the main treatment for high Pitta (fire), since it cleanses heat from the small intestine and liver, as well as the colon. But, for this therapy Pitta must be drawn into the gastrointestinal tract by diet, herbs, oil massage and sweating therapy. Otherwise purgation may not be helpful.

Purgation is an important way of eliminating heat and toxins from the body. It helps purify the blood as well as the digestive tract. It drains down the excessive fire rising upwards in many infectious or delirious conditions of the head and brain.

Kapha (Water) Type Constipation

Kapha constipation is usually due to the system being clogged with mucus. There will be heaviness, lethargy, tiredness and other signs of high Kapha. Stools will be copious, whitish or with phlegm. The tongue will be pale and fat with a white or mucus coating. The abdomen may be bloated, along with a feeling of dull pain and edema.

The main cause is sluggishness or congestion of the colon. Provoking factors include too much heavy or mucus forming foods, excessive sleeping, sleeping during the day, sedentary life style, and other Kapha increasing actions.

It may also occur as a complication of Kapha (phlegm) disorders in the upper body; stomach and respiratory disorders with excess mucus draining down through the digestive system. Hence while treating the constipation, other more primary anti-Kapha therapies, expectorant or emetic therapy, should be considered.

Treatment

Anti-Kapha diet should be followed avoiding especially heavy, constipating food including sugar, cheese, yogurt, bread, pastries, potatoes, pork. Often fasting is good, for one to three days. Increased physical and mental activity is needed, aerobic exercise and less sleep.

Light laxative and purgative herbs are indicated. Bitter laxatives can be used — aloe, rhubarb and senna. These herbs also help remove fat and reduce weight. Hot spices, ginger, cayenne and black pepper are needed.

Three grams of powdered rhubarb root along with two grams of dry ginger can be taken in one cup of warm water before sleep for more severe cases.

Bulk laxatives and laxative oils should not be used as these increase Kapha and will promote stagnation.

Cleansing enemas with spicy and expectorant herbs such as ginger, calamus and bayberry are also helpful.

Ayurvedic formulas include Triphala 2–6 gms. along with Trikatu 1–3 gms., taken with aloe juice or warm water before sleep, or the Digestive Stimulant (no. 1) with the Colon Tonic (no. 5).

Intestinal Gas and Colic

Intestinal gas, or colic pain, indicates bad digestion and the formation of Ama. It is characteristically a high Vata (air) condition but can be brought about by poor digestion in any of the humors. It usually involves some bloating or distention, along with abdominal sensitivity or migrating abdominal pains. Most abdominal pain is related to gas or indigestion.

The causes are mainly dietary, though nervous and emotional upset can trigger it as well. It is brought about by eating foods that are difficult to digest: beans, cabbage family plants and raw onions are too dry or gas causing; sweets, ice cream, and oily foods are too heavy. It can be caused by wrong food combinations such as eating sweet foods or juices with starchy, salty or protein meals, by combining dairy with sour fruit or with bread, meat or fish, or by overeating. Our cultural habit of eating sweet desserts after meals causes fermentation and gas. Psychological factors are mainly excess worry, strain and stress.

Gas and distention is often a secondary condition or precursor of constipation or diarrhea. The downward moving air (apana) is obstructed. It usually indicates poor functioning of the digestive fire as well.

General Treatment

Simple and moderate eating is required; not eating too much, or too frequently, or combining too many foods at the same meal. Sweet taste should be avoided or taken, in moderation, by itself. Spicy, carminative (gas-dispelling) herbs are indicated. These include cardamom, fennel, ginger, peppermint, orange peel, bay leaves and most cooking spices.

Ajwan, Indian wild celery seed, is very good, along with a little rock salt. Cardamom and fennel in equal parts are excellent for most indigestion, gas and abdominal pain, one-half teaspoon of the powder infused in one cup of water taken before meals. Asafoetida, valerian, nutmeg and camomile have analgesic properties for intestinal pain. Castor oil, with a little cayenne or asafoetida, can be applied to the abdomen for pain, also.

Most digestive formulas are good, like Trisugandhi, Trikatu and the Digestive Stimulant (no. 1).

Vata (Air) Type

Indications are gas and distention, with variable appetite, constipation, insomnia, palpitations or nervousness. There may be severe or migrating abdominal pain. The cause is mainly too much light or dry food — beans, cabbage, raw onions, potato or corn chips, peanuts, or excess salads; excessive worry, fear, anxiety and other such high air psychological factors also may be involved.

Treatment consists of an anti-Vata and anti-Ama diet, watching proper food combination, and avoiding too much sweet food, such as cookies, cakes, pastries and ice cream. Dry pastries, cookies, and dry fruit aggravate Vata by their dry quality. Herbs prescribed are spicy, carminative herbs - asafoetida, ajwan, ginger, fennel, cumin, cardamom, calamus.

Typical Ayurvedic formulas are Asafoetida 8, Lavanbhaskar powder or Trisugandhi powder, 1–3 gms. before meals with warm water. These herbs can be taken after meals as well for overeating.

Chinese herbs include carminatives — perilla leaf, magnolia bark, ginger, citrus peel. Typical Chinese formulas include Magnolia and Ginger combination.

Many common Western cooking spices are good for this condition, including those mentioned above as well as camomile, oregano and thyme.

Pitta (Fire) Type

Symptoms of high Pitta such as hyperacidity, heartburn, diarrhea and irritability will occur along with gas. Treatment again begins with anti-Pitta diet. Gas dispelling herbs and formulas should be combined with bitters. Cooler carminative herbs are indicated — fennel, coriander, cumin, mint, saffron. Good bitters are gentian, barberry, golden seal, katuka. Cardamom and fennel can be taken along with barberry.

The typical Ayurvedic formula is Avipattikar powder, but most bitters are good, particularly if combined with a small amount of dry ginger. The Antacid formula (no. 12) can also be helpful. Coriander, fennel and cumin in equal parts are another good formula.

Kapha (Water) Type

Symptoms of high Kapha will prevail, phlegm, congestion, nausea or vomiting. The herbs and formulas for Vata type can be used with emphasis on the hotter herbs — cayenne, dry ginger, ajwan, calamus and cloves. Trikatu formula is also indicated, with warm water (not honey).

Hemorrhoids

Hemorrhoids are caused by varicosity of the veins around the anus. Initially they may only involve pain or difficult evacuation. In more severe cases prolapse and bleeding can occur. They can be due to any of the three humors, but are most commonly Vata (air) and Pitta (fire). Again, Agni or the digestive fire must first be improved with the right spices. Turmeric is a special spice for reducing swelling and inflammation of the muscle tissue and can be applied locally as a paste or in the form of various Turmeric cremes sold in Ayurveda.

Causes include wrong diet, constipation, diarrhea, wrong posture, sedentary life-style, stress, irritability, excessive worry or excessive sexual activity.

General Treatment

Astringent herbs are used — haritaki, alum, pomegranate, red raspberry and mullein to help tighten the tissues. Haritaki herbal wine is an Ayurvedic specific for this condition. These herbs are good applied topically as a wash, a paste or a suppository.

Purgatives or laxatives may be helpful to ease elimination, when the cause is constipation. Squatting and the use of cold water to clean the anus after defecation may be helpful.

According to Chinese medicine, most chronic prolapse conditions are caused by sinking of the central chi (primary energy). They are treated by tonics — ginseng and astragalus — and special herbs to raise the yang — bupleurum and cimicifuga (black cohosh). The most typical formula used is Ginseng and Astragalus. This chi syndrome does not correspond to any of the three humoral types, but the formulas can be used for many types of chronic hemorrhoids in all of them.

Vata (Air) Type

Vata hemorrhoids involve pain, not only in the rectum, but also in the thigh, back, lower abdomen and urinary bladder. There is loss of appetite. The hemorrhoids are dry, rough, irregular. There is seldom bleeding or swelling of the hemorrhoidal tissue.

Vata hemorrhoids are caused by constipation, dry stool, straining at evacuation. They are more common in the elderly or the bed-ridden. Factors include too much cold, raw, dry, light or astringent food and sedentary life with lack of exercise. Emotional factors include worry, anxiety and fear.

Treatment consists of anti-Vata diet, much like for constipation, with emphasis on warm, moist, oily food. Buttermilk with a little cumin and rock salt is also good. The colon must be lubricated properly. Warm sesame oil can be applied to the lower rectum or taken as an enema (1/2 cup in the evening).

When digestion is weak and a more pronounced tongue coating exists, spices to improve digestion which also improve circulation in the colon should be taken. These include basil, dry ginger, black pepper, cayenne, turmeric.

Ayurvedic herbs include haritaki, amalaki, ashwagandha, shatavari, Triphala, Draksha or Asafoetida 8 formulas. Bulk laxatives like psyllium are also good.

Pitta (Fire) Type

Pitta type hemorrhoids involve redness, swelling, and often, bleeding or discharge of pus. There may be a burning sensation at the rectum or along with the passing of the stool. The stool is usually loose and yellow or greenish in color. Prolapse may occur after frequent or hot type diarrhea. There will be thirst, hunger, irritability and anger.

Causes are too much spicy, sour or salty food, alcohol, and overexposure to the sun or heat. Emotional factors are irritability, anger and aggression.

Treatment is similar to that of Pitta diarrhea. It requires anti-Pitta diet with emphasis on salads and green vegetables. The nightshades, tomatoes, potatoes, eggplant and peppers, should be avoided, particularly where there is rectal bleeding. Pomegranate juice is good. Bitter and astringent tastes are prescribed.

Good herbs are aloe gel, turmeric, cyperus, barberry, katuka, and neem. Turmeric, cyperus and barberry in equal parts can be very effective. Formulas include Triphala with ghee, as well as the anti-diarrhea formulas.

Good demulcents and astringents for bleeding hemorrhoids include mullein leaf, raspberry leaf and marshmallow, or the Ayurvedic herb ashok. Aloe powder should not be used as a purgative as it aggravates rectal bleeding.

Kapha (Water) Type

Kapha type hemorrhoids are large, whitish or pale in color and slimy to touch. They are mainly an accumulation of phlegm or fat and may be associated with polyps or swollen glands in other parts of the body. There will be mucus in the stool, which may also be pale in color. The urine may be milky in color. The patient frequently suffers from colds, cough, runny nose, excess salivation or sweet taste in the mouth.

Treatment is similar to Kapha constipation. Fasting or light anti-Kapha diet is indicated, strictly avoiding all mucus forming foods.

Strong cleansing and stimulating spices can be used like cayenne, black pepper, dry ginger, bayberry, calamus. Good formulas include Trikatu and Triphala taken together with honey.

DISEASES OF THE STOMACH

The stomach is the site of the first stage of digestion. Most digestive disorders either begin here or are first noted here. The stomach is a Kapha (water) organ, and diseases of Kapha most often originate here. It is a sensitive organ and is easily upset not only by wrong diet but also by emotional disturbance or worry. The condition of the stomach often indicates the state of the Kapha in the body, the sense of contentment, nourishment and feeling of abundance in life, as it is like the mother to the rest of the body.

Vomiting
Nausea

Vomiting is an excessive movement of the upward-moving air (udana). Nausea is a milder version of the same. It can be brought about by accumulations of the three humors, by toxins or by psychological factors such as fright or severe repulsion. Causes include bad food or water, bad food combinations, overeating or other dietary indiscretions. Vomiting can be involved with other digestive or respiratory system disorders, so care should be taken to find its cause. It is related to cough and asthma, often occurs with them, and can be treated by many of the same herbs and formulas.

Excess use of emetic therapy or undue promoting of vomiting, (for weight reduction) can cause it, as well as undue suppression of the digestive fire by any factors.

Nausea and vomiting occurs more frequently in Kapha (water) types. Kapha accumulates as phlegm in the stomach, where it blocks peristalsis and causes udana to rise up. Vomiting occurs to clear it out. Any excess eating of Kaphogenic foods, sweets, oils, dairy, meat, or just overeating, may precipitate it.

Differentiation

Vata (air) vomiting is dry type vomiting with thirst, pain in the chest and sides, palpitations, anxiety and astringent taste in the mouth. It is often a nervous reaction.

Pitta (fire) vomiting is the bilious variety with sour fluid, bitter taste in the mouth, burning sensation, thirst and red face.

Kapha (water) type is watery or mucousy vomit with sweet taste in the mouth, excessive salivation, heaviness and labored breathing.

Vomiting can occur in stomach flu or with putrid food in the stomach. It is also common during pregnancy (morning sickness).

In the Chinese system, vomiting, like cough, is often caused by rebellious chi or adverse chi rising. It is treated with herbs, like cardamom or fresh ginger, to regulate the chi. This type and its treatment resembles the Vata type in Ayurveda.

Other factors include accumulation of dampness and internal cold, which is more like Kapha. The herbs used for it are mainly hot spices.

Another causative factor for it in Chinese medicine is heat in the stomach, which is much like Pitta and treated by bitter herbs.

General Treatment

Anti-emetic herbs are administered to stop vomiting. Certain, mainly spicy, herbs have this special potency. As it is most often an acute condition, treatment is often symptomatic.

However, the patient should be examined initially to see if it is a condition of toxins or food poisoning. If so, vomiting should be encouraged by the using emetic herbs such as calamus, licorice and salt (the latter two in large amounts). Often a good old 'finger down the throat' will do, first taking mint tea or warm water, up to one pint, to make the vomiting easier.

The favorite Western emetic is lobelia (with a touch of cayenne). The Chinese prefer the calyx of the persimmon fruit.

Such emetic therapies were more in vogue for cleansing the stomach in poisoning before the invention of pumps to clear the stomach.

If there is a severe Kapha condition, it may also be better to promote vomiting. Otherwise the mucus may be trapped in the stomach and lungs and continue to depress their functions.

Many common spices are good to prevent vomiting. Among the best are fresh ginger, fennel, basil, nutmeg, cardamom and cloves. A simple combination of cardamom and fennel in equal parts, 1 tsp. infused in a cup of warm water with a little honey, is good for stopping almost any kind of vomiting. Lemon juice with a little honey or sugar is also good.

The typical Ayurvedic formula is Cardamom combination. This is particularly good for Kapha and Vata.

Typical Chinese formulas include Minor Pinellia and Hoelen combination, good for almost any kind of vomiting.

These same common spices are among the best Western herbs for this condition.

Specific Treatment

For Vata, anti-Vata regime is indicated. Sleep, relaxation, calm and meditation are important because the causes are usually psychological (hypersensitivity of the mind and nervous system). Cardamom compound can be used taken with warm milk, or cardamom and fennel can be added to honey or warm milk (1/2 tsp. of the powder of each).

For Pitta, anti-Pitta regime should be followed. Mild herbal bitters will be helpful, such as barberry or aloe gel, along with the anti-vomiting herbs, coriander, cardamom and fennel. Strong bitters — aloe powder or rhubarb root — tend to aggravate nausea and vomiting. The main Ayurvedic formula is Avipattikar powder.

Kapha vomiting is due to excess mucus, which should be cleared up with expectorant herbs. Anti-kapha regime is indicated. Trikatu is the best common formula, or Clove combination, taken with honey.

Hyperacidity

Acid or sour taste is a sign of Pitta disorders, usually indicating high Pitta (fire) in the small intestine. There will be heartburn, belching of sour fluids, perhaps nausea and vomiting.

Causes are mainly dietary: too much spicy or sour food, too much greasy food, alcohol or overeating in general. Excess intake of sweets, including pastries, cakes, pies, can also cause hyperacidity; sugar causes fermentation and acid production in the stomach, particularly if wrongly combined with other food types.

Treatment

Anti-Pitta diet is prescribed, with antacid food such as milk or ghee and emphasis on such bland whole grains as basmati rice. Bananas should be avoided as they have a sour post-digestive effect. Sour taste, as in pickles, yogurt, wine etc., should be avoided.

Good herbs are aloe gel, shatavari, amalaki, licorice, marshmallow, gentian, barberry, conch shell — those herbs with mainly demulcent and bitter properties. Antacid formulas include conch shell combination (Shankha bhasma) taken with cool water or aloe gel. The Antacid formula (no. 12) is specific to this condition. A good Chinese herb is oyster shell, which is also antacid.

Hyperacidity can also occur with weak digestion. Food will sit in the stomach and ferment, producing burning sensation. This is more common in Vata (air) and Kapha (water) types. Typical formulas for improving the digestive fire are indicated such as Asafoetida 8 and Trikatu.

Mineral herbs such as oyster or conch shell (and most antacid medicines or baking soda) tend to depress the digestive fire and should be used with care or combined with the spices for weaker digestions.

Ulcers

Ulcers are an inflammation of the mucus lining of the stomach. They involve pain, burning sensation and, when more severe, bleeding. If perforated, they can be life-threatening. They are usually due to psychological factors such as stress, worry or overwork but there are many dietary causes as well, including too much spicy or sour food.

Ulcers, most commonly are a Pitta (fire) condition. Excess acid from the small intestine accumulates in the stomach and burns through the lining, causing inflammation.

It is not always an excess of stomach acid that causes ulcers. Some may be due to high Vata (air) and its characteristic excessive thinking and nervous sensitivity. Sometimes there is a deficiency of the mucus (Kapha) secretions of the stomach. This allows a normal or even low amount of acid to burn through. Ulcers can even be caused by a deficiency of stomach acid; the food stays in the stomach too long and eventually burns through what may be a thin stomach lining.

General Treatment

A bland diet is indicated, with whole grains and easy to digest foods. A milk fast may be advisable. Alcohol and smoking should be avoided. Spices, pickles, vinegar and other strong-tasting substances should be eliminated from the diet until the condition improves. Bananas and nightshades should be taken with care. Most of the therapies are similar to those for hyperacidity but should be followed more strictly.

Demulcent herbs for soothing the stomach lining are indicated — aloe gel, shatavari, licorice, marshmallow, comfrey root, slippery elm. Aloe gel is probably the simplest and most effective home remedy. The Antacid formula (no. 12) is generally good, as it regulates stomach acidity and protects the mucus membranes.

Pitta (Fire) Type

The general treatment prevails. Bland anti-Pitta diet should be taken. Bitters are good, such as, aloe, barberry, gentian, chiretta, katuka. Formulas are Sudarshan powder and Mahasudarshan powder, as well as Shatavari compound.

Good Chinese herbs are coptis, scute, gentian, and gardenia. Formulas include Coptis and Scute combination.

Western herbs are golden seal, gentian, and barberry. An excellent simple formula is equal parts gentian, barberry and licorice, 1 teaspoon of the powder infused in a cup of warm water before meals.

Vata (Air) Type

Excess dry, light or spicy food can aggravate an ulcer condition. Too much cold or raw food can also cause this difficulty by disturbing the digestive fire. Forgetting to eat, irregular or inadequate food intake can cause variability in acid production, making it too low at some times and too high at others.

Vata ulcers involve more pain and less burning sensation. Often the person feels cold, light headed or anxious. Application of heat to the stomach will give relief (if not, it is probably a Pitta condition). Other Vata symptoms — palpitations, insomnia, abdominal distention, gas or constipation — may prevail.

Treatment requires, at first, a bland diet, but spices can be safely used. Typical anti-Vata digestive formulas can be helpful, such as Asafoetida 8, Lavanbhaskar powder or Trikatu, but should be used with care if the tongue is dry, cracked or red in color. They should be taken with warm milk or ghee.

Kapha (Water) Type

Kapha people seldom get ulcers, as they seldom worry. Kapha ulcers are characterized by phlegm and nausea, lack of appetite, dull pain and heaviness. They may be caused by grief, greed or attachment. Strong digestion promoting spices are indicated, including cayenne, dry ginger, black pepper, cloves or formulas such as Trikatu. Demulcents may aggravate the condition.

A cautionary note: if there is any uncertainty as to whether Pitta is involved, or any kind of burning sensation is noted, hot spices should not be used but the general or anti-Pitta therapy followed instead.

DISEASES OF THE LIVER AND GALL BLADDER

The liver is a Pitta (fiery) organ, the site or origin of many Pitta (infectious and inflammatory) disorders. Most liver disorders, such as jaundice and hepatitis, are typical aggravated Pitta conditions. Such Pitta disorders as ulcers and hyperacidity have their origin in wrong function of the liver and gall bladder. Pitta literally means 'bile'; excessive bile production or congestion in the flow of bile usually indicate high Pitta. In Ayurveda, the liver is the seat of fire and easily heats up, causing various inflammatory diseases. The subtle enzymes, the 'bhuta agnis', are located in the liver. They transform digested food particles into the forms of the five elements needed to build up the tissue for the five sense organs in the body.

Moreover, the liver is the site of most Pitta (fiery) emotions. Negative Pitta emotions are irritability, anger, jealousy and ambition; positive ones are courage, confidence, enthusiasm and will power. Disturbances in these emotions can cause liver dysfunction. These factors relate mainly to the solar plexus and to the navel chakra. Pitta constitution individuals, and those prone to liver disorders, need to keep the navel center both clear of blockages and not overly active. This can be done by surrendering one's personal will in life to the higher creative and spiritual will in the heart.

General Care of the Liver

There are many good, generally bitter, herbs for promoting the flow of bile, cleansing the blood, detoxifying the liver and thereby relieving high Pitta. These include common Western herbs — gentian, barberry, dandelion and golden seal. Europeans habitually take digestive bitters to counteract their generally Pitta type constitutions and their Pitta diets (alcohol, red meat and generally hot, greasy, oily, heavy or overly sweet foods) that impair liver function.

Turmeric and barberry in equal parts are very good for clearing liver energy and preventing emotional stagnation. Adding of gotu kola to them calms the liver and mind as well, and helps counter addictions to sugar, fat, and alcohol, which impair liver function.

The Chinese herb bupleurum is also specific for liver care. Many Bupleurum formulas exist in their system for harmonizing the liver including Major and Minor Bupleurum.

Aloe gel is an excellent liver tonic, taken 2–3 tsps. 2–3 times a day. It has both cleansing and building properties. The Liver Tonic (formula no. 8) is excellent.

The most specific Ayurvedic herb for the liver is Bhumyamalaki (Phyllanthus niruri). Modern clinical studies both in India and the West show that as a single herb it is effective in most liver disorders. So far it appears to be the only substance that can treat hepatitis B in carriers, thus arresting the spread of the disease.

Mild spices, such as coriander, fennel, cumin, turmeric, cyperus, mint, lemon and lime, help promote liver energy and improve appetite in conditions of sluggish or congested liver. They can be used as spices in cooking or taken as teas before or after meals.

Many green herbs — dandelion, nettles, chickweed, comfrey leaf — are good for cleansing the liver; chlorophyll in general is good for this purpose.

Cooling nervine herbs, such as gotu kola, skullcap, passion flower, sandalwood and bhringaraj, are best for lowering the liver-deranging fiery emotions.

In terms of diet, the liver is best cleansed with an anti-Pitta approach, emphasizing raw vegetables and green vegetable juices. Sugars, fats and oils should be avoided, except for ghee. Ghee is the easiest oil for the liver to digest and helps restore its enzymatic function. It is a good vehicle for bitter liver-cleansing herbs.

A liver-cleansing regime is often helpful in the spring as part of a general detoxification and blood purification approach. At this time most of the wild green herbs and green vegetables with anti-Pitta properties are easily available.

Hepatitis
Jaundice

Hepatitis is originally an infectious disease, but wrong diet and other mainly Pitta provoking factors can increase the possibility of contracting it. The viral form is the most dangerous and has the more rapid onset. The bacterial form is not as easily transmittable or as quick to show symptoms, but can have very long-term debilitating effects. This disease is mainly caused by bad food and water and lack of sanitation. When severe, it results in jaundice, with yellow discoloration of skin, eyes, urine, feces and mucus.

Symptoms of hepatitis are fever, loss of appetite, nausea and vomiting, pain and tenderness in the liver area or hypochondriac region, yellow discoloration of skin, eyes, nails and waste materials, fatigue, and diarrhea.

Provoking factors include too much oily, greasy food, too much meat (particularly red meat), too many sweets. As the liver is responsible for sugar and fat metabolism, these foods tend to overtax its powers. Smoking, drinking alcohol, and the use of recreational drugs (marijuana, amphetamines) are also very damaging to the liver. A history of infectious diseases such as herpes or mononucleosis can also make one more susceptible. Psychological factors are anger, resentment, depression and suppressed emotions.

Herbal medicines are helpful in both acute and chronic hepatitis, particularly the latter. Western medicine often has little to offer for hepatitis except bed rest; this is recommended under the herbal therapies also, sometimes for a period of several weeks.

Treatment

For acute hepatitis, treatment is strongly anti-Pitta. Anti-pitta diet should be followed, avoiding all hot, spicy, sour and salty food, as well as meat, fish, cheese, oils, fried food, and pure forms of sugar and concentrated sweets. Even milk and ghee should be avoided in acute conditions. Raw green vegetables and sprouts can be taken to cleanse the blood. Mung beans are the best staple food for strengthening liver function, and a monodiet of mung beans can be followed for a week or two to reorient the liver. Then basmati rice can be added to make Kicharee, along with turmeric, coriander and other liver-cleansing spices. Complete rest is recommended, and strong exercise, travel or sexual activity should be avoided.

Mainly bitter herbs are indicated, those with bile clearing, blood cleansing and mild purgative action. Aloe gel is the best general herb, particularly with small amounts of turmeric and coriander. Aloe herbal wine is excellent in most conditions, chronic or acute. Treatment should be followed for at least three months to prevent the condition from becoming chronic.

Ayurvedic herbs are phyllanthus, katuka, aloe, barberry, nishot, guduchi, gotu kola, bhringaraj, and chiretta. Additional formulas are Tikta, 1 tsp. twice a day, Guduchi extract, 1–2 tsps. twice a day; Sudarshan powder, 1–4 gms. twice a day; or the Liver Tonic (no. 8). Phyllanthus, by itself, is excellent. Triphala can be taken as a laxative. Formulas should be taken with aloe gel or juice as the vehicle.

Chinese herbs include coptis, gentian, rhubarb root, bupleurum. Formulas include Gentian combination (strong type), Capillaris combination (for acute jaundice), Rehmannia 6 (weak type).

Western herbs include golden seal, barberry, rhubarb root, cascara sagrada, yellow dock and dandelion. Dandelion leaf has better detoxifying properties in acute stages; the root is more useful in chronic conditions.

Isatis (in Sanskrit nila) is an important Ayurvedic and Chinese herb with well-proven antibiotic properties for infectious hepatitis. Dosage is one ounce of the root or leaves daily, preferably with other liver-cleansing herbs.

For chronic hepatitis, tonics including aloe gel, guduchi extract, amalaki, shatavari and formulas such as Chyavan prash and Shatavari compound are indicated. Oils for rebuilding the liver (once it can digest oil) include sesame, olive and avocado. Chronic hepatitis usually involves anemia and becomes a wasting disease, so iron supplements or Ayurvedic iron preparations are also helpful. For cirrhosis, bhringaraj is the best Ayurvedic herb. Phyllanthus again is excellent, specifically for hepatitis carriers (who may otherwise not exhibit symptoms).

Chinese tonics for rebuilding the liver are dang gui, rehmannia, lycium and he shou wu (fo ti).

Gall Stones
Cholecystitis

Gall stones are caused mainly by congestion and obstruction in the flow of bile. They often occur along with cholecystitis, inflammation of the wall of the gall bladder. With gall stones there is often acute pain in the liver and gall bladder region along with swelling and tenderness.

The condition, particularly with more pronounced inflammation, is mainly a Pitta condition.

Pitta (fire) type gall stones are yellow, green or red in color, with sharp angles. Vata (air) type are black or brown, and dry or rough. Pain may be severe, but inflammation and fever will not be pronounced. Kapha (water) type are round, soft, whitish, like phlegm, and seldom involve significant pain.

Treatment

In acute cases an initial purgation with liver cleansing herbs — aloe, rhubarb root, senna, cascara sagrada, is good. Usually, the more acute the pain and the higher the fever the stronger the purgative action which can be used. However, such acute cases are generally safer under clinical care.

Purgatives should be followed with the liver cleansing and clearing herbs under the hepatitis section. In chronic conditions, the treatment is like that for chronic hepatitis, and strong purgatives should not be used.

Special herbs with stone-removing (lithotriptic) properties include Ayurvedic herbs — pashana bheda, gokshura, katuka, Chinese herbs — desmodian and lygodium, and Western herbs — corn silk, uva ursi, and gravel root. Corn silk tea, one ounce per pint of water along with a tbs. of coriander taken daily, is often effective in milder cases. Most herbs for urinary-tract stones will also help clear gall stones if taken with an herb to conduct the action to the liver area (coriander or turmeric).

Liver-harmonizing formulas such as the Liver Tonic (no. 8) can be taken with strong teas of these stone-dispelling herbs as their vehicle. A good common formula can be made with turmeric, barberry, gravel root, corn silk and coriander in equal parts.

Diet should be as per the constitution, but in acute cases avoid all food the liver has trouble digesting (sweets, oils, fats).

DISEASES OF THE SMALL INTESTINE

Ayurveda recognizes a whole series of diseases of the small intestine that reflect its unique view on health. In Ayurveda, the small intestine is the seat of Agni, the digestive fire. Therefore, the main treatment is to improve Agni with spicy digestive stimulants, as listed under the digestive system generally.

The digestive fire has two actions: it grasps the essence of nourishment from the food; and it kills any bacteria or pathogens in the food. When it dysfunctions, not only will digestion be hindered, but also toxins will enter the body causing low resistance and poor immune function.

The small intestine is called grahani in Sanskrit, meaning 'that which grasps things'. When the small intestine is not functioning properly, the food will not be assimilated or absorbed adequately. There will be chronic indigestion and poor elimination, almost no matter what we may eat or do. We will be plagued with a whole series of digestive system dysfunctions such as constipation, diarrhea, gas, lack of appetite, excessive appetite, fatigue, low energy, low resistance. We may learn to live with dysfunction, as it often does not result in severe diseases, but we seldom feel really good or healthy.

Many of these conditions are associated in Western medicine with other diseases, such as hypoglycemia, candida, food allergies, chronic diarrhea or dysentery, chronic gastritis or intestinitis, etc. Often these are only secondary complications of the poor functioning of the small intestine. Sometimes this condition is dismissed by medical doctors as a mental condition if nothing physically wrong is found in the patient. The Ayurvedic view brings these together as small intestine disorders, making understandable what are otherwise difficult conditions to diagnose, often with contradictory symptoms. For this reason, we are introducing this disease concept here. These conditions are very common in our culture, but have not been classified in the same way or with the same clarity.

Malabsorption

Weakness of the small intestine creates what we could call 'malabsorption syndrome.' It has been equated with 'sprue syndrome', a condition of chronic poor digestion usually occurring in the tropics where the body is unable to deal with the higher bacterial content of the environment. However, this syndrome is also occurring as part of the general deterioration of our natural environment in the West; we are seeing more pollution and new strains of bacteria and viruses to weaken our systems. Probably at least half of us will have this malabsorption condition at some time or another. As a chronic condition, it can be tolerated; and often the doctors can't help us. It is difficult to cure, as the very source of digestion is unbalanced.

From a dietary standpoint, malabsorption can be brought about by any dietary extremes. It is caused by too complex or too irregular a diet: food that is too hot or too cold, too much raw food or too much over-cooked food, too much sweet food, overeating, or too much fasting. Eating too much canned food, junk food or an otherwise devitalized diet can also produce it. Any of these tend to unbalance the digestive fire, particularly if we change quickly from one to another. Hence, dietary extremists frequently end up with this condition.

Malabsorption is often the result of other chronic digestive system disorders such as diarrhea, dysentery, and constipation. It can be brought on by excess use of purgatives and colonics, or the taking of too many medicinal or recreational drugs, stimulants and antibiotics. Individuals who are overly stressed or hypersensitive will also be at risk.

Symptoms include variable appetite, unpredictable digestion, poorly formed stool with undigested food particles and foul smell, alternating constipation and diarrhea, and abdominal pain usually centered in the umbilicus. Spots or ridges on the fingernails or poor formation of nails is common. Malnourishment will show up as emaciation, often no matter what or how often the individual may eat. There will be debility and weakness of the muscles and bones, and a tendency towards low fevers or low grade infections. Unlike diarrhea and dysentery, there will be no dehydration. Colonics, purgatives and enemas will tend to make the condition worse.

While malabsorption can occur in any of the three humors, it is more common in Vata (air) types, given their irregular habits.

Many of these conditions are classified in Chinese medicine under 'chi' (primary energy) disorders, primarily chi deficiency but sometimes as complicated with chi stagnation. Symptoms include weakness, fatigue, lack of strength, shortness of breath, lack of appetite, poor assimilation, chronic diarrhea, and poor resistance.

Differentiation

Vata (air) type malabsorption syndrome is characterized by intestinal gas, abdominal distention and migrating pain, dry skin, cracked tongue, anal fissures, hemorrhoids, more chronic low weight and a tendency towards arthritis. The stool will be watery, frothy and passed with noise or gas alternating with hard, dry stool. Palpitations, anxiety and insomnia will occur, with feelings of faintness, ungroundedness and depression.

Pitta (fire) type is indicated by inflammation, ulceration or burning pain in the intestines. Diarrhea of yellow color will be more common; also a tendency to anemia, with emotional symptoms of anger and irritability.

Kapha (water) type symptoms include mucus in the stools, dull aching pain in the abdomen, heaviness, congestion in the lungs, less weight loss, and a tendency towards edema and diabetes.

General Treatment

The diet should be simple, avoiding the extremes mentioned above. Heavy and hard to digest food should be avoided. The best food, generally, is buttermilk (takra). It is best to prepare one's own, as most commercial buttermilk is overly salted. Make fresh yogurt, not too sour, add an equal amount of water and churn or blend for a few minutes. This creates the kind of buttermilk which Ayurvedic medicine prescribes. The whey or liquid part left over from yogurt or curds is also good. After a buttermilk fast of a few days, add Kicharee or other whole grains, followed gradually with other foods, thus reeducating, in time, the whole digestive system. Many simple starches are good at an early stage including kudzu (pueraria starch), basmati rice, lotus seed flour and potatoes.

Special spices to improve absorption are indicated, usually combining pungent and astringent tastes. These include nutmeg, cardamom, long pepper, cloves, fresh ginger, cinnamon, fennel, cumin, bayberry, cyperus, haritaki, chitrak. Herbal wines such as Draksha or Cyperus compound wine are excellent.

The Herbal Absorption formula (no. 9) is devised for this purpose, and taken with buttermilk. Pitta types having malabsorption and acidity can take it with aloe gel.

Specific Treatment

Vata types should follow the anti-Vata diet with the spices mentioned above. Whole grains and Kicharee are good; avoid too much cold or raw food and raw juices. Buttermilk can be taken with fresh ginger or nutmeg. Draksha or a little wine can be taken with meals. Formulas include Nutmeg compound, Cardamom compound or Garlic compound, as well as Vata's standard digestive formula of Asafoetida 8. These can be taken with buttermilk.

Pitta should follow an anti-Pitta diet, avoiding all fried and greasy food. Buttermilk can be taken with fennel and coriander, with herbal bitters or with formulas such as Tikta or Avipattikar powder.

Kapha should follow anti-Kapha diet, avoiding such typical items as cold water, ice cream, cheese, and pastries. Buttermilk should be taken with dry ginger or such formulas as Trikatu or Clove compound.

In more chronic and debilitated conditions, tonics such as ashwagandha, bala, ginseng and astragalus can be used. Chinese Chi tonics, the Four Gentlemen for mild conditions, or Saussurea and Cardamom compound for more severe conditions, can be helpful.

MISCELLANEOUS DIGESTIVE SYSTEM DISORDERS
Food Allergies

Allergens are subtle, high energy particles that have the capacity to irritate the nervous system. Food allergies may result initially from overexposure to these allergens. In the long run, however, allergic reactions are usually due to a hypersensitivity of the nervous system itself and indicate some internal weakness. Their causes are often emotional including stress, anxiety and worry. Allergies also result from our toxic environment, junk food, bad air, noise and other forms of environmental pollution.

Allergies occur when the immune system is depressed. Taking drugs and anti-biotics or exposure to chemicals lowers our immune function. Poor nutrition as a child can create a weakened immune system. The immune system is transferred through the mother's milk, particularly that given immediately after birth. Hence, when the baby is taken from its mother's bed at birth, which is the common practice in all hospitals, weak immune systems and allergies become more common. If children are not breast fed at all, the risk is increased.

Food allergies are more common in Vata (air) constitution individuals, as they possess the most sensitive nervous systems. Allergies show that, on some level, the individual is rejecting food, and feels not properly nurtured in life. Food allergies are more common where there is low vitality; the energy is not sufficient to give adequate resistance to environmental forces. Food allergies are not uncommon in Kapha (water) types with their low state of the digestive fire.

Symptoms of food allergies include bloating, gas, indigestion, diarrhea or constipation, congestion, headaches, skin rashes. These usually occur after eating various 'provoking' type foods — milk, wheat, soy, corn, nightshades (tomatoes), peaches, strawberries, etc. These foods may be either generally hard to digest (milk and wheat), or contain various hard to digest substances such as the alkaloids in the nightshades.

Vata (air) people most commonly become allergic to Vata-aggravating foods — beans, soy and corn.

Pitta (fire) people most commonly become allergic to tomatoes and other nightshades and to sour fruit such as peaches and strawberries.

Kapha (water) people have more allergies to Kapha-increasing foods — dairy and wheat.

General Treatment

Contact with allergens should be limited, but the immune and digestive systems should also be strengthened to allow us to endure them. It is not always possible to identify which foods are provoking the allergic reactions. Nor, if they can be identified, is it possible to avoid them altogether. Some people are so sensitive they will be allergic to almost anything.

Initially, a strict diet, according to one's constitution, should be followed, additionally avoiding all known allergens as much as possible. It is important, however, not to become paranoid or overly self-protective in avoiding allergens, as the emotions themselves are often more damaging to the immune system, in the long run, than are the particular foods. It is important to be watchful rather than fearful. A positive attitude in life is one of the best treatments for this condition.

Herbs and formulas to increase the digestive fire and to regulate digestive function are indicated. These are the same as those for improving digestion for each humor: Asafoetida 8 for Vata, Avipattikar or the Antacid formula (no. 12) for Pitta and Trikatu for Kapha.

Other treatment is much like that for the Malabsorption syndrome. Hence, spices like nutmeg, cardamom, bay leaves, fennel, cumin and ginger are good, as is the Absorption formula (no. 9). For Pitta, herbal bitters or Ayurvedic herbs like guduchi are excellent. Food allergies indicate we are not able to assimilate these particular foods, so it is largely a kind of malabsorption syndrome.

Long term treatment, once the allergic sensitivity is relieved, is tonification, or supplementation, with such herbs as ginseng, ashwagandha and shatavari. In avoiding the foods we are allergic to, we must be careful not to follow a too-reducing diet, as the long term treatment is not reducing at all.

Candida

Candida is an infestation of the candida albicans yeast. It usually starts in the g.i. tract but can enter the blood and lodge itself in various organs. Treatment is similar to a parasitical condition (see below). Symptoms include chronic low energy, low grade fevers, variable digestion, weak immune system, and food allergies. Many of the conditions listed as signs of candida are common to many weak digestive system complaints or other auto-immune disorders. It is helpful to have a medical test to check for the existence of the pathogen.

Candida is usually caused by weakness of the digestive fire. It is usually an Ama, or toxic, condition caused by the accumulation of an undigested food mass in the intestines. It can occur in any of the three humors but is most commonly a Vata (air) or Kapha (water) condition, as they tend more to low Agni.

Causative factors include eating too many sugars, taking stimulants or drugs, excess use of antibiotics, depressed immune system, frequent colds, flu or yeast infections, hypersensitivity of the nervous system, emotional factors such as worry and fear, as well as the general toxic state of our environment.

General Treatment

According to Ayurveda, conditions such as candida are symptomatic of an internal weakness or disharmony. The treatment principle is not just to try to kill off the pathogen (in this case the yeast), but to strengthen the internal energy. This involves normalizing digestion and then taking herbal tonics to strengthen the immune system. Such herbs include ashwagandha, bala and kapikacchu in Ayurveda or ginseng, astragalus and schizandra in the Chinese.

While it is important initially to avoid any yeast-containing or yeast-promoting foods and to take anti-fungal herbs, this will not take care of the internal weakness and can have a long term effect similar to antibiotic drugs. This regime can further weaken the immune system. It is particularly dangerous in Vata constitutions, as such reducing diets aggravate Vata. Such treatment methods are still based on a view of the problem as external in origin. Though the methods are naturalistic, the way of thinking is still allopathic.

An anti-Ama or detoxifying diet is indicated, mainly the avoidance of heavy, damp and mucus-forming foods including sugar, dairy, breads and fruit. Cold water, ice, and cold or raw foods should be avoided.

Hot spices with anti-parasitical powers are useful, such as cayenne, asafoetida and prickly ash. Garlic alone, 3–5 cloves a day, can be helpful. Garlic not only helps destroy the yeast but also protects and builds up the digestive power. Spices like cardamom, bay leaves and calamus, which help digest sweet and mucus-forming foods, are important; or the formula Trisugandhi powder.

Special anti-fungal herbs and anti-parasitical herbs are useful: valerian, wormwood, mugwort, saussurea, vidanga or the special anti-candida herb from South America, pau d'arco.

Vata (Air) Type

Symptoms are insomnia, lower back pain, dry skin, nervousness, restlessness, feeling spaced out, ringing in the ears, and depression. There will be chronic gas, abdominal bloating, and constipation, with erratic or variable energy.

Anti-Ama (detoxifying) diet can be followed, initially, for two weeks or so. For the long run a predominately anti-Vata diet is indicated, with emphasis on complex carbohydrates like whole grains, including Kicharee. Sugar, including sweet fruit juices, and yeast foods should be avoided. Food should be cooked with spices or curried. Dairy should be avoided except for buttermilk and ghee. Salads and raw food should not be taken. Beans should definitely not be eaten, or cabbage family plants and mushrooms. The best spices are asafoetida, garlic, basil, ajwan, cayenne.

Formulas include Asafoetida 8 and Garlic compound tablets.

Pitta (Fire) Type

Indications are fever, thirst, burning sensation, hyperacidity, and acute infections. Treatment involves anti-Pitta diet, but avoidance of sugars. Raw food and greens, or chlorophyll juice, will be particularly good. Bitter detoxifying herbs are indicated — aloe, katuka, chiretta, neem, barberry. Chinese bitters — coptis, scute, phellodendron and gardenia are useful, as are Western bitters like golden seal, barberry, gentian, wormwood and pau d'arco.

Formulas include Tikta, Sudarshan powder and Mahasudarshan powder. As the liver is often involved, the Liver Tonic (no.8) and other liver-regulating herbs are good.

Kapha (Water) Type

There will be accumulation of phlegm, frequent colds and flu, swollen glands, edema, heaviness, dullness and excessive sleeping. Treatment is an anti-Kapha diet avoiding all heavy, oily or greasy food such as meat, fish and dairy, as well as all sweets. Whole grains — corn, millet or rye — are good, as is mung beans.

All hot spicy herbs listed above are good. Formulas include Trikatu and Clove compound taken with warm water (not honey). Trisugandhi formula is also good, or cardamom, bay leaves and dry ginger in equal proportions.

Parasites

Intestinal parasites are not as uncommon as we think, though with the improved sanitation of Western countries they are not the major problem here they once were. Main causes are impure food and water, travelling in unsanitary areas and weak digestion.

Parasites are more common in Kapha (water) and Vata (air) constitutions and are usually associated with Ama, undigested food. Long term parasite infestation causes wasting away of tissues and aggravates Vata.

Pitta (fire) types seldom suffer from parasites because their digestive fire is usually high. Even when contracted, the parasites are burned up in the process of digestion.

In Ayurveda parasites are classified according to the medium in which they reside. Vata caused parasites reside in the stool, Kapha caused in the mucus or mucus membranes, and Pitta caused in the blood.

General Treatment

Initial fasting or anti-Ama (detoxifying) diet is prescribed. Sweets, meat and dairy products should particularly be avoided. Usually a purgative is given, then a course, 3–5 days, of anti-parasitical herbs. Purgation is given again and the stool is examined to see if the parasites have been dispelled. This usually works better in acute conditions.

In chronic conditions, tonic and nutritive herbs have to be given to balance out the depleting effect of the parasites.

Parasite growth is often encouraged by low Agni (weak digestive fire) and they, in turn, cause low Agni. The use of hot spices to promote digestion — cayenne, black pepper and asafoetida — is a major part of anti-parasitical treatment.

Bitter taste is also indicated in treating for parasites, owing to its cleansing and reducing properties. Good bitters for worms include wormwood, tansy, golden seal, rhubarb and aloe powder. The last two are good purgatives for parasites.

Other herbs have anti-parasitical action through a special property (prabhava) and may not be unpleasant tasting. An example is pumpkin seeds, which can be eaten freely during a fast to help dispel worms. Some strong anti-parasitical herbs can be toxic, like pinkroot and male fern, and must be used with care (though they are less toxic than many Western drugs for the same purpose).

The main Ayurvedic herb for parasites is vidanga, which is effective even for tapeworms. Pomegranate, particularly the root bark, is good for tape, round or pin worms. Other herbs are holy basil, katuka, betel nuts and cyperus.

Additional Western herbs are santonica (all kinds of worms), wormseed (round, hook or tape worms), rue.

Specific Treatment

Vata (air) type indications are gas, constipation, abdominal pain and bloating, insomnia, anxiety and other high Vata symptoms.

Additional treatment involves anti-Vata diet with limited intake of rich foods. Garlic and hot spices can be taken.

Formulas include Vidanga compound, Garlic compound and Asafoetida 8. Castor oil can be used as a purgative. Where malnutrition exists herbs such as ashwagandha, bala and ginseng should be taken.

Pitta (fire) type indications are fever, burning sensation, diarrhea or loose stool and other high Pitta signs. Pain in the gall bladder and liver area is common.

Additional treatment involves anti-Pitta diet with a lot of raw food, vegetable juices and greens. Spices should be avoided and digestive bitters taken. The bitter side of the general therapy is used.

Formulas include Vidanga compound taken with aloe gel or juice. Bitters are strong pure bitters — coptis, chiretta, katuka, gentian and golden seal.

Kapha (water) indications are phlegm, nausea, fatigue, feelings of dullness and heaviness, lack of appetite and poor digestion.

Additional treatment involves anti-Kapha diet with free use of spices, as hot as one can bear, for instance, cayenne and garlic in liberal amounts. All sugar and dairy must be avoided.

Formulas include Vidanga compound, Trikatu or Asafoetida 8. Aloe powder or rhubarb root can also be used as a purgative.

METABOLIC DISORDERS

These are more general digestive system disorders characterized by long-term imbalance of body weight.

Obesity

Obesity is the carrying of excessive weight, usually in the form of fat. The amount of weight that is considered excessive often depends upon the culture. Modern Western culture values thinness (a Vata or air type frame). Many eastern and traditional cultures have valued heaviness (a Kapha or water type frame), indicating affluence or plenty to eat.

Overweight may not be a disease, therefore, but a condition of holding more weight than the cultural standard. It should be noted that attempts to stay artificially thin may be unhealthy and may aggravate Vata, the biological air humor. Overweight truly becomes a disease when extra weight held is quite high and leads to other health problems (hypertension, diabetes or arthritis).

Still, according to Ayurveda, it is better to be too thin than too heavy. It is easier to build up a person who is too thin than to reduce one who is too heavy. A heavy body is a good breeding ground for toxins (Ama) and may reduce the life expectancy.

Causes of overweight include overeating, eating too much heavy or cold food, too frequent meals, excessive sleeping, and lack of exercise. Hormonal imbalances may exist. Emotional factors include attachment, sentimentality and clinging. Lack of self-esteem can be an important factor. Sometimes the extra weight becomes a security factor, put on for greater protection in dealing with the world. Generally, the digestive fire will be weak in this disease of low or slow metabolism. It is usually a Kapha (water) disease in Ayurveda.

Weight-reducing and appetite-suppressing drugs may also suppress the digestive fire and, over the long-term, further weaken the metabolism. They will also increase Vata (air) and thereby aggravate nervous-type obesity.

General Treatment

Overweight requires a lightening (langhana) or reducing method, with light diet, fasting, spicy herbs to improve digestion, mild laxatives to keep the bowels clean. Sometimes tonic herbs provide a deeper kind of nourishment which we may be looking for in excessive eating. Guggul and myrrh are good general herbs, as also shilajit. One gram of guggul or 1/2 gram of shilajit taken two to three times a day with ginger and honey can correct most forms of obesity over a period of several months. Aloe gel with ginger or turmeric is another good combination. Nervines are useful to calm the tendency towards excessive eating. Best is gotu kola.

The Herbal Reduction Formula (no. 13), taken with honey, is a specific formula for this condition.

Strong reducing therapies should not be started in the winter season, as they can lower heat and resistance. Usually long-term mild reducing therapies will be more successful than short-term crash methods.

Kapha (Water) Type

Overweight is more common in Kapha constitutions. Their metabolism is slow, and they easily put on weight. Their appetite is continuous, and they often eat as a means of relieving stress or tension. They can become attached to or addicted to the joys of cooking and eating. In addition, they may suffer from hypo-thyroid or other hormonal conditions that cause them to hold weight.

Their excessive weight consists largely of water and fat. It is usually related to weak function of the pancreas and kidneys, and the pulse and energy level may be low. The individual is generally flabby, pale in complexion with moist skin. There will be excessive phlegm or saliva. Subcutaneous fat deposits may develop along with benign tumors.

Treatment is primarily dietary, following an anti-Kapha diet for an extended period of time. Sugar and sugar products should be avoided as much as possible. Salt intake should be reduced. Dairy, sweet fruits, breads, pastries, meats, fish and oily foods should be taken as little as possible. Sprouts, yeast and other enzymatic agents should be taken to help in the process of digestion. Food should not be taken before 10 am. or after 6 pm. Hot spices should be taken to raise the metabolism, along with fasting, unless there is debility. Fruit juice fast should be avoided, with spice teas or vegetable juices taken instead. All cold drinks should be avoided. As the condition is a long-term metabolic imbalance which the system has become used to, these measures should be employed gradually, allowing a slow, natural speeding up of organic functions that will not shock the system.

While it is preferable to eat less in quantity, it is even better to eat a different quality of foods — more vegetables, preferably steamed without oil or salt, beans and whole grains, and less of the heavier foods. Mung beans are excellent.

Excessive sleeping, or sleeping during the day, should be avoided. Exercise, particularly of an aerobic nature, should be undertaken. However, if the patient is weak, exercise should not be taken to the point of excessive sweating, shortness of breath or fainting.

Herbs include: hot spices to increase the metabolism — cayenne, black pepper, ginger, garlic and turmeric; bitter herbs to reduce fat — katuka, barberry, gentian, myrrh. Barberry is considered a rejuvenative for fat tissue, both eliminating excess fat and producing better quality tissue. The usual combination of turmeric and barberry is also useful here for obesity. Guggul or myrrh (preferably as a tincture) is specific and can be taken along with spices or bitters.

Ayurvedic formulas include Trikatu or the Digestive Stimulant (no. 1). Mild laxatives such as the Ayurvedic Triphala, aloe gel or cascara sagrada are good. Strong purgatives may not be good; they tend to lower the metabolism further. Trikatu and Triphala together with honey are excellent. A similar effect can be gained combining the Digestive Stimulant (no.1) with the Colon Tonic (no. 5). A specific formula is the Weight Reduction formula (no. 15).

Mild diuretics — plantain, corn silk or gokshura can be helpful, as well as herbs or formulas for improving kidney function such as shilajit. Nervine herbs such as gotu kola and calamus combined or skullcap counter the habit side of the disease.

Chinese formulas include Citrus and Craetagus, which is, generally, good for overeating and food stagnation (Ama) conditions. Additional Western herbs are alfalfa, dandelion and chicory roots.

Vata (Air) Type

Vata caused obesity is characterized by irregularity in weight. Periods of overweight fluctuating with periods of normal weight, or even underweight, may occur. Weight gain or weight loss may be sudden or unpredictable. Appetite will also be variable. Excessive amounts of sugar or carbohydrates taken to help calm the nerves will contribute to obesity.

Psychological factors are fear, anxiety, worry and nervousness. Extra weight will give greater feelings of security or stability.

The most difficult form of obesity is a combined Vata-Kapha type with a nervous mind (Vata) and a slow metabolism (Kapha). Mental habit and physical weakness combine in ways that are difficult to counteract. Under such conditions it is better to aim at reducing Vata (calming the nerves) than reducing Kapha (applying restrictive diet).

Treatment involves anti-Vata diet but with emphasis on complex carbohydrates. Foods to be taken include whole grains and starchy vegetables. Pure sugars should be avoided. Spices should be used with discretion; fewer of the hot spices (pepper and cayenne) and more of the spicy-sweet ones (fennel, cardamom, coriander).

Ayurvedic formulas include Asafoetida 8. Herbs to calm the mind and allay nervous habits are good, including gotu kola, calamus, jatamansi, nutmeg and valerian, or formulas like Sarasvat powder. Guggul or myrrh are helpful here also.

Pitta (Fire) type

Pitta obesity is usually caused by overeating. The appetite is high and the digestion is usually good, so there will be a tendency to eat more. As fire types can best digest sugar, they can also become addicted to it. They will also tend to eat more red meat. Weight will involve a good development of muscle and not just flab.

Treatment involves anti-Pitta diet. Meat, fish, oily or greasy food should be avoided, as well as sugars and pastries. One should take raw salads along with green herbs and chlorophyll. Digestive bitters are specific, as well as bitter laxatives.

Ayurvedic herbs include aloe, katuka, barberry, turmeric. Formulas include Sudarshan powder, the Liver Tonic (no. 8) and other liver-regulating formulas. Chinese formulas include Major Bupleurum combination. Helpful Western herbs are barberry, gentian, dandelion, cascara sagrada and Swedish Bitters formula.

Gems for Saturn, such as blue sapphire or amethyst, are helpful for obesity along with gems for Mercury like emerald, peridot and jade. Ruby or garnet for the Sun can be helpful when the condition is due to chronically low digestive fire.

Underweight

Underweight can also be a disease, though in our culture it is not always recognized as such. Lack of body weight can cause poor resistance, low vitality, nervousness and insomnia. There will be lack of appetite, depression, malaise, and psychological instability.

There may be wasting away of the tissues including loss of hair, falling of teeth, weakness of the bones and lack of sexual vitality, as well as other signs of premature aging.

Causes are frequently constitutional. Undue suppression of the digestive fire — too much fasting, dieting, or too much eating of light, cold or raw food, irregular eating habits, etc. — can contribute. Other factors include overwork, too much exercise and excessive sexual activity. Psychological factors are worry and grief (often following loss of a loved one), excessive study or too much mental activity.

Low weight may also be involved in convalescence from a severe disease that has depleted the body tissues. It may occur more commonly in the elderly or in children. Treatment involves an increasing or tonification therapy. Heavy, rich nutritive diet is taken along with tonic, building herbs.

Underweight is usually a Vata condition, as air types tend towards lightness. Vata individuals often forget to eat or their irregular eating habits cause long term suppression of the digestive fire. Use of stimulant drugs such as amphetamines can bring this condition about also.

Treatment

An anti-Vata diet is usually best. Meat and fish are helpful or other heavy foods like root vegetables, whole grains, nuts, dairy, oils and sugar. Meat or bone marrow soup may be necessary in the beginning or a mild starchy grain gruel (rice, mung beans or oats).

Spices are indicated but not necessarily in the beginning treatment. The hotter spices in particular, may cause further depletion of vital fluids by their drying nature, and overstimulate what is usually already a hypermetabolism.

Tonic herbs are essential: ashwagandha, shatavari, bala, licorice prepared in milk. Ayurvedic formulas are Ashwagandha compound, Shatavari compound, Dhatupaushtic compound, Chyavan prash. These can be taken with milk or draksha.

Additional Western herbs include comfrey root, slippery elm, marshmallow, and saw palmetto. Chinese herbs are ginseng, astragalus, dang gui, and rehmannia; formulas include Ten Major Tonic and Woman's Precious Pill.

Pitta (Fire) Type

Underweight can also occur as a high Pitta condition in which persons literally burn themselves up. Often there is high fire in the mind with excessive thinking and an overly critical nature. The condition may follow a severe febrile disease, blood loss or hepatitis. Anemia and poor liver function are usually involved.

Treatment is similar to that for Vata with an anti-Pitta diet that emphasizes building-type foods. All spices are to be avoided. Salads and raw vegetables should not be taken in excess, as they are not strengthening enough but cooked vegetables are good. A milk fast may be advisable in the beginning. Ghee is excellent. Whole grains such as wheat and rice are good and mung beans in specific. Raw sugars can be used in moderation.

Ayurvedic herbs include aloe gel, gotu kola, and shatavari. Guduchi is excellent. Formulas include Chyavan prash, Brahma rasayan, and Shatavari compound.

Chinese herbs include ho shou wu (fo ti) and formulas include Women's Precious Pill (can be used by men also). Additional Western herbs are comfrey root, marshmallow, slippery elm, American ginseng, and licorice.

When underweight, gems for Jupiter such as yellow sapphire, yellow topaz or citrine are best, along with gems for Mercury such as emerald, peridot and jade. Green color, that of Mercury, is good for regulating metabolism: for increasing weight in those too thin; for decreasing it in those too fat.

Anorexia

Anorexia can become a severe condition connected to over-dieting and underweight. The digestive fire may be suppressed to the point where no food can be taken in or held in the stomach. There can be repeated vomiting to the point of dehydration. Causes are usually emotional traumas or chronic undereating.

While nausea, vomiting and mild anorexia are usually symptoms of a Kapha (water) disorder, severe anorexia with pronounced weight loss is mainly a high Vata (air) condition involved with fear, nervousness, insomnia, pain in the chest and abdomen and palpitations. There may be a feeling of constriction in the throat, along with difficulty swallowing, possibly with a feeling of choking.

Even Vata people can become anorexic or lose their appetite if they eat too many sweet or Kaphogenic foods, particularly at the beginning of meals, like sugars, ice cream, milk, cheese or yogurt. Vata types like the calm they feel by excess eating of sugars and carbohydrates, but it can derange them further. Periods of overeating of carbohydrates may alternate with periods of lack of appetite and undereating, thus deranging the whole digestive process and leading ultimately to severe anorexia.

Treatment

Spices to regulate digestion and stop vomiting — cardamom, fennel and fresh ginger — are required. Ayurvedic formulas include Cardamom compound or Asafoetida 8, but remember that the taste of asafoetida may be hard to take.

A mild bland diet is best such as Kicharee (equal parts rice and mung) or meat soup (preferably chicken). Coffee, tea and all drugs and stimulants must be avoided. The rest of the treatment is like that for underweight, with tonics like Chyavan prash and Ashwagandha compound.

In addition, calming and grounding nervine herbs should be taken including valerian, nutmeg, ashwagandha or sandalwood. Rest and a

calming and supportive environment are required. Two parts ashwagandha and one part gotu kola are excellent taken with 1/2 part of
cardamom and fennel. One to two teaspoons of the powder is infused in
a cup of water with a little honey and sipped every 2–3 hours until the
system is calmed.

Sesame oil massage is very helpful, particularly to the head and feet
(but not to the abdomen). Sandalwood oil to the head often restores
balance and calm.

2
DISORDERS OF THE
RESPIRATORY SYSTEM

The lungs and stomach are the primary sites of Kapha, the biological water humor. Phlegm is produced in the stomach, accumulates in the lungs, and then travels throughout the rest of the body producing various diseases.

Most respiratory disorders, therefore, are Kapha disorders. Kapha or water types tend towards colds, flus, sore throat, swollen glands, bronchitis, asthma, pneumonia and other diseases of the respiratory system.

We must, however, consider the role of the other humors as well. The lungs are an important site of air, Vata. Here the energy of the life-force (prana) is taken into the body. Many respiratory disorders involving lack of strength, shortness of breath, wasting away of tissues, and dehydration, such as consumption or tuberculosis, tend to be Vata diseases. On the other hand, most of the severely infectious conditions of the respiratory tract (as of all the systems) tend to be Pitta conditions.

Whenever there is poor digestion there tends to be accumulation of mucus, regardless of the humoral condition involved. Mucus does not necessarily indicate high Kapha, but it does indicate low Agni. So improving the digestive fire is a major treatment for respiratory system disorders. Causes of respiratory disorders include wrong diet, overexposure to the elements, seasonal changes, poor posture, poor breathing practices, excess or deficient exercise, and bad air. Psychological factors include attachment, grief and fear.

Treatment requires not only right herbs and diet but also Yoga practices including Pranayama (breathing exercises). Local applications of herbs are gargles, herbal oils or decoctions through the nose (nasya), and smoking, as well as applying herbal oils or pastes to the head, back or chest.

A good lung tonic can be made with two parts elecampane root, two parts comfrey root, and one part each cinnamon, ginger and licorice. For Kapha (water) types, cloves or calamus can be added. For Pitta (fire), burdock root can be used instead of elecampane. For Vata (air), ash-wagandha or ginseng can be added.

Or the Lung Tonic (no. 3) can be taken, with a tsp. of honey for Kapha; honey and ghee, two parts to one, for Vata; and honey and ghee, one part to two, for Pitta.

Emetic Therapy*

The main Ayurvedic treatment for Kapha disorders is emesis or therapeutic vomiting (Vamana). It is one of the strongest herbal treatment methods and requires some caution. It is often preferable to go to a Pancha Karma clinic or be under the supervision of a qualified Ayurvedic prac-titioner for this treatment. Once the art of vomiting is learned, however, it is possible to do it for oneself. Regular or daily therapeutic vomiting to cleanse the stomach and lungs is important for maintaining health and promoting longevity, particularly for Kapha types. The same effect can be achieved over longer periods of time with anti-Kapha diet and expec-torant (phlegm-dispelling) herbs.

Pranayama

Pranayama, Yogic control of the breath, should be considered as a primary therapy for long-term treatment of lung disorders. These breath-ing practices can correct most lung problems including long-term allergies and asthma. Breath control increases energy, gives strength and promotes circulation. Exhalation should be twice the length of inhalation. There should be no forceful attempt to hold the breath. For Pranayama to be effective, right posture or asana must be first achieved; otherwise the lungs will be contracted and proper breathing will be difficult. Pranayama, should not be attempted in acute conditions of asthma without the help of an experienced teacher.

For most Kapha (water) disorders, alternate nostril Pranayama should be practiced. Breathing in through the right nostril and out through the left is called 'solar pranayama'. The breath should be retained primarily after exhalation. For Pitta, or inflammatory conditions of the lungs, one should breathe in the left nostril and out through the right (lunar pranayama).

For Vata (air) conditions, either alternate the two types of breathing or breathe in and out through both nostrils (as with Soham pranayama). However, where there is more dryness in the lungs or dry cough with

---

*   See section in 'Herbal Therapies'

insomnia, lunar pranayama is better. Retention of breath should be after inhalation.

'Soham' pranayama, mentally chanting the mantras 'so' on inhalation and 'ham' (pronounced 'hum') on exhalation, is a good balanced Pranayama. It develops perception and the primary vitality, Ojas. 'So' naturally deepens inhalation and improves Prana, the primary air. 'Ham' naturally increases exhalation and removes excess Apana, the downward moving air. Soham pranayama is good for all constitutions.

COMMON COLD
FLUS

The common cold is still our most common disease. It is often the first stage of other diseases, indicating a breakdown in our bodily defenses which may allow further conditions to arise. There are many different rhino-viruses that are behind it.

Colds and flus are usually Kapha (phlegm) diseases and the symptoms are of that humor. There is accumulation of mucus, runny nose, sore throat, congestion, cough, body ache, headache and chills with mild fever.

Causes include exposure to cold air or wind, cold, damp or mucus forming food, and seasonal changes, as well as most Kapha-increasing factors.

General Treatment

An anti-Kapha and anti-Ama (detoxifying) diet is prescribed. Diet should be light, warm and simple: for example, whole grains and steamed vegetables in moderate quantities. Avoid dairy products, especially cheese, yogurt and milk. Heavy, oily and damp food should not be taken: meat, nuts, breads, pastries, candies and sweet fruit juices. Fasting is often helpful if the individual is not too weak.

Lemon and ginger juice can be taken with warm water and honey. Fresh ginger or other spice teas, cinnamon, basil and cloves, are good. Tonic herbs like ashwagandha, shatavari or ginseng, should be avoided owing to their heavy nature.

Herbal treatment uses diaphoretic, expectorant and anti-cough herbs. The peripheral circulation needs to be restored and the cold dispelled. After drinking warm spice tea, the patient should go to bed under a warm blanket and be brought to a mild sweat. Other sweating methods such as dry sauna or steam box can be used. The patient should only be mildly sweated; profuse, should be avoided.

Typical Ayurvedic herbs include ginger, cinnamon, long pepper, licorice, basil, cloves, mint. The main formulas Sitopaladi powder or

Talisadi powder taken with honey or ghee. The Lung Tonic, (no. 3) can be taken in the same way.

In Chinese medicine a cold is called a 'surface wind-chill syndrome', and treated with warm spicy surface-relieving herbs, like ginger and cinnamon. Formulas include Ma Huang decoction, a strong diaphoretic, and Cinnamon branch decoction, mild diaphoretic.

Additional good Western diaphoretics are sage, hyssop, thyme, osha, bayberry.

Differentiation

Although colds are generally of a Kapha (water) nature, they can be of a Vata (air) or Pitta (fire) nature.

Vata type colds involve dry cough, insomnia, scanty phlegm, hoarseness or loss of voice. A few drops of sesame oil can be placed in the nose with an eye dropper. Herbs include not only the spices and warming diaphoretics mentioned above but also demulcents: such as licorice, comfrey root, shatavari and ashwagandha. Sitopaladi powder can be taken with warm milk or along with Shatavari compound or Ashwagandha compound.

Pitta (fire) colds involve high fever, sore throat, red face, yellow or blood-streaked mucus. Treatment is with cooling diaphoretics such as mint, burdock, yarrow, elder flowers and chrysanthemum — what Chinese medicine calls 'spicy-cool surface-relieving agents'. The Chinese patent medicine, 'Yin qiao san', is excellent for this and most other types of colds.

For colds with high fever (usually a Pitta condition) a good formula can be made with equal parts basil, sandalwood and peppermint, 2–3 tsps. of the herbs infused per cup of water, and taken every two to three hours.

COUGH

Cough is also usually a Kapha (water) disorder. It is caused by accumulation of mucus, or by irritation to the mucus membranes of the respiratory tract. Treatment concentrates on bringing out the phlegm, not just suppression of the cough, which is what most allopathic anti-cough drugs and syrups do.

Cough may be due to the other humors as well. Treatment is largely the same as for a cold. In addition specific cough-relieving herbs are used.

Ayurvedic herbs and spices for cough are cloves, cinnamon, ginger, sumac, long pepper, bibhitaki, and calamus; turmeric powder by itself is good. A good home remedy is equal parts honey and lemon juice in teaspoonful dosages. Vasa is a special Ayurvedic anti-cough remedy. It is often given as an herbal jelly or an herbal wine.

Typical Ayurvedic formulas for cough include Clove combination, Sitopaladi powder, Talisadi powder, 1–6 gms. three or four times a day. Draksha can be taken in tablespoon dosages. Catechu is a good astringent for cough and sore throat in Kapha and Pitta conditions. Other astringents like alum root can be used the same way, but they may aggravate Vata (dryness) conditions.

Differentiation and Treatment

Kapha cough involves expectorating thick or slimy mucus of clear or white color and an infrequent cough. A distaste for food, feeling of heaviness, and sweet taste in the mouth with excess saliva or feeling of nausea will be symptoms. The patient will complain of cold, and the lungs may be full of phlegm.

Treatment involves anti-Kapha diet, avoiding dairy and other mucus-forming foods. Ice, cold water and fruit juices should not be taken. Hot spicy herbs, particularly long pepper, dry ginger or chitrak as a milk decoction, are helpful as is Trikatu compound.

Pitta type cough involves expectorating yellow phlegm, sometimes streaked with blood. There will be a burning sensation in the throat and chest, along with fever, thirst and dryness of the mouth. The mouth will taste bitter or pungent.

Treatment is much like that for Pitta type colds. Ghee can be used to soothe the throat. Powdered lotus seed with honey is helpful. Licorice combination can be used. Western herbs are mullein, horehound and coltsfoot.

Vata type cough is usually a dry cough with little expectoration. Cough will be frequent, painful and with a particular sound. Pain in the chest and heart, or a headache is typical. There will be dryness in the mouth, hoarseness and perhaps nervousness, anxiety or insomnia. (This is like 'yin-deficient' cough in Chinese medicine).

Treatment involves anti-Vata diet. Anti-cough and demulcent herbs are prescribed, licorice, marshmallow, comfrey root, shatavari and ash-wagandha. Formulas include Cardamom combination and Draksha, plus what is indicated under the common cold.

Other Herbs for Cough

Chinese herbs for cough include apricot seeds, coltsfoot, loquat leaves, fritillary, and pinellia. Loquat and fritillary cough syrups are particularly good for dry cough. Ophiopogon combination is specific to dry, hacking, night cough.

In Western herbalism there are other additional cough-relieving herbs; horehound, wild cherry, yerba santa, grindelia, thyme, spikenard, osha and mullein. Syrups or candies made from these are helpful (sugars soothe the throat).

Usually anti-cough herbs are used for their specific action. They are not used energetically, so the energetics will depend upon the other herbs in combination. One or two anti-cough herbs can be added to formulas for treating various kinds of respiratory disorders, depending on the condition.

SORE THROAT

This is usually a complication of the common cold and receives similar treatment. Sore throat with congestion and phlegm is a Kapha (water) condition.

Sore throat with dryness, hoarseness and constipation is a Vata (air) condition. Sesame oil or ghee, particularly made with calamus or licorice, should be applied to the throat.

Severe, swollen sore throat and strep infection is usually a Pitta (fire) condition. It requires the use of antibiotic, blood and lymph cleansing herbs such as katuka, golden seal, yellow dock or isatis.

Gargling with astringent herbs is recommended, particularly for Kapha and Pitta types. Use alum, turmeric, sumac, sage and bayberry. If there is dryness in the throat demulcents like licorice or slippery elm are required.

Other Ayurvedic herbs are cloves, haritaki, bibhitaki, zedoaria, and formulas include Sitopaladi and Talisadi.

Typical Chinese herbs for severe sore throat include honeysuckle, forsythia, isatis and platycodon.

Special Western herbs include echinacea and mullein. Echinacea tincture, 10–30 drops every few hours, is excellent for severe sore throat.

LARYNGITIS

Laryngitis is the loss of voice that comes with many respiratory disorders. Kapha (water) type is characterized by phlegm blocking the throat and the larynx.

Treatment involves anti-Kapha diet and expectorant herbs. Good spices for the throat include cloves and calamus; useful herbs are bayberry, bibhitaki, zedoaria. These herbs can also be smoked. Formulas include Clove compound.

Pitta (fire) type is indicated by severe sore throat, yellow mucus, and fever. Bitter herbs are used: katuka, turmeric, barberry, prepared or taken with ghee.

Vata (air) type is characterized by dry throat and low voice. It is more apt to be chronic. Treatment involves the use of anti-Vata diet and demulcent herbs like shatavari or marshmallow. Ghee or sesame oil can be applied in drops to the throat. Simple licorice tea is good.

For improving the voice and speaking ability, Calamus ghee is excellent, 1 tsp. three times a day.

BRONCHITIS
PNEUMONIA

Bronchitis is an infection of the bronchi of the respiratory passages. It is treated as a more severe form of the common cold or cough and can present varieties relative to the three humors. Such expectorants and diaphoretics as bayberry, cloves, ginger, calamus, nutmeg and licorice are still effective. Cooling anti-cough agents like vasa, gotu kola or mullein are good in the higher febrile stage, as is the special Ayurvedic lung tonic vamsha rochana (bamboo manna).

Pneumonia can be similarly differentiated but is more dangerous as the fever tends to be higher. Deer horn ash (Shringa bhasma) is specific for pneumonia. Gypsum ash (Godanti bhasma) is effective for the high fever stage of these diseases, as is the Chinese formula Gypsum combination.

In such acute conditions antibiotic herbs are useful: echinacea, goldenseal, katuka and isatis, taken every two to three hours in dosages of three to five grams of the powder or twice that in decoction. The Herbal Febrifuge (no. 7) is good, taken with honey. Antibiotic drugs may be necessary when the condition is severe.

In convalescence from weak lung conditions, including tuberculosis, Chyavan prash is excellent, or other lung tonics like comfrey root, slippery elm, shatavari, ashwagandha or ginseng preferably taken as milk decoctions.

ASTHMA

Asthma is a more severe form of cough condition that involves gasping, wheezing and difficult breathing. Causes include allergies, complications of other lung diseases, and hereditary factors. It is mainly a Kapha (water) syndrome and treatment is like other Kapha lung disorders; though differentiation of humoral types also exists. Bronchial asthma can be from any of the three humors but is most often Kapha in nature. Cardiac asthma is usually Pitta (fire), and renal asthma is usually Kapha (water).

Differentiation

Vata type asthma is characterized by dry cough and wheezing. Additional symptoms are thirst, dry mouth, dry skin, constipation, anxiety and craving for warm drinks. Attacks occur predominantly at Vata time, dawn and dusk. Pitta type asthma is characterized by cough and wheezing with yellow phlegm. Other symptoms are fever, sweating, irritability and need for cool air. Attacks are at Pitta time, noon and midnight.

Kapha type asthma is characterized by cough and wheezing with abundant clear or white phlegm. The lungs will be full of water, producing a raling sound. Attacks are at Kapha time, morning and evening. They are relieved by smoking of herbs.

General Treatment

Care must be taken to differentiate syndromes, as the condition can change quickly. Acute wheezing is treated by bronchodilators such as ephedra, lobelia or vasa. Lung tonics like ashwagandha or ginseng may aggravate this condition, as they tend to close or consolidate the energy of the lungs. Acute asthmatic attacks can be dangerous and should be treated by a professional. In clinical situations in Ayurveda asthma is mainly treated with emetic therapy. Milder symptoms can be treated with diet and herbs.

Long-term treatment often requires tonification to rebuild the energy of the lungs. Tonics should be taken between acute attacks. In Ayurveda such herbs include ashwagandha, shatavari, bala, gotu kola and licorice. Formulas are Chyavan prash, Ashwagandha compound, Shatavari compound.

In Chinese medicine, for radical treatment, such tonic formulas as Rehmannia 6 plus Ophiopogon and Schizandra can be used in chronic conditions. Human placenta can be used as a single herb.

Special Ayurvedic treatment involves smoking bronchodilating and antispasmodic herbs such as cloves, bayberry, ephedra, tobacco, marijuana, and datura. The latter toxic substances, however, require special attention.

For allergic type asthma, turmeric powder is helpful. It should be warmed in butter with raw sugar and taken frequently in teaspoonful doses during acute attacks.

Differentiation and Treatment

For Kapha (water) types, treatment involves anti-Kapha diet, avoiding all mucus-forming foods, as well as yogurt and sour fruit. Hot spices can be used freely: cayenne, mustard, ginger and pepper. A milk decoction of long pepper taken daily is said to correct chronic asthma. Mustard or ginger paste can be applied to the chest.

Important Ayurvedic herbs are long pepper, calamus, bayberry, and ephedra. Formulas include Trikatu, Sitopaladi, Talisadi compound and Clove compound.

Important Chinese herbs for this condition are ma huang and apricot seeds. A typical formula is Major Blue Dragon.

Good Western herbs include mullein, bayberry, sage, and thyme.

For Vata (air) types, anti-Vata diet is prescribed along with spices. Sour fruit juices are good, like lemon or lime.

Ayurvedic herbs include those for Kapha along with tonics for the lungs, as Vata conditions always tend towards wasting of the tissues.

For Pitta (fire) types, anti-Pitta diet is prescribed along with cooling herbs like coriander, gotu kola or burdock. Vasa is particularly good and Brahma rasayan works well as a long term restorative food.

HAY FEVER
ALLERGIC RHINITIS

Hay fever is another condition of autoimmune derangement and also relates to hypersensitivity of the nervous system. It is usually a Vata (air) disorder, as Vata types are the most sensitive, but Pitta (fire) and Kapha (water) types exist. Pitta is involved in the more severe allergies with toxic blood and symptoms of fever, red eyes and rashes. Hay fever most often occurs in a weaker or more debilitated constitution.

In acute conditions treatment is similar to that for the common cold, with a detoxifying diet. Dairy and other mucus-forming foods should be avoided. Between attacks, however, it is important to strengthen the immune system and the lungs, particularly for Vata constitution individuals, with diet more according to constitution. For this tonification therapy important Ayurvedic herbs are ashwagandha and bala; Chinese are ginseng and astragalus; and Western is comfrey root. Chyavan prash is a good general tonic to take or the Energy Tonic (no. 2). Brahma rasayan is excellent for both expectorant and nervine action.

Vata type hay fever involves cough with little phlegm, headache, insomnia, restlessness, anxiety.

Pitta symptoms are burning eyes, thirst, fever, yellow nasal discharge, and skin rashes.

Kapha symptoms are abundant clear or white phlegm, dullness and heaviness.

Treatment

All kinds of hay fever require special herbs to clear the sinuses, open the head and dispel phlegm. Basil tea (particularly holy basil or Tulsi from India) is good, taken with honey. Coriander and cilantro (coriander leaf) are best for Pitta. For Kapha, the old standby, Trikatu is good, or dry ginger powder as a snuff.

Ayurvedic herbs include calamus, gotu kola, ginger, cloves, camphor (in very small amounts), ephedra, and bayberry. Calamus ghee applied in the nose is excellent. Gotu kola oil or ghee is similarly used for Pitta conditions.

Chinese herbs include magnolia flower, xanthium (cocklebur), mint, angelica, wild ginger, and chrysanthemum.

Additional Western herbs are peppermint, sage, eucalyptus, wintergreen, bay leaves, and mullein flowers.

When Pitta is involved, bitters and blood cleansing herbs such as echinacea, barberry, dandelion and burdock must be added.

Essential oils, like menthol, eucalyptus or camphor, or ginger paste can be applied to the temple or root of the nose (avoiding the mucus membranes). Sandalwood oil to the forehead is good when there are hot or febrile sensations.

For red, itchy eyes, ghee, particularly that made with Triphala can be applied to the eyelids. Triphala ghee is best, and ghee by itself is helpful. Camomile, eyebright or chrysanthemum in lukewarm infusions can be used to wash the eyes.

A good formula for hay fever can be made with gotu kola, calamus, angelica, wild ginger and licorice in equal parts as powders. Vata and Kapha types can take this with honey, Pitta with aloe gel or with the addition of other bitter herbs. Or the Lung Tonic (no. 3) can be taken with the Brain Tonic (no. 6).

3
CIRCULATORY SYSTEM
DISORDERS

HEART DISEASE

According to Oriental medicine, the heart, not the brain, is the seat of consciousness. It is the site of the Atman, the true or Divine Self. An old European adage states, 'As a man thinkest in his heart, so is he'. This thought is also found in the *Upanishads*, the great ancient scriptures of India. How we feel in our hearts is the measure of who we really are. What we think in our heads is often no more than a superficial impression, passing momentarily through us via the senses. Hence, heart diseases reflect deep seated issues of identity, feeling, and consciousness. Heart disease is perhaps the main cause of death in this country. This is largely because the heart is denied in our culture which aims at personal achievement rather than communion with others. Many of us literally die of broken hearts or spiritual starvation.

Heart diseases include heart attacks, stroke, angina, arteriosclerosis, and hypertension. Heart attacks, the end result of most heart diseases, are often preceded by palpitations, insomnia, numbness or severe pain in the chest or middle back that radiates down the arms. Other indications are cyanosis (blue color of lips and tongue), loss of consciousness, fever, cough, hiccup, shortness of breath and vomiting.

Causes of heart disease include wrong diet, physical or emotional trauma, congenital or hereditary factors, suppressed emotions or excess strain and anxiety. It may occur as the complication of other diseases (rheumatic diseases or liver disorders). As the heart is an organ of emotion, emotional causes should always be considered first. These include difficulties in work or relationship, usually indicating that on an inner level we are not in touch with our own hearts. They may show insensitivity to the hearts of others.

Heart disease can occur with any of the three humors. In the Ayurvedic association of Pitta (fire) with the blood, heart disease, particularly heart attacks and strokes, is commonly a Pitta disorder. The red faced, angry, ambitious, hard driving executive, who suddenly dies of a heart attack, is typically a Pitta person who denies his true heart.

Vata (air) type heart disease is more common in the elderly, where there is drying out of tissue and hardening of the blood vessels. Kapha (water or phlegm) type occurs mainly from overeating and the accumulation of mucus, fat and cholesterol which obstruct heart functioning.

American and European diet which concentrates on animal fats and heavy oily food, and life-styles which are competitive and ambitious, or sedentary make us culturally prone to heart attacks.

General Treatment

The first thing for the heart always involves an extended period of rest or reduced activity, both physical and mental. Strain and worry should be set aside. Patients must get back in touch with their real hearts and what they really want to do in life. Yogic asanas and meditation are good, with no forceful efforts at control of the breath or the mind. Heavy exercise and travelling should be avoided.

Arjuna (Terminalia arjuna, a relative of the Triphala herbs) is a special powerful Ayurvedic herb for all kinds of heart diseases. As Ayurveda's heart medicine par excellence, it tonifies the heart and lungs, stimulates blood circulation, strengthens the heart muscles, stops bleeding and promotes the healing of tissues. It is good for all three humors (a 'tridosha' medicine). It is usually given with ghee or in the form of a medicated ghee. All people with heart weakness can benefit by this herb, regardless of the nature of their disease.

One to three grams of arjuna powder can be taken daily. Or the Heart Tonic (no. 11) can be taken, with honey for Kapha, with ghee for Pitta and with milk and ghee for Vata. Arjuna combines well with ashwagandha and guggul as an all-around heart tonic. Another useful Ayurvedic and Western herb for heart pain and high cholesterol is elecampane.

Another good heart tonic for all three humors is saffron, usually prepared in a milk decoction, 1 gm. per cup. It is a special tonic and rejuvenative for Pitta and for the female reproductive system.

A special Chinese herb for heart diseases is salvia (dan shen), a kind of sage. It improves circulation, strengthens the heart and calms the emotions. It is excellent for angina pain, acting like a natural nitroglycerin (taken with a small amount of cardamom and sandalwood). It is helpful both before and after heart attacks and is good for thinning the blood. It is particularly useful in Pitta and Kapha conditions, but can be used on Vata with warm spicy herbs like cinnamon.

The best Western heart tonic is hawthorn berries. It improves circulation, strengthens the heart muscle and helps dissolve cholesterol. It is particularly good for Vata and Kapha and increases longevity. It works well as a tincture and makes an excellent herbal wine.

Myrrh is another Western herb, useful (like the Ayurvedic guggul) for cleansing the blood, clearing cholesterol, improving circulation, and strengthening the deeper tissues. As a heart tonic, the tincture can be taken, or it can be decocted in turmeric and carefully strained.

Other good spices for the heart are ginger, cardamom and cinnamon, which are particularly useful on Vata and Kapha conditions. They promote circulation, uplift the emotions and promote joy. Sandalwood is a specific herb and essential oil for calming and cooling the heart.

Many gems and metals, either worn or taken internally as tinctures or specially prepared ashes (bhasmas), are good for the heart. They work on a subtle and long-term level to protect it. Ruby, garnet and gold are heart stimulants. Pearl, moonstone, emerald, jade and silver calm the heart. Yellow sapphire and yellow topaz tonify and strengthen the heart. Purifying drinking water by keeping it overnight in a copper vessel will help prevent arteriosclerosis. Gold stimulates the heart, and silver sedates it.

Differentiation

Vata (air) type heart diseases are indicated by palpitations, tremor in the heart, numbness, tightness in the chest, and throbbing, breaking, or bursting pain in the heart region. There will be insomnia, labored breathing, dry cough and constipation. Often there will be a dark discoloration around the eyes. The individual becomes very intolerant of noise and loud speech. Attacks will be more common following overwork or excessive exercise. Psychologically, there will be restlessness, fear, even fright, anxiety and sometimes fainting, after which the symptoms will worsen.

Pitta (fire) type disease symptoms are burning sensation in the region of the heart, and a feeling of smoldering heat. There will be spontaneous sweating, fever and a general feeling of heat all over the body. The face will usually be flushed, with red or bloodshot eyes. There will be dizziness, sometimes fainting, and the eyes and skin will become pale and yellow. Vomiting of bile or sour fluids may occur, along with loose yellow stool. There may be nosebleeds or a tendency to bleed easily. Emotionally, anger and irritability will prevail, with outbursts of temper which cause an aggravation of symptoms.

Kapha (water) type heart diseases are indicated by a feeling of heaviness and stiffness in the region of the heart. There will be congestion in the chest, accumulation of phlegm, cough, excess salivation, lack of appetite, nausea and perhaps vomiting. Fatigue and excessive sleeping are symptoms, and mentally the patient may feel dull and lack clarity. Emotionally, there will be greed and attachment and an unwillingness to let things go.

In short, most nervous heart conditions are Vata; most inflammatory heart conditions such as myocarditis, endocarditis, pericarditis, are Pitta; most congestive heart conditions or cardiac edema are Kapha.

Specific Treatment
Vata (Air) Type

An anti-Vata diet should be followed, avoiding dry, light and artificial foods and irregular diet. Fish is good, as well as oily vitamins such as A, E, and D. Garlic can be used freely, particularly as a milk decoction. A small amount of red wine or the herbal wine Draksha can be taken with meals. The patient should rest, relax, be quiet, spend time in nature, meditate, and do sitting Yoga postures.

It is helpful to wear a ruby or garnet set in gold, on the ring finger of the right hand to strengthen the heart. Sandalwood oil can be applied to the forehead or chest when palpitations or pain occur. The mantra 'sham' is good to help calm the heart. The mantra 'ram' can be used to strengthen the heart.

Important herbs are ashwagandha, garlic, arjuna, cinnamon, cardamom, sandalwood, guggul, elecampane, and licorice. A milk decoction of ashwagandha, 3–6 gms. of the herb and 1 tsp. of ghee per cup, can be taken 2–3 times a day.

Formulas include Ashwagandha compound, or more specifically, Ashwagandha ghee or Ashwagandha herbal wine, as well as the Arjuna preparations. Garlic compound is excellent.

Additional helpful Western herbs include comfrey root, solomon's seal, hawthorn berries, and myrrh.

Additional Chinese herbs are dang gui, rehmannia, zizyphus, ginseng, astragalus and formulas like Ten Major Herbs.

Pitta (Fire) Type

Treatment requires anti-Pitta diet, avoiding particularly alcohol, hot spices, too much oil or greasy food, red meat, and too much salt. Exposure to sun and strong exercise should be limited. Emotionally, strain, anger, hatred, resentment and violent urges should be set aside. One should cultivate peace, love and forgiveness.

An emerald set in silver, and worn on the middle finger of the right hand, is helpful. Pearl and moonstone are also recommended. Sandalwood oil should be applied to the third eye and to the chest. The mantra 'sham' is indicated for its cooling and calming action.

Good herbs are arjuna, saffron, sandalwood, shatavari, and gotu kola; bitters such as aloe gel, katuka, and barberry. Katuka or barberry can be given in equal parts with licorice and taken with ghee (dosage two grams taken after meals). Purgation is helpful in acute conditions. Important formulas include Arjuna preparations, Gotu Kola compound and Brahma rasayan.

Additional helpful Western herbs include motherwort, myrrh, and golden seal. Additional Chinese herbs include salvia, coptis and formulas such as Coptis and Rhubarb combination, particularly for acute conditions.

Kapha (Water) Type

Kapha type is caused by the development of high cholesterol through a Kapha-increasing diet. Anti-kapha diet should be followed avoiding sugar, dairy, cheese, butter, eggs, fatty meats, lard, and salt. Draksha herbal wine can be taken.

Like Vata, Kapha types can benefit from wearing a ruby or garnet set in gold. Camphor, mustard or cinnamon oil can be applied to the chest. Chanting of Om is helpful for its clearing and opening action.

Expectorants (phlegm dispelling herbs) should be taken, or mild emetic therapy. Good herbs include arjuna, calamus, cardamom, cinnamon, guggul. Equal parts elecampane and long pepper (cayenne can be used as a substitute) taken with ghee is good for Kapha heart disease, with one gram (two '00' capsules) taken after meals. Licorice should be avoided as it increases cardiac edema.

Formulas include Arjuna preparations and Trikatu or the Digestive Stimulant (no. 1) taken with honey.

Additional Western herbs include cayenne, myrrh, bayberry, and motherwort.

Western herbalists have found cayenne to be good for reviving the heart after attacks. It is excellent for Kapha heart disease and useful in Vata. It will aggravate Pitta, however, and should only be used for short-term heart revival in their case. According to the Ayurvedic practice, cayenne would be better taken in ghee. Chinese and Ayurvedic practice uses purified aconite in a similar way.

Motherwort is another famous heart herb used in the West and in China. It has cooling and diuretic properties, making it good for Kapha and Pitta and for cardiac edema.

HYPERTENSION

Hypertension is high blood pressure. It is one of the main complications and causes of heart disease. Most of its indications and treatment are as under heart diseases with the addition of more specifically nervine herbs: gotu kola, calamus, valerian, skullcap, and jatamansi. The Heart Tonic (no. 11) can be combined with the Brain Tonic (no. 6), or the latter taken alone with honey or ghee as per the humor.

The special Ayurvedic herb sarpagandha (Rauwolfia serpentina) regulates the blood pressure, but it is toxic and not yet approved for import.

Differentiation and Treatment

Vata (air) type hypertension is irregular in nature. The blood pressure may rise suddenly and fall suddenly. The pulse will be irregular or erratic both in rhythm and strength. Increase in blood pressure will follow worry, strain or overwork, nervousness or insomnia. It is frequently involved with nervous system disorders.

Treatment is as under heart disease. Mainly tonification therapy is given. Garlic is particularly good. Nutmeg in milk decoction can help as can Saraswat powder. Long term tonification through Ashwagandha preparations is usually required. A good formula can be made with equal parts ashwagandha, valerian and gotu kola, taken with ghee.

Pitta (fire) hypertension is indicated by flushed face, red eyes, often violent headache, sensitivity to light, nose bleeds, anger, irritability and burning sensation. It is often a complication of liver disorders and much of the treatment is the same.

Bitters are helpful including aloe gel, barberry and katuka. Purgation is indicated with bitter herbs such as aloe, rhubarb or senna. Gotu kola is specific here for calming the mind. Formulas include Gotu Kola preparations, Brahma rasayan and Saraswat powder. Gotu kola and skullcap in equal proportions work well.

Kapha (water) hypertension is constant in nature. There is usually obesity, tiredness, edema, and high cholesterol. Dairy, butter, eggs and high fat foods should be avoided. Good herbs are cayenne, myrrh, garlic, motherwort, and hawthorn berries. Licorice should be avoided. Formulas include Arjuna preparations and Trikatu.

ARTERIOSCLEROSIS

This is a condition of high cholesterol and clogging of the arteries. Both Kapha (water) and Pitta (fire) types are due to fat accumulations. Vata (air) type is owing to hardening of the arteries.

Treatment is as for heart diseases, generally, and for hypertension, which usually follows from arteriosclerosis.

Garlic is a good herb for high cholesterol in Kapha and Vata constitutions; with honey for Kapha, in a milk decoction for Vata. Calamus and turmeric are excellent, as is elecampane. Aloe gel with turmeric or safflower or the Ayurvedic katuka are good for Pitta. Other good herbs are myrrh, saffron, motherwort, hawthorn berries and the Ayurvedic guggul, which is excellent for clearing cholesterol. Chinese herbs are he shou wu (fo ti) and salvia.

HYPOTENSION

Hypotension or low blood pressure is not a specific disease but it is involved in many chronic conditions and often occurs in debility, anemia and malnutrition. It is related to weakness of the digestive fire, requiring treatment on that level. It is most common in Vata (air) types, who tend towards poor circulation. In Kapha (water) it occurs because of congestion and stagnation, phlegm clogging, and reduced blood flow. In Pitta (fire) it is mainly associated with anemia or damaged liver function.

To counter hypotension, circulatory stimulants are indicated: turmeric, cinnamon, ginger, cayenne, garlic, aconite, black pepper or cardamom.

For Vata garlic or Garlic compound are good. For Kapha types Trikatu should be taken. Pitta should take saffron or turmeric in aloe gel.

Wearing of ruby or garnet (not for Pitta constitution) is important, as the condition is often chronic and requires long term remedial measures. These stones increase circulation. Pitta types should use yellow topaz or yellow sapphire.

BLEEDING

Bleeding, or hemorrhage, is due to a variety of causes. It may occur because of injury. Disease factors that cause bleeding include fever, infection or humoral imbalance. Minor bleeding includes most nose bleeds and slight amounts of blood in the phlegm or stool.

Internal bleeding suggests serious complications, like infection and tumors. One should have a medical examination as to its origin, even if we choose to treat it with natural methods.

Bleeding is mainly a Pitta (fire) disorder. It is called 'rakta-pitta' in Sanskrit, which we could translate as a condition of heat or bile in the blood. When the blood is overheated it flows more easily, the veins and arteries become fragile, and bleeding occurs.

Causes of bleeding are mainly those which aggravate Pitta, such as over-exposure to heat or sun, excessive exercise or travelling, overeating of spicy, sour or salty foods. Anger or a too aggressive life style can bring it on. In weaker types, it can be caused by malnutrition and dehydration.

Moreover, long-term or chronic bleeding results in anemia and malnutrition. Fever can cause bleeding; and blood loss, in turn, can bring fever.

Differentiation

Vata (air) caused bleeding is dark red, frothy, thin or dry. It is usually from the lower orifices, the anus and urethra, and is considered more difficult to treat.

Pitta (fire) caused bleeding is dark, purple, black. It may be mixed with bile. It can be from either the upper or lower orifices.

Kapha (water) caused bleeding is thick, pale, oily, slimy and may be mixed with mucus. It originates mainly in the lungs and stomach. Kapha caused bleeding is usually from the upper orifices, mouth, nose, eyes and ears. It is more easily curable.

General Treatment

Immediate treatment requires the use of astringent and hemostatic herbs to stop bleeding. Most spicy herbs should not be used, as they promote the flow of blood. Local application of ice or cold water by its contracting action stops bleeding. A cool shower is often sufficient to stop bleeding from the nose.

A little alum powder (a mineral) applied to the site will stop most bleeding; or the powder of any herb with a large amount of tannin, such as white oak bark or alum root. Common herbs and weeds — self-heal, yarrow, plantain, chickweed or blessed thistle — can be made into a paste and applied directly to the site. In Ayurvedic common usage, turmeric powder is applied locally, particularly for injuries. Fresh turmeric root helps wounds heal naturally without scarring. Aloe gel can be used in the same way.

Good Ayurvedic astringents include aloe, manjishta, saffron, alum, turmeric, arjuna, ashok and the Triphala formula.

Good Chinese herbs are pseudoginseng, agrimony, cattail, and mugwort. Pseudoginseng, a ginseng relative and also rather expensive, is good for any kind of bleeding. Yunnan bai yao, a Chinese patent medicine made from it, can be used internally or externally.

Additional Western astringents and hemostatics include arnica, yarrow, self-heal and mullein.

Pitta (Fire) Type

Treatment requires keeping the patient cool. An anti-Pitta diet should be followed, avoiding hot, spicy food and sour and fermented food. Pomegranate juice is good. Strong exercise or exposure to heat should not be allowed. Anger should be released as much as possible. Milk is good, particularly for bleeding from the lungs, and can be taken with a little turmeric.

The general treatment applies here. Aloe gel is excellent, internally or externally.

Vata (Air) Type

Vata bleeding is caused by dryness of the mucus membranes or blood vessels. It may accompany dry cough or constipation. When large amounts of blood are involved, more severe Vata disorders are indicated.

Treatment for mild conditions requires demulcent and tonic herbs to strengthen the mucus membranes: shatavari, licorice, ashwagandha, bala and their compounds. Hemostatics are added to these. Triphala is good for most lower orifice bleeding, particularly taken with a hemostatic tea, like red raspberry or agrimony, as a vehicle.

Kapha (Water) Type

For Kapha conditions, bleeding is due to blockage of the vessels by phlegm which drives the blood the wrong way.

Most hemostatics can be used, as above, along with hot spices such as cayenne, ginger and the Trikatu formula.

EPISTAXIS OR NOSE BLEED

Nose bleed requires additional local application of herbs. An infusion of astringent herbs can be applied to the nose with an eye dropper. For a Vata (dryness caused) condition sesame oil should be applied nightly in the same way. For Pitta type (with red face and feeling of heat or fever) sandalwood oil can be applied to the forehead. Teas such as coriander, vetivert, sandalwood or gotu kola are good, as is the treatment under Pitta liver disorders. Kapha requires additional expectorants like sage, hyssop, turmeric or elecampane.

ANEMIA

Anemia is called 'pallor disease' in Sanskrit (panduroga), as it causes the body to turn pale. There is a deficiency of blood, in quantity or quality. It is a Pitta (fire) disorder, usually classified with such liver disorders as jaundice and hepatitis. Physiologically, it is thought to be caused by bile entering into and thinning the blood; this is the general movement of Pitta in its disease development. It can also be caused by high Vata or high Kapha (in which case these humors are treated).

For Vata (air) types, anemia is usually part of a pattern of general deficiency and malnourishment. For Kapha (water) it is part of a pattern of obesity, edema and congestion.

Symptoms are pale and lifeless appearance, lack of energy, low grade fever or burning sensation, irregular elimination, yellowish and scanty urine, indigestion, vertigo, fainting and fatigue. For women, there is scanty or pale menstrual flow or absence of flow altogether.

Causes are wrong diet, eating of too much pungent, sour and salty food (these tastes in excess aggravate both Pitta and the blood), alcohol, or malnutrition. Anemia may follow traumatic injury, pregnancy, excessive menstruation, or other conditions of excess bleeding. It may be brought about by febrile diseases, the heat of which damages the quality of the blood, or by liver disorders, which impair the liver's ability to build up the blood. Excess sexual indulgence, which depletes Ojas and thereby weakens all bodily fluids, can result in anemia.

Women are prone to anemia owing to their monthly blood loss via menstruation. The majority of women can benefit from diet or herbs to improve the blood, particularly right after the menstrual cycle is over.

Differentiation

Pitta (fire) caused anemia is due to bile thinning the blood. There will be burning sensation, fever, and thirst. The skin and nails will be pale with a yellowish tinge, and bodily discharges will turn yellow.

Kapha (water) caused anemia is due to excess mucus blocking proper digestion and thinning the blood. The face, eyes, skin and urine will be white, with excess phlegm and salivation. There will be edema, often overweight, excess sleeping and heaviness of the limbs.

Vata (air) type involves dry skin with a darkish tinge, anxiety, tremors, insomnia, constipation and possible dehydration.

General Treatment

Nutritive diet is indicated with foods, herbs and supplements to build the blood. Good foods include red meat, bone soups, milk and sesame seeds (black). Some fruit is good for building the blood, particularly the juice of pomegranate or black grapes. Sugars are helpful, especially jaggery and molasses.

Iron supplements are indicated, as well as vitamins A and E. However, as iron preparations weaken the digestion, they should be taken with herbs to improve digestion such as ginger or cinnamon.

The Ayurvedic tonic jelly Chyavan prash is excellent; 2–3 tsps. twice a day, with warm milk. Turmeric ghee is good or ghee to which turmeric powder is added.

The bowels should be regulated with laxatives as in most liver disorders (laxatives help stimulate liver function by draining out excess bile through the large intestine). In this more delicate condition, use mild laxatives such as aloe gel, Triphala or cascara sagrada.

Important Ayurvedic herbs are aloe gel, amalaki, haritaki, saffron, shatavari, manjishta, and punarnava. One-half to one gram of saffron in warm milk can be taken daily with ghee.

Special Ayurvedic iron preparations are excellent: humanized, non-toxic iron oxides are prepared by repeated incineration of iron, as well as cooking it in various herbal substances. Most common are Iron ash and Navayas compound. Good formulas without iron are Shatavari compound, the Energy Tonic (no. 2) and the Woman's Tonic (no. 4).

Red coral, garnet and ruby are good gems to wear for improving the blood, particularly for Vata and Kapha constitutions. Pearl or moonstone is good for Pitta and Vata.

Chinese treatment involves special blood tonic herbs such as dang gui, rehmannia, fo ti, and lycium. Formulas include the Four Materials for simple blood deficiency and Woman's Precious Pill for combined blood deficiency and weak digestion (evidenced by loose stool, lack of strength and shortness of breath). The latter is commonly available as a patent medicine in Chinese and other herb stores.

The favorite Western herb is yellow dock, which contains large amounts of iron in its root. Prepared with blackstrap molasses, it becomes a good blood tonic, particularly for Pitta and Kapha type conditions. Its blood cooling, bile moving and laxative properties are also helpful.

Specific Treatment

The general treatment is similar in all three humors. Diet and spices, however, vary considerably.

For Pitta type raw salads, green vegetables, sprouts and common green herbs such as nettles, dandelion leaf, and red raspberry leaf are good. Chlorophyll helps cleanse bile from the blood, thereby improving its quality, particularly in Pitta conditions. Milk and ghee are good. Bitters, aloe gel, barberry, and katuka, are helpful for controlling liver function.

Vata should take more rich food including dairy, red meat and oils, like ghee or sesame. They should avoid raw food and raw vegetables, as these are not nutritive enough. Ghee made with Triphala is good taken along with raw sugar. Herbal wines like Draksha are excellent.

Kapha should concentrate on improving digestion and getting rid of phlegm. Spices with circulatory stimulant properties should be used: cayenne, cinnamon, saffron, turmeric or the Trikatu formula taken with honey.

4

DISEASES OF THE URINARY TRACT
AND WATER METABOLISM DISORDERS

The kidneys are a very important organ in Oriental medicine. Their action is closely related to the nervous system and the reproductive organs. They are as important to water metabolism as the colon is to food (metabolism of the earth element). Just as wrong eating habits damage the stomach and the g.i. tract, wrong drinking (not only drinking alcohol) damages the kidneys and the urinary tract.

The kidneys are weakened by drinking either too much or too little water, by excessive sexual activity, by alcohol, by taking diuretic drugs, by antibiotics, and by not heeding the urge to urinate. Excess consumption of calcium or of foods like spinach which contain oxalic acid are additional factors. Too much travelling or excessive thinking weakens kidney function. Fear and fright damage the kidneys on a psychological level. The kidneys weaken with old age, as well as being delicate in sensitive or traumatized children.

Cleansing the Kidneys

Toxins can accumulate and lodge themselves in the kidneys and urinary tract, particularly when the kidneys are not filtering the blood properly. Symptoms include lower back pain, sciatic pain, difficult or painful urination, urinary tract infections, swollen prostate, or kidney stones. An occasional kidney flush can be a helpful preventative measure, much like an occasional flushing of the colon. Again, it should mainly be done during the warm season.

One can fast for a day, then drink a quart to a gallon of water the following morning. Add mild diuretic herbs — coriander, parsley, lemon grass, horsetail or corn silk, or the Kidney Tonic (no. 10).

Too much use of diuretics, however, can weaken the kidneys. Diuretics aggravate Vata (air) by overstimulating the kidneys. Too much water, particularly cold or ice water, will weaken the kidneys and usually increase Kapha (water).

It should be remembered that the human body is composed not primarily of water but of plasma, an oily solution. Drinking too much water, particularly distilled water, can drain essential substances from the plasma and leave the body depleted.

Water not only brings fluid into our body, it also brings Prana, the life-force. Hence, water devitalized by chlorination or distillation will not energize the life-force properly and this can contribute to many health disorders. Fresh spring water is preferable. The quality of our water can be improved by putting it in a copper vessel overnight. Aeration of water gives it more Prana, such as pouring it back and forth between two cups before we drink it.

The best Ayurvedic herb for tonifying and strengthening the kidneys is shilajit, a special mineral pitch exuded by various rocks in India. It improves kidney and bladder function, improves sexual vitality, strengthens the nervous system, reduces tumors, is antiseptic and helps dissolve stones. It is good for all three humors and is an important rejuvenative (rasayana). It is useful for urinary tract disorders, whether cleansing or building actions are needed. The purified mineral can be taken in dosages of 500 mg. to 1 gm. twice a day or Shilajit compound can be used. It can be used for any of the conditions below and is excellent for diabetes.

DIFFICULT URINATION (DYSURIA)

Most kidney disorders reveal themselves through some abnormality or difficulty in urinary function. Difficult or painful urination can be caused by any of the three humors. We use the symptom to diagnose and treat underlying poor kidney function.

Vata (air) caused dysuria is indicated by severe pain in the lower back, rectum and urinary channel. Urination will be frequent but scanty, with sharp or colicy pain. Constipation, insomnia and other high Vata conditions will prevail.

Pitta (fire) dysuria involves dark yellow or red urine. Urination is frequent, often profuse, with burning sensation. There will be feverishness, irritability and other high Pitta signs.

Kapha (water) involves pale or milky urine, often passed with mucus. There will be a feeling of heaviness in the lower abdomen and a dull pain in the kidney region.

General Treatment

Diuretic (urination promoting and soothing) food and herbs must be taken. The best general diuretic for all three humors is Tribulis terrestris (gokshura in Sanskrit), the common goatshead or puncture vine whose little stickers are a nuisance in our lawns and fields. Its action is sure but mild, and it has tonic properties for the kidneys which prevent it from aggravating Vata.

The best general diuretic herb from Chinese Medicine is the mushroom hoelen (fu ling). It is mild and has tonifying action, particularly for the spleen and heart.

There are many good Western herbal diuretics as well, like common cleavers and plantain, as the diuretic property is very common in the herbal kingdom. Sarsaparilla is one of the best, and also has tonic properties.

Specific Treatment

For Kapha the typical anti-Kapha diet is indicated, avoiding cold drinks, fruit juice, dairy, cheese, oils and fats. Hot spices and diuretics are indicated, like cubebs, cinnamon, juniper berries along with parsley, uva ursi or cleavers. Formulas include Trikatu and Sandalwood compound or the Kidney tonic (no. 10) with warm water.

Treatment for Pitta is much the same as for urinary infections, avoiding spices, oils, sour fruit, etc. Cooling diuretics are indicated: tribulis, punarnava, uva ursi, pipsissewa, horsetail, burdock or plantain. Formulas include Sandalwood compound or the Kidney tonic (no. 10) with cool water.

For Vata demulcent-diuretic herbs should be used, which soothe the mucus membranes and aid in urination. These include gokshura, bala, marshmallow, licorice and sarsaparilla. Formulas include Gokshura guggul or the Kidney tonic (no. 10) with milk.

EDEMA

Edema is regarded as a classic symptom of high Kapha, excess water in the system, but it can occur in the other humors as well. Kapha types tend towards edema, particularly as they get older.

Kapha (water) type edema has more pronounced swelling, with moist and white skin. When pressed, the tissue tends to hold the shape of the imprint for a time.

Vata (air) type edema is indicated by dry skin and visible veins. The tissue is spongy and comes right back up when pressed.

Pitta (fire) type edema is associated with swelling, redness and burning sensation.

Treatment

As edema is usually a long standing condition, dietary therapy is particularly helpful. Good diuretic foods include grains like corn, barley and rye, vegetables like celery, carrot, parsley and cilantro, fruit like cranberries and pomegranate. Most beans are diuretic, particularly aduki beans.

One cannot relieve edema merely by taking large amounts of diuretic herbs or drugs. These can weaken the kidneys further by overstimulating them.

Mild diuretics are best — gokshura, corn silk, hoelen, lemon grass, coriander and formulas such as Gokshura guggul or the Kidney tonic (no.10). Vata can take such herbs with milk or warm water, Pitta with aloe gel or cool water, and Kapha with honey.

Shilajit is important for edema, particularly in weak types, 1–2 gms. twice a day with water or milk.

URINARY TRACT INFECTIONS

Urinary tract infections involve difficult, frequent or burning urination, possibly with pain, bleeding or discharge of pus in the urine.

Acute infections are usually due to high Pitta (fire). To treat them effectively the diet should be strongly anti-Pitta, avoiding alcohol, spices (except coriander) and nightshades, particularly tomatoes. Cranberry, coconut or pomegranate juices are often good. Sexual activity should be curtailed.

General Treatment

Typical Ayurvedic herbs for burning urination are sandalwood (a natural urinary antiseptic), shilajit, coriander, punarnava, lemon grass and fennel. For urinary pain gotu kola can be used. Formulas include Sandalwood compound and Gokshura guggul or the Kidney Tonic (no.10) taken with aloe gel.

Typical Chinese formulas are Dianthus combination (strong diuretic action), Polyporus combination (moderate) and Anemarrhena, Phellodendron and Rehmannia (weak, with tonic action).

Western herbs are uva ursi (strong), pipsissewa (moderate), horsetail, plantain and spearmint. A good formula can be made with pipsissewa, plantain, marshmallow, coriander, lemon grass and gotu kola in equal parts.

Specific Treatment

Vata (air) urinary tract infections will be chronic, low grade and irregular. Herbs should be taken to tonify the kidneys — ashwagandha, bala and shatavari — along with mild diuretics. Ashwagandha compound can be taken with Gokshura guggul or the Rejuvenative tonic (no. 2.) can be taken with the Kidney tonic (no. 10). Sarsaparilla and corn silk are good Western herbs for this condition.

Kapha (water) type infections will be due to excess mucus in the kidneys. All dairy products and fats should be avoided, but spices can be used. Good herbs include cinnamon, cubebs, juniper berries and parsley. Standard anti-Kapha formulas can be used, such as Trikatu, along with shilajit, a more specific diuretic.

STONES IN THE URINARY TRACT

Urinary tract stones can be caused by any of the humors. The main factors are Kapha (phlegm) which accumulates in the urinary tract and Vata (wind) which dries it out, creating the stone. They are related primarily to wrong diet, but other factors can come into play as well.

Strong diuretics and stone-dissolving (lithotriptic) herbs are specifically indicated in acute conditions. These include corn silk, gravel root, Ayurvedic pashana bheda and shilajit, and Chinese lygodium and desmodian. They can be taken as teas along with demulcents such as marshmallow or licorice to deal with burning or pain. Large amounts of water, sweet or astringent (not sour) fruit juices and herb teas should be taken to help flush out the stones.

Purgation is helpful, particularly when the pain is acute. Castor oil or rhubarb root can be used. Constipating food like most beans and cabbage family plants should be avoided. Guggul, myrrh and gotu kola are helpful for pain relief.

Differentiation

Kapha (water) stones are mainly composed of calcium. They are soft, smooth and white, and are passed without severe pain. Usually urine will be pale or white and in large quantity.

Pitta (fire) stones are yellow or red in color and composed mainly of oxalates. They are sharp and painful. There will be dark yellow, red or burning urine, often mixed with blood or pus.

Vata (air) stones are brown or black in color and composed mainly of phosphates. They are rough, dry, and irregular and cause severe pain throughout the lower abdomen and thighs. Urination will be difficult, scanty and irregular and may be associated with extreme pain.

Specific Treatment

Pitta types should avoid the nightshades, tomatoes, eggplant, peppers and potatoes, along with spinach, chard, onions and other foods that increase oxalic acid. Cilantro juice can be taken.

Purgation with bitter herbs like rhubarb is often helpful. In addition, strong cooling diuretics should be used such as uva ursi, corn silk, gravel root, tribulis or pashana bheda.

Vata should avoid food that is too light or dry, including dry grains like corn. Tonic and demulcent diuretics-sarsaparilla, sandalwood, marshmallow, and ashwagandha are good as well as the milder diuretics, corn silk and tribulis. Purgatives such as castor oil or Triphala can be used.

Kapha should avoid dairy, cheese, fats and oils. Strong bitter and pungent diuretics can be used: uva ursi, juniper berries, cubebs and gravel root.

Two ounces of corn silk infused in a pint of water taken daily is helpful for most urinary tract stones. It can be taken with a smaller amount of lemon grass.

DIABETES

Diabetes is a disease of profuse urination in Ayurveda. Not specifically a urinary tract disorder, it is a dysfunction of the water system and a water metabolism imbalance. Twenty such diseases are listed according to the three humors that cause them, but diabetes as we commonly know it, relates mainly to two types, diabetes insipidus and diabetes mellitus.

Diabetes is a severe disease, difficult to treat and with many complications. Natural remedies cannot often cure it, particularly that of juvenile onset, but they can alleviate many of its side effects and improve the quality of life and energy. For juvenile onset, and once the pancreas function is totally lost, the condition is generally not reversible.

Differentiation

Diabetes manifests itself as excess thirst and excess urination. Initially, it is primarily a Kapha (water) disease involved with obesity and excess consumption of sweet, kaphogenic foods. Kapha increases in the stomach due to low pancreas function, then enters the other tissues, causing frequency or turbidity of urination.

Long-term diabetes involves thirst and wasting away of tissues, and is or becomes primarily a Vata (air) disease. This is true in diabetes mellitus, the most common type of diabetes. Vata accumulates in the large intestine and travels to the pancreas, deranging pancreas function.

Pitta (fire) can also cause diabetes. It accumulates in the small intestine, then travels to the liver and pancreas upsetting their functions.

Wrong diet is often a causative factor in diabetes, with excessive consumption of sugar, sweets, dairy products, alcohol, fat, and breads. It can be caused by obesity, excessive sex, sleep in the day time, lack of exercise, worry, stress and anxiety, or it may be hereditary. Psychologically, diabetes is a disease of desire, thirst, and lack of contentment in life.

General Treatment

The best general herb and common spice for regulating pancreas and liver function, particularly useful in the initial stage of diabetes, is turmeric, taken as a powder, 1–3 gms. two to three times a day with aloe gel.

The main Ayurvedic herb in more severe or long-term conditions is shilajit, usually taken in the form of Shilajit compound. Another important Ayurvedic herb is gurmar (Gymnema sylvestre). It is the subject of modern scientific research throughout the world for its anti-diabetic properties. Sushrut, one of the greatest ancient Ayurvedic doctors, ascribed to it the property of destroying the taste of sugar (gur-mar means sugar-destroying). It is able to reduce excess sugar in the body. It is usually taken along with shilajit and is part of Shilajit compound.

Guggul and myrrh are useful for the obesity that is often behind the problem. Vasanta Kusumakara, a special mineral preparation, is helpful in severe cases.

Though sugar should be generally avoided, pure, unheated honey can be taken.

In gem therapy, Jupiter stones, yellow sapphire or yellow topaz, are helpful for improving sugar metabolism and for protecting the life. They are usually set in gold and worn on the index finger of the right hand.

Specific Treatment

For Kapha (water) types, long term anti-Kapha diet is the main treatment. Bitter melon is a good food for diabetes. Bitter taste is indicated as it helps control sugar and fat metabolism and liver and pancreas function. Good bitter herbs include aloe, gentian, katuka, neem, barberry, turmeric, golden seal, and myrrh. Black pepper, cayenne and ginger and other pungent herbs are helpful for weight reduction. Useful Ayurvedic formulas include Chandraprabha and Shilajit, as well as Trikatu.

Vata (air) type diabetes involves emaciation, thirst, dehydration, extreme hunger, insomnia, low energy and burning sensation in the hands and feet, as well as high blood sugar and profuse urination.

Anti-Vata diet is indicated, avoiding too much sugar and sweet juices. Complex carbohydrates, nuts and dairy can be helpful. Meat can be useful, particularly bone marrow soup. Ghee is very helpful and should be taken 1–2 tsps. 2–3 times a day, particularly calamus or ashwagandha ghee.

Oil treatment is essential, particularly the application of warm sesame oil to the head or forehead in a series of drops (shiro dhara) at least two nights a week. (This can also be helpful for Kapha types).

Herbal treatment aims mainiy at tonification using herbs such as shilajit, ashwagandha, bala and shatavari and their formulas, as well as Chyavan prash.

Important Chinese herbs for tonification therapy in diabetes are ginseng, astragalus, dioscorea, pueraria, schizandra, trichosanthes root, rehmannia, lycium and the formulas Rehmannia 6 and Rehmannia 8.

Good Western herbs for tonification include comfrey root, solomon's seal and American ginseng in strong decoction.

Pitta (fire) type or Pitta stage diabetes involves fever, acidity, bleeding, ulcerative sores, red, yellow or bluish urine, irritability and hypertension.

Treatment is anti-Pitta. Bitter herbs are indicated as under Kapha, along with cooling demulcent tonics such as shatavari, aloe gel or marshmallow for weaker types. Gotu kola ghee is good. The Liver Tonic (no. 8) is helpful.

Chinese formulas include Major Bupleurum for liver excess type and Gypsum combination for lung and stomach heat type.

5
REPRODUCTIVE SYSTEM
DISORDERS

Ayurveda stresses maintaining the health and vitality of the reproductive system. This is not simply to allow for a better sex life. It is to afford greater vitality for the body as a whole and for the nervous system specifically. Sexual energy can become creative energy and help facilitate mental or spiritual work. Hence, many yogis use herbs for the reproductive system for their general energizing effect. Such herbs enhance Ojas, our underlying vital essence; they do not irritate the sexual nerves or promote unwanted sexual activity.

Most diseases are based upon or involve some wrong use of sexual energy, as sexual energy is the primary energy of the body and mind. Most psychological disorders are based upon an inability to form right relationships and are largely sexual in origin. Hence, the right use of sexual energy is the key to health.

Our highly sexually oriented culture is suspicious of any weakening of the sexual drive. Lack of interest in sex, even in men, however, is usually not a sign of disease. It can be a sign of the development of higher consciousness, with the awakening of detachment. It may be a sign of good health. Toxins in the system irritate the nerves, creating a large sexual appetite or a sexual drive not easy to satisfy. In a body free of toxins the sexual drive is mild and easy to satisfy.

It is natural for interest in sex to decline with age. Constant preoccupation with sex is not necessary; nor is it the highest human good. This does not mean there is anything wrong about sex; it has its place in nature. The guilt and shame about sex we find in Western religions of Judaism, Christianity and Islam causes more problems than it solves.

Sex is often used as a substitute for other things, particularly for lack of creative living, in which case sex is not in its right place.

On the other hand, increased sex drive is not necessarily a sign of poor health or lack of spiritual development. The awakening of the subtle energies of the mind, stimulating the lower chakras, often increases both the sexual drive and mental creativity. This, however, can still cause some health disorders if not managed properly; or if not transmuted, it can be difficult to deal with.

Moreover, abstinence from sex can be a causative factor in disease. If the energy is merely repressed, vitality can stagnate and weaken. Hence, sexual abstinence usually requires some use of asana, pranayama and meditation to turn it into a positive force.

Excessive sexual activity causes Vata (air) and Pitta (fire) disorders, as it depletes the essence of water from the body. It makes us more susceptible to infectious diseases. Toxins transmitted through sexual secretions can circumvent our defensive system and directly lodge in our deepest tissues. Sex without love depletes the vitality and deranges the emotions.

According to Ayurveda, masturbation can cause diseases because there is not the emotional and energy exchange that helps maintain balance in the system. Disrupting balance, it aggravates Vata. Over-stimulating the imagination, it can make us vulnerable to negative psychic or astral forces.

Ayurveda also sees homosexual activity as more likely to cause disease than heterosexual activity. It does not create a natural balancing of the system as the two physical and emotional bodies are of the same polarity.

Vata constitutions have the greatest interest in sex but the lowest vitality for it. They are more likely to have different or deviant sexual patterns. Kapha types have the best sexual vitality with continuous but moderate interest. For them the family life as a whole is important. Pitta falls between the two; the drama and passion are the main things for them.

Seasonally, sexual activity is more appropriate in the winter and spring when Kapha is high. It is more depleting in the summer and fall, in Pitta and Vata seasons. It is better done at night than during the day, and when the moon is waxing than when it is waning.

Sexual Abstinence (Brahmacharya Chikitsa)

Abstinence from sex is important in the treatment of many diseases. It is helpful whenever there is debility, emaciation or underweight, or in convalescence, and is a major part of tonification therapy.

Abstinence is valuable in treating mental and nervous system disorders as the sexual fluid lubricates and nourishes the nerve tissue. Sexual activity often increases rajas and tamas, disturbance and dullness in the mind, and reduces sattva, mental clarity, needed to treat mental disorders. Hence, the system of Yoga has always emphasized 'brahmacharya', control of one's creative energy through transmutation of the sexual force, as one of the main factors for spiritual development.

Abstinence from sex naturally occurs in acute disease conditions, as in fevers. Disease lowers our interest in sex and causes us to preserve our vitality.

Increased sexual activity, on the other hand, is used to treat Kapha diseases such as obesity.

DISEASES OF THE MALE REPRODUCTIVE SYSTEM

Reproductive system disorders are given less emphasis in men but should not be overlooked. Men should consider treatment of the reproductive system and sexual habits as a primary factor for health.

SEXUAL DEBILITY

Sexual debility is lack of sexual vitality or inability to perform adequately sexually. Symptoms include low energy, fatigue, tiredness, lack of sexual motivation, and impotence. Nervousness, palpitations, spermatorrhea, nocturnal emissions and premature ejaculation may occur. Sometimes weak kidney indications, frequent urination or lower back pain, will happen.

Sexual debility can be caused by overwork, too much exercise, stress, or trauma. It may be a complication of underweight and malnourishment where there is insufficient energy. Or it can be caused by overweight which slows down and dulls the reflexes. Emotional factors are fear, difficulties in relationship, feelings of rejection. For a strong sex drive the male ego has to have some confidence; failure or lack of success in life can cause it to weaken. According to Ayurveda, sexual debility is frequently caused by excessive sex, the product of sexual exhaustion.

In Ayurvedic terms it is more commonly a Vata (air) condition. Abstinence from sex is an important initial treatment. Rest and relaxation is helpful.

Treatment

Tonification therapy is generally required, with anti-Vata diet and foods to increase semen. These are dairy products, ghee, nuts, lotus seeds, garlic, onions, okra, jerusalem artichokes, shellfish and meat.

Special tonic herbs for the male reproductive system are indicated: ashwagandha, shatavari, bala, cuscuta, and licorice. Kapikacchu (Mucuna pruriens) is one of the best Ayurvedic herbs in this respect. Important formulas are Ashwagandha compound and Chyavan prash, as well as the

Energy tonic (no. 2). These can be taken with milk and ghee. See also Male Sexual Vitality formula (no. 17).

Additional Chinese herbs are he shou wu (fo ti), lycium, astragalus seeds and formulas such as Rehmannia 6.

Good Western herbs include saw palmetto, comfrey root, and marshmallow.

Sexual debility can also be a Pitta (fire) condition where Pitta burns out the semen. Treatment is also tonification. Aloe gel is good, as is shatavari or Shatavari compound taken with milk, sugar and ghee.

Kapha type sexual debility is characterized by lack of interest in sex, obesity, excess mucus causing congestion and sluggishness in the system. Sugar is often used as a sex substitute.

It is treated by aphrodisiac stimulants such as long pepper, garlic, cloves, damiana, and yohimbe. Formulas include Trikatu and Clove combination taken with honey. Guggul and shilajit are also useful here (and can be helpful for the other humors).

MALE STERILITY

Inability to produce enough or good quality of sperm to bring about conception results in male sterility. Sexual function may otherwise be normal.

A tonification therapy similar to that for sexual debility can improve sperm count, as above. Key foods are dairy products, ghee, sesame oil, garlic, and onions. Good herbs are ashwagandha, kapikacchu, bala, and long pepper. Indian clinical studies show that ashwagandha is quite effective in raising sperm count. It can be taken as a simple milk decoction. Pungent, bitter and astringent tastes should generally be avoided as they cause depletion of sperm.

ENLARGED PROSTATE

Prostate enlargement is common in old age with weakening of sexual function. It can happen in younger men through excessive sexual practices or from undue suppression of ejaculation. Modern medical treatment generally regards it as an infection and uses antibiotics.

The best general Ayurvedic herb is gokshura, particularly when combined with ashwagandha. Shilajit is useful. The Western herb saw palmetto is effective, particularly for the Vata type.

Most commonly it is a Vata (air) condition and comes in the Vata stage of life (old age). Symptoms include lower back pain, low energy, constipation. Treatment involves anti-Vata diet and spices like garlic and onions. Other good herbs are bala, kapikacchu, guggul and marshmallow.

Formulas include Ashwagandha compound, Gokshura guggul and the Kidney tonic (no. 10).

Pitta (fire) type involves infection, swelling and fever. The urine will be dark yellow or red. Treatment is similar to that for urinary tract infection, with the addition of cooling and diuretic herbs like uva ursi, echinacea or punarnava, to tonic herbs like ashwagandha or formulas such as Chyavan prash. Lemon grass tea can be taken regularly.

Kapha (water) type is due to water retention and excess phlegm. Treatment is similar to that for edema. Hot spicy diuretics can be used: cinnamon, ginger, cloves, cubebs, and juniper berries. Again, shilajit is important, as is guggul.

VENEREAL DISEASES

In the sexual act we bring into contact the deepest tissue level of our bodies. This allows reproduction to occur; it can also allow toxins to be transmitted directly into the most interior tissues. We can be invaded by pathogens, potentially devastating in their effects, which could otherwise be easily fought off. The greater the variety of our sexual partners and practices, the more likely we are to contract such venereal disorders. Venereal diseases can become epidemics and threaten the health of a whole culture, which is what we are seeing in our world today.

GENITAL HERPES

Like any highly infectious condition, this is largely a Pitta (fire) disorder, particularly in the acute phase. But it can involve the other humors as well, particularly where there is debility or toxins (Ama) in the system. Genital herpes involves heat in the liver that is transmitted downwards along the liver meridian through the urino-genital region. The blood is usually impure, and excess bile may clog the system. In addition there will be accumulated stress, anger or anxiety.

Pitta type herpes is indicated by fever, thirst, red, swollen or painful lesions, irritability and other Pitta signs.

Vata (air) type herpes involves dry skin, constipation, lesions will be painful and hard but not red or inflamed. There will be lack of energy and insomnia.

Kapha (water) involves weeping or oozing lesions with little redness or pain, and other phlegm accumulations in the system.

Sarsaparilla is a good herb for venereal disease in any of the three humors; it has good anti-viral properties.

Gotu kola helps to calm the mental unrest of the condition and has excellent cleansing properties for the urino-genital system.

Treatment for Pitta

In acute conditions, when the lesions appear, or in Pitta constitutions, treatment should be an anti-Pitta with a blood-cleansing diet. Avoid hot spices, alcohol, sour food, excess salt, and excess sugar. Raw vegetables, salads and vegetable juices should be taken in season. Coriander is the best spice to use, and cilantro or parsley is good. Mung bean or kicharee fast helps during acute attacks.

Stress should be reduced, with adequate rest and relaxation. Sexual activity should be moderated. During acute attacks, sandalwood oil should be applied to the head and coconut oil to the body. Pancha karma treatment can be followed, with emphasis on purgation.

The sores can be washed or douched with such cooling herbs as gentian, golden seal, sarsaparilla, and alum.

Herbal treatment is cleansing the liver and blood. Diuretics and purgatives are helpful for their cleansing action. Mainly bitter taste is indicated.

Good Ayurvedic herbs are aloe gel, barberry, gentian, sarsaparilla, sandalwood, gokshura, punarnava, shatavari, manjishta, and katuka.

A typical Ayurvedic formula for acute conditions would be 3 parts manjishta, 2 parts shatavari, and 1 part each of katuka, gokshura, sarsaparilla, and lemon grass. Rhubarb may be added if constipation exists. Typical Ayurvedic patent medicines are Sarsaparilla compound or Sandalwood compound, preferably taken with aloe gel. Tikta and the Liver Tonic (no. 8) are also good.

In chronic conditions or between attacks one can take Chyavan Prash, Brahma rasayan or gotu kola tea.

Chinese treatment consists of heat-clearing therapy with Gentian combination, usually with the addition of special anti-viral herbs such as isatis or honeysuckle, during acute attacks.

Between attacks, tonification with Rehmannia 6 or Anemarrhena, Phellodendron and Rehmannia formula is given.

Additional good Western herbs for acute attacks are echinacea, golden seal, plantain, uva ursi, pipsissewa, and marshmallow.

Vata (Air) Treatment

Herbs such as sarsaparilla, aloe gel, turmeric, barberry, sandalwood and gotu kola are required, with typical tonics like ashwagandha, bala, shatavari and licorice. Combination blood cleansing and tonification therapy is indicated. Diet should be anti-Vata, avoiding hot spices.

Formulas include Sarsaparilla combination with milk or ghee and Ashwagandha compound when more severe weakness exists.

Kapha (Water) Treatment

Use liver cleansing herbs, aloe, barberry, turmeric and gentian along with hot spices, cayenne, dry ginger, long pepper, and cloves.

Formulas include Sarsaparilla combination with Trikatu.

OTHER VENEREAL DISEASES

Other infectious venereal diseases, syphilis and gonorrhea, can be treated like herpes, with a similar differentiation of humoral syndromes. Sarsaparilla compound is especially good for syphilis. For women, cleansing emmenagogues such as aloe gel, myrrh, saffron, safflower and other menstruation-regulating therapies are good, as per symptoms.

AIDS

According to Ayurveda, AIDS is primarily a disease of low Ojas, the vital sap of the body, the essence of the reproductive system that maintains the autoimmune system. The AIDS virus can only affect us if our Ojas is already low. Factors that deplete Ojas include excessive sexual activity, poor diet, junk food, use of drugs, too much thinking or worrying, and lack of sleep.

As Ojas is the essence of Kapha (water), symptoms of low Ojas usually involve both high Pitta (fire) and high Vata (air). There will be anxiety, restlessness, irritability, vertigo, insomnia, palpitations, and chronic fevers.

Ojas relates to sattva, so a sattvic life-style should be followed (see section). Sattvic herbs for the mind like gotu kola, calamus and sandalwood are helpful. Yogic postures and breathing exercises, particularly lunar pranayama, are important.

Treatment

Both anti-Pitta (anti-fire) and anti-Vata (anti-air) regimes should be combined. Spicy, sour, bitter and astringent tastes should be avoided. Food should strengthen Ojas and be sattvic in nature: sesame seeds and oil, almonds, chick peas, milk, yogurt, and ghee (clarified butter). Sesame oil should be applied externally, with sandalwood or Brahmi oil applied to the head.

It is important to abstain from sexual activity or at least reduce as much as possible. Anal sex, above all, should be avoided as it drains Ojas from the system. (It overly-stimulates apana, the downward moving air, and drains away prana, positive vitality.) Masturbation should also be avoided; it is very reducing to Ojas. (The lack of emotional interchange drains energy from the nervous system.)

Typical Ayurvedic herbs for building Ojas include most strong tonics and tonics to the reproductive system such as ashwagandha, shatavari, gokshura, bala, and kapikacchu. Shilajit is excellent, taken 1–3 gms. twice a day with milk and ghee. Formulas include Ashwagandha compound, Shatavari compound, Chyavan Prash, or the Energy Tonic (no. 2).

The Ayurvedic special preparation, diamond ash (hira bhasma) is important. A Mercury compound, Makaradhwaj, is also good for restoring vitality but should not be taken in acute infections.

Mantras for increasing Ojas include Om, Shum and Shrim. Gems to wear include Jupiter stones (yellow sapphire, yellow topaz, citrine) and Venus stones (diamond, clear zircon).

The Ojas-increasing herbs should be combined with diuretics, gokshura or sarsaparilla, for cleansing the genito-urinary tract and with gugguls or myrrh for cleansing the deeper tissues. Triphala guggul is good. Guduchi is excellent for clearing deep seated fevers and strengthening the immune system. Much of the treatment for other venereal diseases is useful here as per symptoms.

Brahma rasayana, gotu kola herbal jelly, has cleansing and clearing effects. Saffron, in milk decoction, is an excellent herb for most AIDS conditions.

A typical Ayurvedic AIDS formula could be made with gotu kola, sarsaparilla, ashwagandha, shatavari, gokshura, sandalwood and coriander. Guduchi, guggul and shilajit can be added if available.

According to Chinese medicine, this disease is largely one of kidney essence deficiency. Usually, it is more a yin than yang, deficiency but it may be both. In addition the immune system or chi is weak, with internal accumulation of dampness and heat.

Typical Chinese formulas for AIDS include Rehmannia 6 or Rehmannia 8 plus Astragalus. Other heat-clearing and blood-moving herbs may be added including salvia, red peony, isatis.

Good Western tonics for AIDS include American ginseng, marshmallow, solomon's seal and saw palmetto. A Western formula can be made with gotu kola, sarsaparilla, American ginseng, marshmallow, plantain, sandalwood and coriander.

GYNECOLOGICAL DISORDERS

Ayurveda has a special branch of gynecological medicine for the treatment of diseases of the female reproductive system. These diseases are primarily reflected in menstrual disorders. Other, more severe, conditions can develop from the hormonal imbalances that derange the menstrual cycle. In this chapter we also discuss pregnancy and fertility.

The menstrual cycle is a good key to the health of a female. It can also be used to determine physical constitution. Regular menstruation, preferably starting with the full moon, absence of pain or tension, smooth flow, and balanced emotions, are signs of good health. However, most women suffer some difficulties with menstruation at one time of life or another.

Menstruation and Constitution

Vata (air) constitution women generally have scanty menstrual flow. The blood is darkish-red or brownish and it is usually a little dry or old. Menstrual cramping may be severe with lower back pain or headache. Feelings of depression and nervous sensitivity may increase, with fear and anxiety, difficult sleep or insomnia. There will be lessening of vitality and resistance may be lowered. The vaginal wall will be dry. Constipation, gas or abdominal distention may occur. Periods are most often short, irregular and variable, lasting only 3–5 days.

Pitta (fire) type women usually have excess menstrual flow because of Pitta's association with the blood. Blood color is dark, red or purple; the flow is profuse and warm, with possible clotting. There may be fever or burning sensation, along with flushed face or red eyes. Skin rashes or acne may occur. Emotional states include anger, irritability and short temper. Diarrhea or loose stool of predominately yellow color may occur. Periods are typically of medium duration, 5–7 days.

Kapha (water) exhibits moderate flow, but the period will last longer, a week or more. The blood will be pale, light red, with possible mucus, and the flow will be continuous. There will be feelings of heaviness and tiredness with desire to sleep more. Some nausea or possible vomiting with excess phlegm and saliva is possible. The breasts tend to swell and there may be edema, particularly in the lower legs. Sentimentality and nostalgia are more prevalent.

Dual types will show a combination of the symptoms of two of the humors.

Menstrual flow can be deranged by many factors. These include poor diet, stress, overwork. Excessive physical exercise, particularly too much aerobic exercise, can cause difficulties. Our modern cultural emphasis on thin bodies is a factor; without adequate fat the body cannot produce enough blood for easy menstruation. A premenstrual regime of quiet and rest should be followed avoiding any strong exercise (mild asanas are good).

Treatment of Menstrual Disorders

Mild menstrual difficulties are treated with the same therapies as balancing the humor predominant in the constitution. Most gynecological disorders involve delay or difficulty in menstruation. Hence, therapies to promote and regulate menstruation are usually indicated with emmenagogue herbs: turmeric and saffron in Ayurvedic medicine or pennyroyal and motherwort in Western herbalism. Antispasmodics (for relieving muscle spasms) and nervines (to relieve cramping pain and calm the mind) are helpful, such as fennel, asafoetida or valerian. Special tonics for the reproductive system are important where there is debility.

Tonics for Women

As blood loss frequently involves weakening of the vitality, herbal tonics are important supplements for the majority of women. They can be used like vitamin or mineral supplements. Typical preparations are Shatavari preparations, the Female Reproductive Tonic (no.4), the Ayurvedic herbal jelly Chyavan prash, or the Chinese patent medicine, Women's Precious Pill.

Shatavari, Asparagus racemosus, is the main Ayurvedic female reproductive tonic. It is highly nourishing, soothing, and calms the heart. Aloe gel is also very helpful and very balanced in its action, cleansing as well as nourishing. Dang gui, Angelica sinensis, is the main Chinese tonic. It combines menstruation-promoting, blood-building and antispasmodic properties.

It should be noted that excess use of such strong emmenagogue herbs as pennyroyal, tansy or rue can derange menstruation or cause excessive menstrual bleeding. This type of herb is usually contraindicated during pregnancy. They are sometimes used to help promote abortions but seldom are sufficient and can cause side effects.

One of the actions of spicy or pungent taste is to move stagnation and increase the circulation of blood. Hence, many common spices can be used for promoting menstruation and often bring in antispasmodic properties as well. Turmeric is the best general spice but many others are good — cinnamon, ginger, cayenne, black pepper, basil, dill, fennel, cardamom and asafoetida. One-quarter to one-half teaspoon of these spices should be taken in 1–2 tsps. of aloe vera gel twice a day for most mild menstrual difficulties.

Or the Female Reproductive Tonic (no. 4), can be taken 2–3 tablets, three times a day the week or two before menstruation, with warm milk or warm water for Vata, with aloe gel or cool water for Pitta and with honey for Kapha.

Please note sections for more specific problems.

PMS

PMS (premenstrual syndrome) has come to signify many of the difficulties associated with menstruation such as absence or delay of menstruation, early menstruation, premenstrual headaches, menstrual cramping, swollen breasts and so on. Specifically, it indicates the emotional or nervous problems associated with menstruation including irritability, rapid shifts of moods, depression and anxiety, along with their complications.

As a psychological condition, Yoga therapies can be helpful with herbs and foods to promote sattva (harmony of mind). Gemstones, which have a special action to calm the mind, are useful. Pearl or moonstone, gemstones for the moon, are good for PMS as they calm the mind and heart and strengthen the female reproductive system. Pearl is the woman's gemstone, generally, and strengthens the feminine nature physically and psychologically.

PMS can be caused by any of the three humors, as an indication of general imbalance; but as primarily a psychological or nervous condition, it is more commonly a Vata (air) disorder. Emotional or mental agitation upsets the normal secretion of hormones regulating menstruation. Provoking factors include poor nutrition, stress, overwork, travelling, difficulties in relationship and suppressed emotions.

General treatment is like that for the female reproductive system generally, as above.

Differentiation

Vata (air) type PMS is characterized by anxiety, depression, insomnia, constipation, headache and severe cramping pain. There will be nervousness, agitation, feeling spaced out and perhaps dizziness, fainting or vertigo with ringing in the ears. Moods may shift rapidly; the person will be very hard to please. Anxiety and feelings of abandonment may occur. The individual will complain of feeling cold, with thirst and dry skin. She may even feel like she is dying or have suicidal feelings, but once the period starts to flow freely most of the symptoms will disappear. The period may be delayed or irregular. The flow is usually scanty, brown or black and the period lasts only a few days, the usual Vata menstrual pattern. Pain is worse at sunrise or sunset (Vata time).

Pitta (fire) PMS is distinguished by anger, irritability, argumentativeness, with temper and possible violent outbursts. There may be diarrhea, thirst, sweating or fever, and the individual will feel hot, particularly in the upper half of the body. There will be more acne or possible skin rashes. The blood flow is usually abundant or excessive and may contain clots. The period will tend to come early and there may be spotting between periods. Symptoms are worse at noon and midnight (Pitta time).

Kapha (water) type PMS is indicated more by tiredness, heavy feeling, crying, feeling sentimental or needing to be loved. Emotional changes will not be as severe. Susceptibility to colds or flu and mucus discharges will increase. There will be lack of appetite and some nausea. There will be more swelling of the breasts or edema. The period will tend to be late. Menstrual flow will be whitish or pale, thick, mixed with clots or mucus. Symptoms will be worse in early morning or early evening (Kapha time).

Specific Treatment

For Vata, an anti-Vata diet is good, with tonic food like garlic and cooked onions. Spices to promote menstruation, such as turmeric, combined with antispasmodic spices such as nutmeg, can be taken in warm milk before sleep. Warm sesame oil should be applied to the head and lower abdomen. It can be applied to the vagina or a douche can be made with demulcents like shatavari. All stimulants — like coffee and tea, tobacco, alcohol and drugs — should be strictly avoided.

Use of red gem stones is indicated — red coral, garnet, ruby or bloodstone build the blood and white stones like pearl or moonstone increase body fluids.

Herbal treatment consists of sweet and spicy tastes with herbs like aloe gel, shatavari, ashwagandha, licorice, turmeric, cyperus, dill, fennel, valerian, jatamansi and asafoetida. Formulas include Shatavari compound, Ashwagandha compound, Asafoetida 8 or the Female Reproductive Tonic (no. 4).

A good simple formula is 3 parts shatavari, 1 part each of turmeric, cinnamon, valerian, and licorice.

Chinese herbs are dang gui, rehmannia, white peony, and ligusticum. Important formulas include the Four Materials and Bupleurum and Tang Kuei. The latter is the basic PMS formula in Chinese medicine, sold as Bupleurum Sedative Pill. It is also good for Pitta.

Western herbs include emmenagogues, nervines and tonics such as pennyroyal, rosemary, camomile, valerian, false unicorn, and comfrey root.

For Pitta an anti-Pitta diet should be combined with menstruation-promoting spices such as turmeric, coriander, fennel, saffron and safflower, but hot spices should be avoided.

Good gems are pearl, moonstone and red coral. The use of fragrances and incense — jasmine, rose, sandalwood and gardenia — is also very good (or a simple gift of flowers).

Ayurvedic herbs include aloe gel, shatavari, turmeric, cyperus, saffron, manjishta, lodhra, gotu kola and bhringaraj. Important formulas include Shatavari and its various preparations and Aloe wine.

A practical formula would be three parts shatavari, and one part each of turmeric, cyperus, and gotu kola.

Chinese herbs are salvia, motherwort, peach seeds, safflower, bupleurum, cyperus, and mint. Formulas include Bupleurum and Peony.

Western herbs are nettles, yarrow, red raspberry, black cohosh, skullcap, and betony. Simple dandelion tea is often effective.

For Kapha the anti-Kapha diet should be followed. Heavy or oily foods should be avoided: spices and light vegetables can be used freely, including all hot spices.

Ayurvedic herbs include aloe gel, turmeric, cyperus, cinnamon, black pepper, long pepper, ginger, and calamus. Formulas include Trikatu or Clove compound.

Chinese herbs are ligusticum, safflower, hoelen, alisma, and the Tang Kuei and Peony formula.

Western herbs include pennyroyal, rosemary, myrrh, cayenne, ginger, cinnamon and most typical emmenagogues.

AMENORRHEA

Amenorrhea is delay or absence of menstruation. As a premenstrual difficulty, much that is listed under PMS is applicable here. As a long term or frequent condition, it is mainly a deficiency disease and usually due to Vata (air).

Causes are exposure to cold, poor nutrition, anemia, emaciation, dehydration. Displacement of the uterus, hormonal imbalance, emotional trauma and other factors may be involved. It may result from severe or wasting diseases such as diabetes. Amenorrhea may be involved with constipation or caused by the same factors that produce it.

Treatment

Herbs to promote menstruation are specific, often along with tonics to rebuild the reproductive system. Myrrh by itself is often good for amenorrhea, particularly taken as a tincture.

An anti-Vata or tonifying diet is primarily indicated using dairy, meat, nuts, oils, whole grains and other nourishing foods. Iron supplements or Ayurvedic iron ash preparations are important. Warm sesame oil can be applied to the lower abdomen or used as a douche. A mild laxative can be taken such as Triphala, aloe gel or castor oil in lower dosages.

For amenorrhea due to cold, many spicy herbs can be used — ginger, turmeric, black pepper, cinnamon, rosemary, or the formula Trikatu. Fresh ginger and pennyroyal in equal parts, ounce per pint of water, 1 cup three times a day, is a good Western herbal treatment for this condition, which is usually easy to treat.

Ayurvedic herbs for Vata-type delayed menstruation include asafoetida, cyperus, myrrh, ashwagandha, shatavari, kapikacchu, black and white musali. Formulas are Shatavari compound and Ashwagandha compound, better taken with fresh ginger tea.

A good simple formula is shatavari and ashwagandha two parts each, and turmeric and ginger one part each, using one teaspoon of the powder per cup of warm water.

Or the Woman's Tonic (no.4) can be taken along with the Energy Tonic (no. 2).

In Chinese medicine absence of menstruation is considered due to stagnation of blood, which may be allied to blood deficiency. Chinese herbs are ligusticum, salvia, dang gui, motherwort. Formulas include Persica and Rhubarb (strong) and the Four Materials (weak).

Additional Western herbs are typical emmenagogues such as wild ginger, tansy, rue, squaw vine. These work better with a demulcent and nutritive like comfrey root, marshmallow, or American ginseng if there is debility.

Kapha (water) type delayed menstruation is due to congestion and sluggishness in the system. It can also be treated by strong warming spices — ginger, cinnamon, cayenne, black pepper — or Trikatu or Clove combination formulas. Most typical emmenagogues are also good, such as pennyroyal.

Motherwort is a good Chinese and Western herb for this condition, as well as for Pitta.

Pitta (fire) type delayed menstruation is usually mild and can be treated by turmeric or saffron in warm milk. Other good herbs are rose, cyperus, dandelion and other cooling emmenagogues.

In more severe cases it is related to blood or liver disorders, which should be the primary focus of the treatment.

DYSMENORRHEA

Dysmenorrhea is difficult menstruation, usually with cramping pain. Much that is said under the previous categories is relevant here.

Dysmenorrhea is more common in Vata (air) types and may be due to dryness in the uterus, lack of proper secretions, or spasms of the smooth muscles of the uterus. It is often associated with bloating, gas or constipation. In Pitta (fire) and Kapha (water) types it is a congestive disorder caused by a blocking of stagnant blood. In Pitta types it is associated with burning sensation and loose stool or diarrhea. In Kapha it is appears with edema or congestion of phlegm.

Treatment

Antispasmodic, muscle relaxing, analgesic, and pain relieving herbs are used along with emmenagogues. Cyperus is a special Ayurvedic and Chinese herb for menstrual cramping pain and can be used for all types. Myrrh or guggul are also useful.

Vata type involves severe colicky pain, constipation, dry skin, headache, anxiety, palpitations, abdominal distention and gas.

Treatment consists of typical anti-Vata diet. Heat or warm sesame oil should be applied to the lower abdomen. Sesame oil or shatavari can be used as a douche.

Herbs are turmeric, nutmeg, asafoetida, ginger, valerian, and jatamansi. They function better with demulcents such as shatavari or licorice, which possess a soothing and cortisone-like effect. Formulas include Asafoetida 8, as well as the Shatavari formulas.

Other good Chinese herbs are corydalis, salvia, and ligusticum; dang gui and white peony help relieve spasms of the smooth muscles of the uterus.

Good Western herbs are camomile, lady's slipper, and evening primrose.

For Pitta and Kapha types note the sections on PMS and on amenorrhea. Pitta dysmenorrhea requires cooling nervines like gotu kola, skullcap, passion flower, and hops. Kapha needs spicy nervines and antispasmodics — ginger, calamus, myrrh, guggul, cinnamon and nutmeg.

MENORRHAGIA

Menorrhagia is excess menstrual bleeding. The period is often prolonged and bleeding or spotting may occur between periods. It is usually due to high Pitta (fire) which heats up the blood. It may be involved with other bleeding disorders, such as blood in the stool.

Causes include overeating of hot, spicy, sour or salty food, smoking or drinking (alcohol), unresolved anger, resentment or hostility. This condition may be caused by abortions, by incomplete miscarriages, by cervical erosion, endometritis, polyps and tumors. IUD contraceptives can bring it about, as well as birth control pills. It can sometimes indicate infection or cancer and should be examined carefully.

General Treatment

Anti-Pitta diet is required with avoidance of all hot and oily food. The patient should be kept cool and should avoid exercise and exposure to heat and sun. During bleeding, an ice pack can be applied to the lower abdomen.

Astringent and hemostatic herbs should be given, such as red raspberry or manjishta. If the condition has persisted, tonics should be given as well. Once the bleeding is reduced, the tonics can be given by themselves as per the treatment of anemia.

Important Ayurvedic herbs include ashok, lodhra, ashwagandha, arjuna, shatavari, aloe, amalaki, bhringaraj. Shatavari and manjishta are excellent in equal proportions. Ashok wine is indicated. Formulas include the Heart Tonic (no.11).

Chinese herbs include mugwort, gelatin, pseudoginseng, with formulas like Tang Kuei and Gelatin.

Additional Western herbs are agrimony, nettles, yarrow, self-heal, and mullein.

More information can be found in the section on 'Bleeding Disorders', particularly for Vata and Kapha types.

LEUCORRHEA

Leucorrhea is an abnormal discharge from the vagina. The vagina has a natural acid environment that protects it from unfavorable pathogens. If this is not maintained, various bacteria, fungi or protozoa can proliferate. Douches of sour taste such as vinegar, yogurt or herbs with acidophilus supplements are effective for this reason.

In Ayurveda, leucorrhea is most commonly a Kapha, excess mucus condition, but can be caused by the other humors. It is the humor that is treated rather than the specific pathogen.

Vata (air) type leucorrhea will be brown, sticky and dry, with more severe pain.

Pitta (fire) type is yellow, foul smelling, perhaps purulent or mixed with blood, with more burning sensation.

Kapha (water) type is white, mucoid, thick, profuse, with feelings of dullness and heaviness.

Causes are mainly those which increase Kapha; eating too much sweet, sour and salty, heavy and greasy foods such as dairy and sugars. Lack of cleanliness, excessive sex, use of antibiotics, infections, or venereal diseases contribute.

Treatment

The most specific form of treatment is douche. Otherwise treatment is according to the humor. Ayurvedic herbs for douche are alum, turmeric, aloe gel, and licorice.

For Vata yogurt can be used as a douche or demulcent herbs such as shatavari and licorice. Ashwagandha, shatavari and their preparations should be taken internally.

For Pitta use bitter herbs: aloe powder, katuka, alum, coptis, golden seal, and gentian. For internal use, aloe gel, turmeric and barberry are indicated for cleansing the blood, or the Herbal Febrifuge and Blood Purifier (no.7).

For Kapha bitter and pungent herbs are combined for douche: aloe powder, alum, calamus, prickly ash, and ginger. For internal use, Trikatu can be taken with honey.

Good Western herbs include wormwood, tansy, rue, alum root, oak bark, usnea, golden seal, and echinacea.

Two ounces of a combination of such herbs should be decocted in a pint of water for twenty minutes, then strained and applied as a douche morning and evening. Golden seal, sarsaparilla and prickly ash in combination with a small amount of alum are good in acute conditions.

MENOPAUSE

Menopause, the change of life in women, can be a time of health disturbances with the shifting of hormones. Treatment requires special herbs for strengthening or rejuvenating the female reproductive system, along with herbs to help regulate the hormones and calm the emotions.

As menopause is associated with the movement into old age, the Vata (air) stage of life, symptoms are primarily of high Vata with increased nervousness, anxiety, insomnia and depression.

The general treatment is similarly anti-Vata. Many herbs which tonify the female reproductive system become helpful again, including aloe gel, shatavari, saffron, kapikacchu, ashwagandha, taken in milk decoctions, if possible, or in their different preparations like Shatavari compound. Chinese tonic herbs such as dang gui, rehmannia, white peony, lycium and Woman's Precious Pill are good.

Aloe gel is specific for maintaining the youthfulness of the female reproductive organs. Chyavan prash is useful here for its general rejuvenative effect.

Pitta (fire) type menopause appears as anger, irritability, and short temper, with more frequent or pronounced hot flashes. Treatment is anti-Pitta, including aloe gel and shatavari tonics, or a saffron milk decoction, or Shatavari compound.

Kapha (water) involves feelings of heaviness, sleepiness, lack of motivation, weight gain or holding of water. Treatment is anti-Kapha. Hot spices are used like the Trikatu formula along with aloe gel.

HYSTERECTOMY

The uterus has functions other than reproduction; it is also an organ of emotion and creativity. When it is removed, feelings of emotional imbalance and insecurity can arise. Along with hormonal imbalance, the system will tend to become devitalized. The metabolism may be deranged and excess weight will be put on.

These factors primarily serve to increase Vata. Depression, ungroundedness and anxiety may increase. The other humors can increase as well, usually according to what is predominant in the general constitution. Pitta types will experience more anger, irritability and heat sensations. Kapha will accumulate more water and phlegm, feel more tired or sentimental.

General treatment consists of tonics to the reproductive system: shatavari, aloe gel, saffron and their preparations or Chyavan prash. Chinese tonic herbs such as dang gui, rehmannia, and white peony again are helpful. Herbs that balance the mind and calm the emotions are helpful — gotu kola, calamus, bhringaraj, jatamansi or Brahmi rasayan. Chinese mind-calming herbs, zizyphus and biota, are good as well as Western nervines, skullcap, valerian and lady's slipper.

Immediately after surgery, herbs are used to promote healing: turmeric and arjuna are best (see section on Post-surgical treatment).

BREAST OR UTERINE CYSTS AND TUMORS

Cysts are not uncommon in the breast or uterus. A significant percentage of women will get them. They are more common in women who do not have children. Most are benign but malignancy does develop in some cases. Malignant tumors are hard to the touch and possess definite boundaries.

Tumors can be due to any of the three humors, but they are most common in Kapha (water) types, owing to the extra weight. Kapha tumors, usually benign, are often subcutaneous fat or mucus accumulations. They involve swelling, dampness and congestion. If large, they can be safely removed through surgery, if necessary. As the breast is a fatty organ, it easily gets such cysts or tumors.

Vata (air) type tumors are characterized by pain. They are dry, variable in size and location. Vata individuals are prone to fear and are more likely to imagine that any swelling or cyst is cancer.

Pitta (fire) tumors are distinguished by inflammation, infection, swelling and hot sensation.

Treatment

Anti-Kapha regime is indicated for most benign tumors. Fat-reducing herbs are indicated combining pungent and bitter tastes. Good herbs are black pepper, cayenne, turmeric, calamus, katuka, golden seal, and barberry. Formulas include Trikatu taken with honey. Honey, itself, has a fat and tumor reducing property. Triphala or other laxatives are helpful as well.

Special herbs for reducing breast tumors include turmeric, saffron, safflower, dandelion, violet, and cyperus. Saffron milk decoction is good; use a higher dosage of saffron, 1–3 gms. per day, for short periods of time.

For the other humors, treatment is as for dysmenorrhea. See also section on Cancer for other anti-tumor approaches.

Milder forms of these same treatments can be used for swollen breasts, either premenstrual or during breast feeding.

PID, ENDOMETRITIS AND ENDOMETRIOSIS

In their acute forms, PID (pelvic inflammatory disease), endometritis and similar conditions are Pitta (fire) disorders showing accumulation of heat and stagnant blood, with infection and inflammation. Often, the liver has to be treated and the blood cleansed (see section).

Treatment requires anti-Pitta diet and regime, avoiding all spices but turmeric, coriander and saffron, also refraining from salt, alcohol and refined sugar, and all oils but coconut and sunflower. Good herbs include shatavari, aloe gel, sarsaparilla, gotu kola, dandelion, myrrh, echinacea. Strong bitters like katuka, golden seal, gentian or uva ursi can be added to these. Shatavari and manjishta in equal proportions works well. Other treatment follows menstrual symptoms (usually Pitta type menstruation). The Woman's Tonic (no. 4) is good taken with aloe gel or the Herbal Febrifuge (no. 7).

In chronic conditions shatavari can be taken with aloe gel, one teaspoon of the powder per one tablespoon of the gel twice a day on an empty stomach.

Endometriosis tends more towards Kapha, with the excess growth of the uterine membrane. This is more the case when there is little infection. Anti-Kapha, anti-tumor and general detoxifying and reducing approach is useful with typical herbs like guggul, myrrh, turmeric and dandelion. Black pepper and katuka or golden seal can be taken with honey.

DURING PREGNANCY

During pregnancy, a mild nutritive therapy should be followed. Herbs which are strong or extreme in their action, as well as emmenagogues, purgatives and toxic herbs, should be avoided.

Herbs for improving the deeper tissues should be used including shatavari, ashwagandha, bala, white musali, and kapikacchu.

Tonic formulas such as Shatavari compound, Ashwagandha compound and Chyavan prash are indicated, or the Energy Tonic (no. 2), preferably taken with milk and ghee.

POST-PARTUM

Immediately after delivery, herbs should be used to cleanse the uterus and promote uterine circulation. These include emmenagogues, saffron, safflower, myrrh and pennyroyal, but taken only for a few days up to a week in most conditions.

Mild nutritive therapy should be continued throughout the period of breast feeding. Use dairy products, particularly for Vata (air) and Pitta (fire) constitutions.

Herbs to increase the breast milk include shatavari, marshmallow and licorice, prepared in milk decoctions. Chinese herbs such as dang gui and rehmannia are good. Herbs to facilitate the flow of the breast milk include fennel, dandelion and nettles. Sage is good for stopping the flow of milk when it is excessive or when breast feeding time is over, or a paste of mung bean flour can be applied to the breast.

MISCARRIAGE
HABITUAL ABORTION

Miscarriage, or habitual abortion, has several causes. More commonly it is a Pitta (fire) condition of excessive movement of the downward moving air (apana). Kapha (water) types are usually fertile but may have a false or ectopic pregnancy. Vata (air) types are more likely to be unable to conceive in the first place.

General treatment for miscarriage involves anti-Pitta diet, with avoidance of spicy and oily foods. Dairy products are helpful, particularly milk. The patient needs adequate rest and relaxation, avoiding travel and exercise. Exposure to sun and heat should be limited.

Herbal therapy aims at tonification and calming the emotions. After a miscarriage, care must be taken first to move out all stagnant blood and heal the uterus with emmenagogue herbs such as aloe gel, myrrh, turmeric, and manjishta. After a week or two follow this therapy with tonification therapy.

Ayurvedic herbs are shatavari, ashwagandha, aloe gel, manjishta, and gotu kola. Formulas include Shatavari compound and Ashwagandha compound, and Chyavan prash.

Good Chinese herbs are mugwort, eucommia, loranthus, with formulas like Tang Kuei and Gelatin combination.

Additional good Western herbs are red raspberry and false unicorn.

INFERTILITY

Infertility is usually associated with poor nutrition or lack of proper development of the reproductive organs. It can also be caused by accumulation of fluids or stagnation of blood.

Generally, Kapha (water) types are the most fertile and Vata (air) types the least fertile. Pitta (fire) types fall in between.

An astrologer can be consulted for the best times for fertility, usually when the moon is waxing and in fertile signs. The woman's fertility can also be determined astrologically.

Treatment

Tonification therapy is generally best with anti-Vata, pro-Kapha diet using nourishing and strengthening foods: dairy products, particularly milk, meat, fish, nuts and oils such as ghee or sesame. Treatment requires mainly the tonic herbs for strengthening the female reproductive system.

Typical Ayurvedic female tonics again are good — shatavari, ashwagandha, aloe gel, saffron, licorice. Formulas include Shatavari compound, Dashamula, and Phalaghrita.

Chinese herbs are dang gui and rehmannia. Formulas include Woman's Precious Pill and Four Materials.

Additional Western herbs are comfrey root, marshmallow, saw palmetto, and false unicorn.

Where it is more a congestive disorder or due to sluggish function, as in those overweight (Kapha types), energy moving and circulation promoting herbs must be employed. Cinnamon, saffron, ginger, myrrh and formulas such as Trikatu and Triphala together with honey are useful. Pitta can use saffron, aloe gel and shatavari.

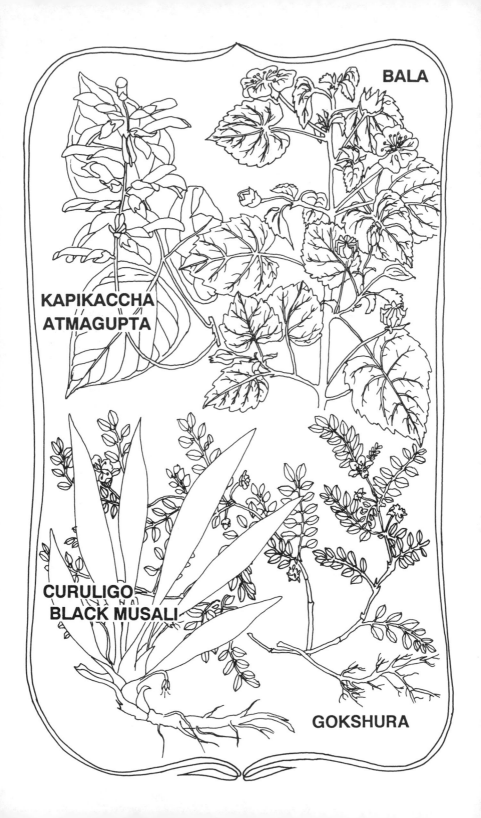

6
FEBRILE AND
INFECTIOUS DISEASES

Ayurvedic medicine traditionally has been used to treat febrile diseases such as malaria, septicemia, pneumonia, bronchitis, and infections of all kinds. As antibiotic drugs begin to fail, these natural methods may again become important. While they may not be as strong or as effective in acute conditions as drugs, they are often more useful in chronic conditions. Moreover, their side effects are less. Natural therapies are less likely to weaken or suppress the immune system; in fact, after treatment our resistance may be stronger. We are not rendered more vulnerable to new pathogens, as happens with drugs. Antibiotic herbs do not breed new resistant strains of bacteria. When used at an early stage and with support therapies of right diet, etc., these herbs can be as effective as antibiotic drugs.

The main indication of all febrile diseases is a rise in body temperature. This is generally accompanied by rapid pulse, body aches, absence of sweating, restlessness, insomnia, delirium and lack of appetite.

Febrile diseases usually relate to high Pitta (fire), since aggravated Pitta causes fever and infection. However, fever can be created by any of the three humors or any combination of them. In addition, fever can arise from external causes such as injuries. Vata (air) type fevers come indirectly from an accumulation of gases or dryness in the body fluids. Kapha (water) type fevers are the result of congestion and stagnation of fluids.

In Ayurvedic classification, there are many different types and degrees of fevers. As these relate to more acute conditions that may require hospitalization, we will deal only with the more common conditions here.

Differentiation
Pitta fevers are characterized by high body temperature, burning sensation, thirst, red tongue with yellow coating, red eyes, perspiration, yellow or burning urine, yellow stool or diarrhea and possible bleeding. There will be irritability, restlessness and disturbed sleep.

Vata fevers show irregularity and changeability, along with more severe pain. Onset is variable, the temperature rise changes and the

temperature does not remain the same. Additional symptoms of high Vata
are anxiety, restlessness, constipation, insomnia, pain and stiffness in the
body, and ringing in the ears.

Kapha fevers are low grade with only mild increase in body temperature. There will be loss of appetite, loss of taste, sweet taste in the mouth
and excess salivation. The body will feel heavy, tired, cold and there may
be a cough.

It is important with fever to discriminate Ama and Nirama conditions
— whether or not the undigested food mass (Ama) exists. When there is
a pronounced tongue coating, Ama is indicated and herbs to promote
digestion are needed such as our common spices or the Trikatu formula.

General Treatment

Bitter herbs are indicated for fevers, especially for severe fevers. They
usually contain antibacterial and antiviral properties; many bitter herbs
have proven antibiotic action in vitro against specific bacteria or viruses.
The reducing effect of these bitter herbs is directed first at the pathogen,
which is separated out from the tissues in which it is lodged. In excess,
however, the herbs will have a reducing action on the body itself, so they
should be used with discretion.

Each herbal tradition has its particular panacea bitter herb that functions as a febrifuge and anti-inflammatory. In the West, it is golden seal
or barberry. For the Chinese, it is coptis. In Ayurveda it is chiretta or katuka
and the formula Tikta.

In addition, diaphoretic herbs may be used to help sweat out a fever;
a rise in body temperature works to kill the pathogen. Simple, fresh ginger
tea can be given for this purpose or basil tea (good for all kinds of fevers).
In Ayurvedic medicine, a smaller amount of hot pungent herbs such as
Trikatu (dry ginger, black pepper and long pepper) is added to bitters to
help burn up the fever. Dry ginger by itself is often good, with honey for
Kapha, butter for Pitta and ghee for Vata. Usual dose is one-quarter
teaspoon of dry ginger per teaspoon of the vehicle.

Generally, diaphoretics work better in the initial stage of a fever,
where there is Ama and they are more effective in Vata and Kapha fevers.
Bitters are better for Pitta and Kapha fevers.

Diuretic herbs can be employed to drain the fever downwards (as fire
is relieved by downward action). Purgatives can be used, but they are
contraindicated in initial or new fevers.

In both Ayurvedic and Chinese medicine the mineral gypsum is
employed for lowering dangerously high fevers. The Chinese use the

strained decoction of the crude mineral, and Ayurveda makes a special incinerated ash called 'Godanti Bhasma'.

Food should be avoided during high fevers, particularly heavy or oily foods. If very hungry, whole grains can be eaten, particularly barley, mung, rice or Kicharee. Mung water or mung bean soup is excellent for all manner of fevers, infections and toxic blood conditions. Adequate liquids should be taken, preferably herbal teas. In initial fevers, do not drink cold water; it tends to drive the fever deeper into the body. A cold water sponge bath can be applied to the head and limbs. Rose water sprinkled over the head and sandalwood oil applied to the forehead, are cooling; also try henna and vetivert. In the beginning or acute stage, the patient should rest.

Initial treatment of fevers, as for the common cold, consists largely of hot spicy herbs for stimulant and diaphoretic action. Long pepper or dry ginger can be used, taken with honey, or Trikatu formula with warm water. Other good herbs include bayberry, cinnamon, ginger, cloves, cayenne.

Old or mature fevers, those which have lasted several days, are treated with typical bitter herbs, as well as purgatives, rhubarb or aloe for Pitta and Kapha, Triphala for Vata.

Chronic low grade fevers usually require some tonification to be resolved. Good herbs for these high Vata or chronic Pitta conditions include aloe gel, shatavari, barberry, katuka, amalaki, bala, and marshmallow. Guduchi is a special Ayurvedic herb from which an extract is made that has proven effective for such difficult lingering fevers. Formulas include Shatavari compound; the Ayurvedic herbal jelly, Chyavan Prash, is excellent, 2 tsps. twice a day taken with milk. Sometimes this condition requires herbs to strengthen the immune system such as ashwagandha, bala, ginseng or astragalus.

Specific Treatment

Pitta fevers require primarily bitter herbs. Important Ayurvedic herbs are katuka, chiretta, neem, vetivert, lemon grass, sandalwood, and coriander. Formulas include Sudarshan and Mahasudarshan powders, as well as the Herbal Febrifuge and Blood Purifier (no. 7). After the fever, a bitter purgative like rhubarb root may be good to clear out residual toxins.

Good Chinese formulas are Coptis and Scute (for septic fever) and Gypsum combination for high fever with thirst and delirium.

Vata fevers need bitter and pungent herbs: black pepper, galangal, ginger, garlic, and barberry. Formulas include Sudarshan powder or the

Herbal Febrifuge with Trikatu, 1–2 gms. of each twice a day with warm water.

Kapha fevers require primarily hot pungent herbs, though bitters can still be used. Black pepper or long pepper can be taken mixed with honey. Formulas include Trikatu or Clove compound taken with honey.

INFECTIONS

For infections, bitter natural antibiotics are also used. In Ayurveda, the most common is katuka; chiretta, gentian, barberry, and isatis are also useful. In Chinese medicine, coptis is the main herb, then lonicera, forsythia, isatis, scute, phellodendron, gentian and rhubarb. The usual Western herb is golden seal; other bitters are barberry, gentian, echinacea, dandelion, sarsaparilla, and usnea. Many herbs possess cooling energy and can be used in this way.

Treatment is largely the same as for fever. The condition is mainly high Pitta (fire). We will examine one form of general infection, boils and carbuncles, below.

BOILS AND CARBUNCLES

Boils and carbuncles are local infections, of the skin and hair follicles, by staph and other bacteria. A toxic blood condition, they are characterized by swelling, pain, fever and discharge of pus. They occur more commonly on the back, legs and arms but can erupt anywhere on the surface of the body. Acne is a much milder condition, which can be treated by the same line of therapies.

In Western medicine, boils are thought to arise from external factors. In Ayurveda, internal impurity, considered the cause, indicates the need for cleansing. They are an Ama (toxic) condition, caused mainly by poor diet but can also come from other impure conditions. The liver is the main organ involved, so any overly toxic liver will tend to cause them.

Differentiation

Pitta (fire) type boils are characterized by redness, swelling, thirst and fever; Kapha (water) type, by large amounts of pus, dullness, heaviness and lassitude; Vata (air) type, by pain. The latter are slow to come to a head and may migrate to other points in the body.

Boils generally result from impure food and water, or overeating of spicy, hot, sour and salty foods (Pitta-causing foods). Intake of excess sweet, oily or greasy foods can cause them; sweet taste in excess will acidify the blood. Overexposure to sun or heat, too many saunas or hot baths, and other such Pitta-aggravating elements contribute. Anger, irritability, stress or suppressed emotions are psychological factors. The condition may be brought on by t:avel to a hotter climate with a higher bacterial count.

Western medical treatment is largely with antibiotics. The main danger is that the infection will become septic, spreading through the body and infecting the internal organs. It can even cause death.

General Treatment

In acute conditions a detoxifying and anti-Pitta diet and therapy is essential. Salads, sprouts and vegetable juices, preferably fresh, should be taken. Dairy, breads, sweets, oils, meat, fish and mushrooms should be avoided. All stale, recooked, and canned food, junk food or otherwise devitalized food such as white sugar and white flour should be strictly avoided. No spices should be used except turmeric and coriander. No oil should be applied to the body, but the essential oil of sandalwood or gardenia can be applied to the forehead. Strong or aerobic exercise should be avoided. Herbal bitter taste is indicated, with some use of astringents. Alterative (blood-cleansing) teas can be drunk including alfalfa, red clover, burdock and dandelion. Specific herbal therapy involves the use of natural antibiotic herbs and special herbs to help dissolve pus (suppuratives).

Treatment is both external and internal, applying herbal packs or poultices to the sore. Important Ayurvedic herbs are manjishta, katuka, neem, isatis, turmeric and barberry. Aloe gel can be taken in 2 tsp. dosages three times a day with turmeric. Formulas are the Herbal Febrifuge and Blood Purifier (no. 7) and the Herbal Laxative (no. 5). Ghee can be helpful externally, the older the better (even if it smells).

Chinese herbs include honeysuckle, forsythia, isatis, coptis, scute, and phellodendron. Formulas are Honeysuckle and Forsythia combination for milder conditions and Coptis and Scute combination for severe.

Western herbs are burdock, sarsaparilla, sassafras, and red clover — mild; myrrh, chickweed, dandelion, barberry, golden seal — strong.

Specific Treatment

Vata boils are caused more by exposure to wind, dryness in the blood and by distention and constipation. Laxatives such as Triphala are helpful. Triphala guggul or myrrh tincture is excellent. Sarsaparilla is a good single herb, and garlic often works well.

Kapha boils relate to impurities in the lymph system, and may accompany phlegm diseases. They require the use of expectorants (pus can be a kind of subcutaneous phlegm) and spicy taste. Good herbs include cinnamon, angelica, turmeric, sassafras, and calamus. Most of the Pitta herbs can also be used, along with Trikatu or dry ginger.

SKIN DISEASES

There are many types of skin diseases: psoriasis, eczema, skin rashes, contact dermatitis, etc. In Ayurveda, they are classified succinctly according to the three humors. Any of them can occur in a form relative to each of the three humors. Those caused by external poisons, poison oak or poison ivy, can be treated like the Pitta type.

Skin diseases are more common in Pitta (fire) types, as Pitta can overheat the blood and thereby poison the skin. Skin diseases that involve loss of skin pigmentation, such as leucoderma, are usually Pitta disorders, as Pitta governs complexion.

Factors causing skin diseases include wrong diet, too much use of sour, salty or pungent tastes, too heavy, sweet or oily food, drinking of alcohol, exposure to the elements, and over use of cosmetics. They are similar to boils, carbuncles and other toxic blood conditions in their origin and treatment.

The skin relates to the plasma, to the outer disease pathway and to the blood. Skin diseases, therefore, relate to the lungs and the liver. The use of expectorants and diaphoretics to cleanse the lungs, and alteratives and bitter tonics to cleanse the liver, are important in the treatment of skin diseases.

General Treatment

There are many good herbs for such cleansing. These include common herbs: dandelion, burdock, red clover, plantain, yarrow, and self-heal. Ayurvedic herbs include turmeric, barberry, sandalwood, and guggul. Additional Chinese herbs are honeysuckle, forsythia, isatis, and bupleurum.

These are useful for most acute cases. In chronic cases demulcents and tonics such as marshmallow, licorice, shatavari and gokshura are needed.

Psoralia, Sanskrit bakuchi, is an important Ayurvedic herb for leucoderma and for restoring normal skin pigmentation and is considered to be rejuvenative to the skin, nails and hair. It can be prepared as a medicated oil. Five grams of the powder can be taken twice a day before meals with a little coriander and honey to mask the bitter taste.

Herbs should be taken externally as well as internally. Externally, herbal decoctions can be used as washes; herbal plasters or poultices can be applied, or some herbal oils used.

Ghee is excellent externally for inflammatory skin diseases, rashes and burns. It is best prepared by placing it in a copper vessel along with about half the amount of water. It should be kept for a month, stirring it occasionally with a copper spoon if possible. The ghee will become whitish in color and take on a more pleasant smell. (This preparation, done over a shorter period of time by rapid stirring of water and ghee in a copper vessel is called Shatodhara ghrita and is sold in India). Such ghee is more absorbable to the skin.

Aloe gel is another helpful topical preparation for almost any kind of skin rash. Cilantro juice is good for most allergic skin conditions. Ayurvedic Turmeric cream can be useful, particularly for acne or for improving complexion (but some Ayurvedic Turmeric creams have many essential oils like sandalwood that can irritate the skin in excess, as can any essential oil).

Saffron is a special herb for nourishing the skin, taken as a milk decoction (one gram per cup) and pearl ash (moti bhasma) or pearl powder is also excellent.

It should be noted that skin rashes sometimes get worse before they get better, as the heat and toxins are being dispelled from the body. Hence, one should not terminate a treatment too quickly if the diagnosis appears sound.

Differentiation

Pitta (fire) skin diseases are characterized by redness, swelling, fever, infection and irritability. They are increased by heat and exposure to the sun. Application of most oils will make them worse.

Vata (air) type show up as dry or scaly skin, itching, distention or constipation. They are aggravated by wind and dryness and alleviated by the application of heavy oils, especially sesame.

Kapha (water) type involve oozing or weeping sores, with congestion, edema and itch. They are aggravated by dampness and cold. Oils also tend to aggravate them.

Specific Treatment

Pitta type should follow anti-Pitta diet avoiding possible allergen foods such as nightshades, tomatoes, peaches, and strawberries, as well as sour dairy products. Coconut juice is good, as is cilantro. Exposure to sun and heat should be avoided. The best oils for external application are coconut, or aloe gel. Brahmi or Bhringaraj oil or the herbs in decoction are good for rashes on the head, neck and face. Most typical alteratives, like burdock or red clover, are good. Bitter laxatives, rhubarb or aloe, are helpful. Formulas include the Herbal Febrifuge and Blood Purifier (no. 7) taken with aloe gel or dandelion tea.

Vata should follow anti-Vata diet. Soothing oils such as sesame should be applied to the skin. Laxatives and enema therapy are helpful. Triphala should be taken on a regular basis, 5–10 gms. before sleep. Triphala guggul or myrrh tincture is good.

Kapha should implement an anti-Kapha diet, avoiding all heavy, greasy and oily food, particularly cheese and yogurt. No oils should be used externally or internally. Diuretic herbs are often helpful, like plantain, burdock seeds or pipsissewa. Formulas include Gokshura guggul or Triphala guggul, as well as the Herbal Febrifuge and Blood Purifier (no. 7) with warm water or ginger tea.

7
MISCELLANEOUS
CONDITIONS

TRAUMATIC INJURIES

Herbs have been traditionally used to treat traumatic injuries. But as allopathic medicine is often more effective in this area, herbal remedies are seldom used today, except when allopathic treatment is not available. Common astringents — nature's first aid chest — grow almost everywhere; yarrow, self-heal, mullein, aloe, comfrey, chickweed and plantain are quite available. These herbs were once very important medicinals, highly regarded in the materia medica of earlier times.

Such herbs can be picked fresh, crushed and applied as a poultice to the injured part. They not only stop bleeding but aid in the healing of tissues. Herbal ointments can be made from them or purchased and used as part of a first aid kit. Or they can be mixed with a little honey and applied. The same herbs can be taken internally for internal injuries in the initial phase.

Bitter antiseptic herbs are useful to counter infection — golden seal, echinacea, aloe and myrrh. They are effective both externally and internally.

Once the wound is closed and any fever or infection reduced, herbs to promote blood circulation are used to stimulate healing: cinnamon, ginger, cayenne, sassafras, and saffron. If healing is slow or if tissue damage and blood loss have been extensive, tonics should be taken, like ashwagandha, ginseng or comfrey root.

Aloe gel is nature's best natural topical herb for cuts, wounds, sores and burns. Fresh chickweed has similar properties.

Turmeric is a major herb for soft tissue and muscle injury. In India, fresh turmeric root is applied directly to cuts and wounds, and they are found to heal without a scar. Treat strained muscles and joints with turmeric as well; it is good for sports injuries. Ayurvedic turmeric creams are helpful, not only for nourishing the skin or removing acne and blemishes, but also for promoting healing of injured tissue.

Ashwagandha is a good tonic for broken bones; use five grams per cup in milk decoctions with a small amount of turmeric or cinnamon.

Other useful herbs in this condition are comfrey root and solomon's seal, which provide nutrition to the bone tissue to promote healing.

Myrrh is an important herb for removing stagnant blood and preventing necrosis. Its Ayurvedic relative, guggul, is often used the same way; the formula Triphala guggul is a natural antiseptic and antibiotic that promotes the healing of the deeper tissues in the body. Take 3 pills three times a day, up to one week in more severe injuries; 2 pills twice a day for a longer period of time for milder injuries or injuries that are slow to heal.

Other plant resins, those of various pines, liquidamber, or the sap of various tropical Indian fig trees, have important astringent, antiseptic and healing properties. Such resins can be dissolved in rubbing alcohol and combined with a little camphor for treatment of bruises and sprains.

Castor oil packs are effective for reducing swelling and promoting healing of bruised or damaged tissue. They can be applied with good results for abdominal pain and tumors. Castor oil can be applied on cotton and wrapped or taped around the affected part.

In Chinese medicine, salvia is used to promote healing of damaged tissue and to prevent scarring and adhesions. Siberian ginseng (often mislabelled as 'ginseng'), Eleuthrococcus senticosus, is used for sports injuries and also helps improve performance by strengthening the muscles, tendons, ligaments and bones. Heart tonics like pseudoginseng or arjuna are useful in this way.

Traumatic injury is an external factor, so it is not treated according to the biological humors. Generally, however, any severe injury over the long term will derange the life-force, Prana, and aggravate Vata (air). Initially, Pitta (fire) may be aggravated with fever and infection.

POST-SURGERY

Surgery, like traumatic injury, disturbs the life-force and deranges the basic homeostasis of the body. Anesthetics and antibiotics complicate this condition.

Many people suffer from poor healing after surgery. Scars and adhesions, particularly in the abdominal area, can cause various digestive system disorders such as gas and constipation, as well as lingering pains. This is partly because Western medicine has not given consideration to post-surgical care beyond clearing up infections with antibiotics.

Turmeric, again, is important both externally and internally and helps remove scars and adhesions, 1–3 gms. of the powder three times a day with honey. Another excellent but more expensive herb is saffron; safflower or calendula can be used as a substitute. Marigold is also good.

Aloe gel is good for healing any damage to the female reproductive organs, as well as for the liver and spleen. Myrrh is also helpful for the female reproductive system, and after bone or joint surgery (for which the gugguls, particularly Triphala guggul, are specific). The Triphala formula, itself, is good after colon surgery. Gotu kola, particularly in the form of Brahma rasayan, aids in the healing of nerve tissue. It also helps remove any emotional trauma that may be involved. Calamus works to restore nerve and sensory function and is particularly good for clearing out the effects of anesthetics. Arjuna is helpful after heart surgery.

Chyavan prash is a good herbal food to take when recovering from surgery; it nourishes the blood and the deeper tissue. Ashwagandha in milk decoction helps calm the mind and fortify Ojas. Shatavari helps calm and nourish the heart and restore sensitivity of feeling. Both Ashwagandha and Shatavari compounds can be used or the Rejuvenative Tonic formula (no. 2).

Fennel is a common spice that promotes healing of hernias; use it also for treating lower abdominal pain and post-surgical digestive disorders. Castor oil packs are also good or just occasional massage with castor oil in milder conditions.

ARTHRITIS

Arthritis is one of the most common chronic and degenerative diseases in the world. Yet, modern medicine has little to offer for treating it except aspirin. In Ayurveda, it is called 'Amavata', a toxic air condition. Arthritis is mainly a Vata (air) disease; it involves pain and weakening of the bones (the main Vata tissue in the body). It can also be divided into types or stages according to the three humors.

Causes include both internal and external factors. Arthritis is more common in windy, damp and stormy climates. It is related to low Agni and poor digestion which causes the accumulation of Ama (toxins). Poor colon function allows the toxins to be taken to the joints. It may also be caused by injury. Arthritis is another auto-immune disorder where the body attacks itself, so much that has been said under allergies is applicable here.

General Treatment

First, it is necessary to burn up the toxins by reviving the digestive fire. Short fasting or hot spicy herbs can be helpful: cayenne, cinnamon, dry ginger, galangal. Hot gemstones such as ruby or garnet set in gold can be used. Care must be taken with these hot remedies, however, where there is fever or inflammation. Avoid damp, heavy, Ama-forming foods and irregular eating habits.

Medicated Sesame Oils

Externally, medicated oils help loosen stiff joints, clear toxins, nourish tissues and relieve pain. The special medicated sesame oils of Ayurveda are excellent in this regard.

Mahanarayan oil, whose main ingredient is shatavari, is excellent for improving flexibility, relieving stiffness and stopping pain. It is good for muscular fatigue, treats varicose veins and nourishes the skin. Hence, it is good for dancers or athletes as well. Narayan oil, whose main ingredient is ashwagandha, is effective for muscular and joint pain. It improves circulation in the lower extremities and helps counter the effects of the aging process. Sahachardi oil, whose main ingredient is sahacharda, is specific to rheumatoid arthritis and is effective where there is muscular atrophy or degeneration of the nerves. These oils should be applied daily with a gentle massage. Chandanbalalakshadi, whose main ingredient is Sandalwood, is cooling and good for Pitta type arthritis.

When these oils are not available, warm sesame oil can be used. We can make our own medicated oils by cooking such herbs in sesame oil (for more information see *Yoga of Herbs* pgs. 82–4).

Sweating therapy with saunas or steam boxes is excellent. A hose is connected to the top of a pressure cooker where special herbs are cooking (typically Dashamula compound). Apply the steam to local areas for more direct treatment (nadi sveda). Diaphoretic, sweat-inducing, herbs can be taken: ephedra, angelica, nirgundi, bay leaves or eucalyptus leaves.

Herbal essential oils, camphor, mint and wintergreen, are good for external application. They can be dissolved in rubbing alcohol or combined with tonic herbs like ashwagandha in medicated sesame oil preparations. Wintergreen contains methyl salicylate and can be used in place of aspirin for pain relief.

Cleansing enemas are helpful (with Dashamula decoction), or daily use of Triphala to cleanse the colon.

Important Ayurvedic anti-rheumatic herbs are guggul, castor oil, turmeric, cyperus, galangal, nirgundi and prasarini. Guggul is most specific for cleansing the bone tissue, strengthening the bones and improving flexibility. Cyperus, an herb also used in Chinese medicine, is now used commonly in Ayurvedic medicine for stopping arthritic pain and contractions. Prasarini and nirgundi possess good analgesic properties for rheumatic pain. Prasarini can be used for abdominal pain also, while nirgundi is a good anti-inflammatory agent.

The most effective Ayurvedic formulas are Triphala guggul, Yogaraj guggul and Mahayogaraj guggul (the latter two contain special minerals). Yet recent clinical studies in India show that the simple guggul itself is as effective as these complex formulas if taken in higher dosages, such as six grams a day. The Antirheumatic formula (no. 13), a modern and purely herbal guggul combination, is excellent.

A good formula with Western herbs can be made with angelica, wild ginger, cinnamon and licorice in equal parts. The herbs can be infused or taken as a powder in one teaspoonful doses with honey (as honey possesses a better cleansing action than sugar, milk or ghee). This formula will work quite well in initial arthritis and is better for Vata or Kapha types. Where more Pitta or inflammation is involved, one or two bitter herbs such as katuka, barberry or golden seal should be added.

Chinese herbs include du huo, qiang huo, ligusticum, Gentiana macrophylla, and Siberian ginseng. Ligusticum is the preferable analgesic. Siberian ginseng is used for chronic and degenerative arthritis.

Additional Western herbs are myrrh, chaparral and yucca.

Differentiation

Vata (air) arthritis involves more pain, which is variable, migrating, throbbing and cutting. It will be relieved by the application of heat and aggravated by the application of cold. The skin is dry or scaly, the joints become stiff and crack, and movement is difficult. Deformation of the bones is more likely to occur. There may be constipation, gas or abdominal distention and lower back pain. Nervousness, anxiety, fear and insomnia are common.

Pitta (fire) type involves inflammation, swelling, and fever or burning sensation. Pain is relieved by cold but aggravated by heat. Symptoms include sweating, loose bowel movements, and irritability.

Kapha (water) type shows as swelling and edema around the joints. Pain will be localized, dull, heavy, and aching. It will be relieved by heat and aggravated by cold and by damp weather. The skin will be oily; there may be congestion in the chest or mucus in the stool.

Specific Treatment

Treatment for Vata type is similar to the general treatment with anti-Vata, anti-Ama, detoxifying diet. Gugguls and medicated sesame oils are the basis of the treatment. Galangal is a special herb for this condition. Where there is degeneration and atrophy of the bones, tonics such as ashwagandha are required; take care, however, that tonics do not increase toxicity (the undigested food mass) by their heavy nature. The colon should be kept clean with castor oil or Triphala.

For Pitta type arthritis, additional bitter herbs along with anti-Pitta diet are indicated. Sandalwood oil or paste, coconut oil or Brahmi oil can be applied to the joints. Cold fomentations or ice packs are helpful. Good herbs are guggul. sandalwood, guduchi, aloe, neem, turmeric, saffron and other bitter tasting antirheumatic herbs such as chaparral. The Antirheumatic formula (no. 13) should be taken with aloe gel.

For Kapha, hot spicy herbs are specifically indicated: cinnamon, ginger, mustard, cayenne, turmeric or the formula Trikatu. Hot herbs, mustard, cayenne, or ginger, can be used in pastes, plasters or in rubbing alcohol. Calamus powder is excellent as a dry massage to the affected area. Mustard oil can be used externally with a little cayenne. Sugar, dairy and oily food must be strictly avoided.

GOUT

Gout is a metabolic disorder in which uric acid is deposited in the cartilages of the joints. In the Ayurvedic view it is a condition similar to arthritis, and many of the remedial measures are the same. The big toe is characteristically involved, becoming swollen and very painful. Gout is called 'Vatarakta' in Sanskrit, meaning Vata (air) in the blood. Treatment is to reduce Vata and cleanse the blood.

Causes include eating food that makes the blood toxic: too much salty, sour and spicy food, too rich, too oily, too hot, or improperly prepared food. Avoid meat, sugar, jellies, pastries, beans, mushrooms, yogurt, pickles, acid fruits, and alcohol. Fresh vegetables may be taken freely; also fresh fruit, rice, wheat, potatoes and milk.

Alterative herbs are used: manjishta, guduchi, guggul, myrrh, neem, sandalwood, vetivert. Aloe gel, preferably with turmeric, is a good home remedy, or the Herbal Febrifuge and Blood Purifier (no. 7). Pinda oil or castor oil can be applied externally. Western herbs are dandelion, red clover, burdock and barberry.

CANCER

In Ayurveda cancer is a disease that often involves all three humors, though it typically starts with a predominance of one. The digestive fire and other Agnis are low, allowing a build-up of toxic substances. The cancer represents a negative life-energy, something like a parasite, which has become established in the body. Negative life-energy usually comes from an excess of Apana, the downward moving air. Hence, Apana disorders such as distention, constipation and diarrhea may be the basis of this condition. Cancer cells, lacking oxygen (prana), represent a growth in the body outside the rule of the life-force.

Cancer has many causes including our toxic environment, devitalized foods, sedentary life-style, and lack of spiritual purpose or effort in life. Its basis often is suppressed emotion or emotional stagnation, which causes accumulation of toxic material, and excess humors. In older Western medicine, it was seen as a disease of melancholy or black bile, which also translates as suppressed emotions. Hence, physical remedial measures are usually not enough to restore health.

In the Vedic system cancer is viewed as a psychic disorder, a disruption in the aura allowing the entrance of a negative astral force. Emotional cleansing, mantra and meditation are important to counter this.

Spiritual Therapies

Gem therapy is helpful; gems are able to balance the aura and protect the life. Blue sapphire set in gold is the best gem for antitumor properties. It helps ward off the negative force invading the body, and should be used with other stones which increase the positive life-force. Diamond is most important for sustaining life and longevity. Diamond, yellow sapphire, and yellow topaz are the best stones for increasing Ojas, the energy of the immune system. Ruby, garnet or red coral can aid in reestablishing proper circulation, which removes the stagnation behind the tumor. Emerald and peridot help increase Prana and relieve pain and disharmony.

Special Ayurvedic diamond preparations (hira bhasma) are particularly useful.

Mantra therapy is excellent for cancer. Simple chanting of Om is excellent for opening up the aura and clearing the psychic air. The mantra, Ram, is best to give protection and bring down the Divine healing force. Hum is effective for casting out negative life-energies. Pranayama is important to increase Prana, the positive life-force, regular solar Pranayama for Kapha, lunar for Pitta, alternating for Vata. Practice of Pranayama is an important cancer preventative.

Differentiation

Vata (air) type cancer involves emotional factors such as fear, anxiety, and depression, and also insomnia. The tumors are dry, hard and variable in appearance. The skin will turn grey, brown or dusky in color. There will be distention, constipation and other high Vata symptoms. Colon cancer is often a Vata type.

In Pitta (fire) type there is anger, irritability, resentment or hatred. The tumors will be inflamed, infected and associated with burning sensation or bleeding. Most forms of skin, eye and liver cancer are of Pitta type.

Kapha (water) type cancer involves tiredness, excess sleeping, congestion and salivation. Usually benign tumors appear first and, over time, become malignant. Surgery is an effective treatment if the cancer is found early enough. Lung or breast cancer is often a Kapha type.

Herbal and Dietary Treatment

The herbal therapies for reducing cancer can be put into several categories:

1. Powerful alterative or blood-cleansing herbs. These herbs destroy toxins, counter poisons and reduce infections. The most famous Western anti-cancer herbs are in this category and some eastern herbs — red clover, dandelion, self-heal, stillingia, burdock, sarsaparilla, Indian sarsaparilla and Chinese oldenlandia.

Such herbs are better if used fresh, and they go well with a detoxifying diet. Dosages of one to three ounces daily may be required. They are useful for lymphatic or skin cancer, and are better for Pitta and Kapha varieties.

2. Strong circulatory stimulants or blood-moving herbs. These herbs promote circulation, break stagnation, reduce masses and aid in the healing of tissues. Herbs used in this way include turmeric and its relative zedoaria, saffron, safflower, myrrh, madder and guggul. Additional Chinese herbs are salvia and spargania.

Good for breast or uterine cancer, liver or pancreas cancer, many of these herbs work on all three humors. Dosages of these herbs need not be that high.

3. Immune strengthening tonics. These include: famous Chinese herbs such as ginseng, astragalus, dang shen, white atractylodes, schizandra, ligustrum; and the Ayurvedic herbs ashwagandha, shatavari, guduchi, bala, shilajit, kapikacchu, and black and white musali. Both Chinese and Ayurvedic herbs of this type have proved their immune strengthening effects in modern clinical studies. Western herbs like American ginseng, comfrey root and solomon's seal, have a similar effect.

These tonics are better in debility conditions, which are usually Vata, and to protect the strength of the patient undergoing stronger therapies, whether herbal, dietary, surgical or chemotherapy. Dosages again must be high, for example an ounce or more per herb per day.

4. Special expectorant or phlegm-dispelling herbs. These include kelp, seaweed, Irish moss and the Ayurvedic bhallatak and Chinese herb fritillary.

They are better for thyroid, neck or lymphatic cancer but can be useful in other types as well. Ayurvedically, they are more for Vata and Kapha cancers.

In addition, many strongly bitter or pungent herbs, with their fat-reducing and toxin-destroying properties, can be useful. These include golden seal, coptis, aloe and katuka (bitter) and cayenne, black pepper, calamus and prickly ash (spicy).

A typical anti-cancer formula combines aspects of all these approaches, varied according to conditions. A good general formula can be made with equal parts turmeric, safflower (or saffron in 1/4 part), manjishta, dandelion, self-heal, sarsaparilla and ashwagandha. It can be taken in strong decoction or 3–6 gms. of the powder three times a day; with honey and black pepper for Kapha, with aloe gel for Pitta and with fresh ginger tea for Vata.

Such herbs taken with a strong anti-Ama or detoxifying diet may reduce tumors, whether malignant or benign, if the tumors are not large, have not metastasized and the patient is still strong.

Meat and dairy products should be strictly avoided, as well as too much protein (the cancer cell itself is pure protein). However, a small amount of protein should be taken to insure the secretion of enzymes to help digest it. Cancer is sometimes seen as a disease of a too-high protein diet or of too much meat. Diet should emphasize raw vegetables and juices such as wheat grass, barley grass, celery, and dandelion, and alfalfa and sunflower sprouts as long as the patient has strength. Raw green juices are full of Prana and help cleanse out any negative life-energy. These naturally cold vegetables should be balanced with spices like ginger and garlic to protect the digestive fire.

If the patient is weak, add tonic herbs to protect the energy and immune system, as mentioned above.

Herbs for cancer in the different humors are:

For Vata — calamus, haritaki, myrrh or guggul and the Triphala formula or Triphala guggul. The colon must be kept clean. Asafoetida 8 is also useful.

For Pitta — saffron, manjishta, dandelion, gotu kola and turmeric. Usually, very strong blood-cleansing therapies, and raw vegetable and juice diets can be applied to Pitta types. The Herbal Febrifuge and Blood Purifier (no. 7) may be helpful, or liver-cleansing therapies and formulas.

For Kapha — cayenne, black pepper, long pepper, bhallatak, dry ginger, guggul, myrrh, turmeric and the Trikatu formula. Strong expectorant approaches are mainly indicated.

Above all, the appropriate Pancha Karma treatment (see section) should be sought.

BLEEDING GUMS
DENTAL PROBLEMS

Swollen or bleeding gums can be treated topically with astringents. Usually it is a Pitta (fire or infectious) condition but may be only a local problem.

Treat by applying astringent herbs to the site. These include alum, alum root, turmeric, catechu, myrrh or Triphala powder. Bitters, such as golden seal or katuka, help by their anti-inflammatory action. The powder is applied several times daily, particularly before sleep. Unfortunately most of these herbs taste bad, so spices like peppermint, spearmint or licorice can be used along with them and aid in their efficacy by helping them penetrate deeper into the gums.

Many Ayurvedic toothpastes and tooth powders exist in India, composed with extracts of astringent herbs. A few of them are already being imported into this country. These rubbed into the gums on a daily basis will effectively prevent or eliminate most gum problems. Millions of dollars in dental work in this country could be saved if we learn this different way of dental hygiene. Rubbing the gums with oils like sesame or coconut is also good for maintaining the tone of the gums. Gum massage is essential for health and longevity of teeth and gums.

If the problem is not just local, usually high Pitta will be the cause and hyperacidity or heat in the liver or stomach will be the provoking factor. This should be treated directly.

For bad breath or bad taste in the mouth many spicy herbs are good, taken as teas, such as thyme, peppermint, cinnamon and cloves. Cloves, wild ginger and prickly ash are good analgesics for toothache. Several drops of the tincture should be applied directly to the site.

8
THE CARE OF CHILDREN
AND THE ELDERLY

Ayurveda considers the proper care of children to be the foundation of the health of a culture. One of its eight main branches is pediatrics. Disease propensity is created by the lack of understanding and care for the unique constitution of the child. An ancient Vedic verse states, "The One God has entered into the mind, born at first, he plays within the child." This Divine Child is worshipped in India as the infant Krishna. All parents were to consider their child as Krishna.

It is important to determine the constitution of your child. An Ayurvedic diet and life-style should be prescribed accordingly. To determine this, you can consult the table at the beginning of the book. The same diet is not good for all children, anymore than the same education is. Without understanding the unique nature of the individual (and that of the child may be different from that of the parent), we are likely to impose a restrictive or inappropriate pattern upon our children. This may make it difficult for them to discover in life who they really are and what their real needs may be. We can also examine childhood as a whole from the Ayurvedic perspective.

THE SEASON OF CHILDHOOD
There are different stages or seasons of human life, each with its particular nature and needs. The age of childhood, being the formative age, is the most important. It is more uniform in different people, races and cultures.

Childhood is the stage of life in which Kapha, the biological water humor, predominates. Water is the formative element, the origin of life and is responsible for growth and development. As children are producing new tissues, new water as it were, they tend to produce more mucus. This indicates poor digestion, which allows phlegm to accumulate rather than new tissue to be built up. For this reason children have more diseases of excess mucus and suffer most from disorders involving the lungs, ranging from the common cold to bronchitis and pneumonia. These are Kapha diseases in Ayurveda. Though children may be individually of any of the three humors, the state of childhood will keep the water humor at a higher concentration. Hence, all children can be treated as Kapha, at least until the age of two, sometimes until the age of five.

DIETARY CONSIDERATIONS FOR CHILDREN

Generally, children should have a bland or even diet, avoiding too many sweets, strong spices, overly sour food, or too much salt. A diet of whole grains and complex carbohydrates promotes a calm and harmonious child. It is easy to pervert the tastes of a child, and such a condition can take years to correct, if ever. Tasty foods, used as a substitute for parental love and care, warp the child's sense of affection.

Yet, children need foods that are building, and most of these increase Kapha. We cannot simply treat children by putting them on a water-decreasing or mucus-reducing diet, as this does not afford them adequate nutrition for growth. In this regard dairy products and sugar are good if taken in the right way. According to the sages of ancient India, milk is an ideal food for children when taken properly and balanced with the right spices.

TAKING OF DAIRY PRODUCTS

For proper growth in children, strongly nourishing foods are needed, including adequate amounts of protein. After mother's milk, the natural food of infants, cow's milk can be taken as the major food of most young children. The main exceptions are those whose culture has not used dairy; they may not genetically possess the enzymes to digest it.

For vegetarians it is helpful to add dairy products to the diet for improving nutrition. Dairy products are good meat substitutes and are equally as strengthening as meat without the negative effects and bad karma of taking an animal's life.

However, dairy products are mucus-forming. This is true not only of milk, but also of cheese and yogurt to a greater degree. Though good foods for children's growth, they are apt to aggravate children's diseases. To counter potential side-effects, they should be prepared properly and taken in the right food combinations.

Most dairy products, particularly milk, do not combine well with other foods. Milk combines poorly with bread, sour fruit, beans, nut, fish or meat. It is usually best taken alone or as a meal in itself. It does combine well with whole grains, however, and sweet fruit like bananas. Yogurt does not combine well with milk, sour fruit or nuts, though it combines better with vegetables and can be taken with meals.

Pasteurized milk is a kind of precooked food. It is devitalized and so more mucus-forming. The best way to take milk is to use raw milk, heat it to the boiling point, which renders it more digestible, and then add mucus-decreasing spices. Such are cardamom, cinnamon, ginger and cloves. Cardamom is perhaps the best. A pinch to one-quarter teaspoon of such spices per cup of warm milk, along with a little honey or raw sugar, not only tastes good but also makes the milk more digestible. To take cold pasteurized milk along with a meal of breads or meats makes a toxic combination.

Warm milk is a good mild sedative to promote sleep. Its calming effect can be increased by preparing it with a little nutmeg (up to 1/4 teaspoon per cup for children). Milk is a mild laxative and while good for constipation, it should be avoided in conditions of diarrhea or loose stool.

The mucus-forming properties of cheese can be reduced by taking it with such spices as cumin, mustard or cayenne pepper. Cheese is the most mucus-forming of dairy products and should not be used in excess.

Yogurt, according to the tradition of Indian use for thousands of years, is best taken with meals, mixed with fresh cucumber and such spices as cumin, coriander, cilantro or cayenne pepper. It is heavy, hard to digest and somewhat constipating (making it good for diarrhea in children). Taken properly, it adds good bacteria to the system and also promotes weight gain (according to Ayurveda, yogurt is not a good food for weight reduction as it is advertised).

Buttermilk is the least mucus-forming of dairy products. The more natural forms of buttermilk, to which little salt has been added, are preferable.

Dairy products, it should be noted, need to be supplemented in the diet with whole grains, like wheat or brown rice, with nourishing fruit, like bananas or papayas, or with complex carbohydrates like potatoes, to afford adequate nutrients for growth.

SUGAR

According to Ayurveda, human beings need a certain amount of sugar for adequate growth, as sugars serve to build the body. White sugar however, is not good, as it is overly refined, a dead or tamasic food, and leaches the minerals out of the body. Jaggery (Gur) is the best form of cane sugar. It is made from the crude syrup and is rich in vitamins and minerals. Other raw or natural sugars are good, like maple syrup, molasses, rice or barley malt and unrefined sugar.

Honey is a very concentrated sugar. It is better used in small amounts as a sweetener or as a medicine. It is excellent with herbs, particularly tonics or expectorants, as it is a good flavoring agent and enhances their effects. But as a food and in cooking (except when the baking temperature is not high), it is harder to digest than sugar and similarly can overstimulate the pancreas.

Sugar, even in the form of fruit or fruit juices, does not combine well with most foods and often causes gas and fermentation. Whenever gas or indigestion exists, it is better to avoid sugar in any form until the problem is taken care of.

Ayurveda recommends a certain amount of raw sugars be given to children, particularly with whole grains or milk. Many such Ayurvedic herbal confections exist using sugar, honey, ghee, nuts and tonic herbs. These are good for the debilitated also.

OILS

A certain amount of oil is necessary in the diet. More is needed by children for purposes of growth. But again, oily foods cause mucus and aggravate many childhood disorders. According to Ayurveda, the best oils for the diet are ghee (clarified butter) and sesame oil. Ghee can be taken as a cooking oil or used like butter. It is regarded as much easier to digest than butter and less mucus-forming.

Oils are also useful in massage (though this is a topic in itself). Giving a warm sesame oil massage to a child calms the nervous system, helps promote sleep and nourishes the skin. Above all, it increases the child's feeling of being nurtured and cared for.

SPICES FOR CHILDREN

Many spices are good for children and help regulate metabolism. Hot spices, however, cayenne, hot chilies and black pepper, should be used with care. They are very drying and can irritate the stomach. The stomach must gradually learn to produce more mucus secretions to deal with them. Warm mildly sweet spices such as ginger, cinnamon, cardamom, coriander and fennel are preferable. Other mild but not sweet spices are turmeric, cumin and basil.

For keeping the system clear of mucus and for improving mental function and sensory acuity, such herbs and spices as basil, thyme, sage, hyssop and mint are good. Spices for relieving colic, gas and distention are fennel, cardamom, cumin and dill. These help stop griping, ease the flow of energy and regulate peristalsis in the colon.

HERBS FOR CHILDREN

Children can benefit from various herbal supplements. In Ayurveda, special tonics for children are prepared, and different companies often have their own proprietary medicines. These not only have good nutritive properties but also help regulate growth hormones. Equivalent-type remedies can be made with herbs available here. For improving growth of bone, teeth and hair, use comfrey root, solomon's seal, marshmallow, American ginseng, licorice and sesame seeds. They are best taken in warm milk, with about a teaspoon of the powder of the herb.

Good Ayurvedic herbs for children include ashwagandha, shatavari, amalaki and bala. Formulas include Ashwagandha compound and the Energy Tonic (no. 2). For improving intelligence in children, calamus is excellent taken in small amounts (1/4 teaspoon) in milk with honey. Gotu kola improves the mind, cleanses the blood, and calms the emotions. Gotu kola is particularly good for children who are hyperactive from excess sugar consumption and poor liver function. The medicated ghees of these two herbs are also good.

Ayurvedic herbal jellies such as Chyavan prash or Brahma rasayan are excellent growth foods for children. In Chinese medicine the famous kidney tonic formula Rehmannia 6, now used mainly for the elderly, was originally devised for promoting growth in children.

The general treatment rule for children is that no strong therapies should be used. For example, cayenne, a very hot herb, and golden seal, a very cold one, should not be used frequently or in large quantities. Herbs which are very reducing, like purgatives such as rhubarb root, or very tonifying such as ginseng, should also be used with discretion. Dosage of herbs is less with the child's age. Infants do well with small amounts, a pinch to a quarter/teaspoon of herbs in teas or milk. Children ages 5 to 10 can take one-quarter to one-half the adult dosage.

Spiritual Therapies

For children's diseases dietary treatment alone is often enough, or as supplemented with mild herbs. It is also important to teach them Yoga at an early age. Their bodies are more supple and postures learned while young can be easily retained throughout life. While meditation is difficult for children, it should still be attempted. It works better if combined with walks, hikes or retreats into nature. Myths, stories and animal forms of the Divine, such as Hanuman, the monkey god in the Ramayana, are important for communicating to the subconscious mind of the child. The natural creative imaginative power of the child should be allowed to flower and be attuned to the symbols of the cosmic mind.

OLD AGE

Ayurveda means literally 'the science of longevity'. Its concern has been not merely to treat disease but to maximize the life span and provide for optimal living. This is not just to give us more time to enjoy the things of this life. It is to allow for a longer incarnation in which spiritual evolution, which requires time and patience, can progress.

In ancient India, the later years were considered the appropriate season of life for spiritual growth, the time when worldly obligations to work and family were completed and when the soul naturally begins to long for the transcendent. Much of the disease or imbalance of our culture comes in our failure to recognize the value of the final stage of life and our inability to offer the elderly the appropriate tools for developing the higher consciousness that is awakening within them. These tools of Yoga and Ayurveda are of special importance to the elderly, providing them the basis for this spiritual climax of their lives. It is important that we endeavor to develop spiritual awareness in our later years, as our last stage of life is what determines the nature of our next incarnation.

Even if our bad habits, smoking or drinking, do not kill us, they create a propensity towards them in future lives. Hence, whatever age we are, it is good to adjust our life style to take care of the physical body in the right way. This will insure that a better way of relating to it will be taken into the next life.

Our elders represent the fruit of our culture and in them we can see the final outcome of our cultural values for good or ill. How we have really lived is reflected in how we age and how we die. Our culture as a whole is adolescent-oriented. Hence, we deprive the elderly of their intrinsic value, placing them under a false standard of youth. It is only natural for us to lose interest in the things of the world as we age — things like sex, money, fame and work — and to develop wisdom, detachment and dis-crimination. This is not a sign of decline but of appropriate growth, as the brilliant color of the autumn foliage or the ripening of fruit. We do not insist that leaves remain green; yet we have little appreciation for the beauty and wisdom of our own season of old age.

Old age is the stage of life dominated by Vata, the biological air humor, and its attributes of coldness, dryness, decay and disintegration. At the same time, as our body weakens and our connection with it grows less, there is space for the development of an awareness beyond it. Typical diseases of old age are Vata disorders: dry and wrinkling skin, constipa-tion, falling of hair or teeth, weakness of the bones, cracking of the joints, arthritis, poor memory, and the failure of hearing and of vision.

Whatever is one's constitution by birth, in old age we have to consider anti-Vata (anti-air) treatment and anti-Vata diet. Oil therapy becomes more important; oil enemas, massage, and external application of oils such as sesame and its medicated forms. Internal use of ghee helps maintain mental clarity. Tonification, rather than reduction therapies, become the primary focus along with tonic herbal foods.

Chyavan prash is the best all-around tonic for maintaining health and youth of tissues. It was originally devised for making the old young again.

Brahma rasayan is excellent for retaining memory and revitalizing the brain cells. When it is not available, gotu kola or gotu kola ghee can be taken. Gotu kola is also perhaps the best herb for improving hearing. For promoting visual acuity, calamus is preferable.

Ashwagandha is the main herb for retaining strength of the bones and joints. It is also good for impotence, premature ejaculation, leucorrhea or urinary incontinence.

Guggul is the best herb for arthritic pain, swelling and cracking of the hands, feet and joints. It normalizes the function of Vata. If it is not available, myrrh tincture can be used.

A good tonic for the bones and joints can be made with such commonly available herbs as comfrey root 2 parts, turmeric 1 part, licorice 1 part and cinnamon 1/2 part. This improves circulation and nourishes the bones. Shilajit is important for maintaining kidney and reproductive system function.

For constipation in the elderly, Triphala is best.

For women, the use of aloe gel on a regular basis preserves vitality and renews the reproductive system. Shatavari is excellent, as is adding small amounts of saffron to these tonic herbs or to milk decoctions.

In Chinese medicine, Rehmannia formulas are given to the elderly: Rehmannia 6 for old age debility plus internal heat (Pitta type), and Rehmannia 8 for additional internal cold (Vata and Kapha type).

Gems are important tools for protecting and extending the life. Yellow sapphire and other Jupiter stones are good for maintaining endocrine function and improving longevity, for wisdom and giving one the power to guide others (a position that naturally belongs to the elderly). Gems for Saturn, blue sapphire or amethyst preferably set in gold, can help prevent or reduce arthritis and cancer.

Yogic postures are important for maintaining flexibility of the joints and for preventing arthritis. Pranayama is helpful in maintaining strength and vitality. Sexual activity should be gradually reduced with age to allow for inner rejuvenation.

PREMATURE BALDING OR GREYING OF THE HAIR

Balding and greying of the hair are part of the aging process. They occur earlier in Pitta (fiery) constitutions, sometimes in the twenties and often in the thirties. They do not necessarily indicate old age or ill health, but can occur as a sign of disease, particularly in women. Balding and greying may be caused by stress, emotional trauma, too much thinking and worrying, sudden blood loss, or excessive sexual activity. Drugs or smoking can also bring it about.

Pitta constitutions have delicate hair with early grey. Pitta type alopecia (balding) often follows blood loss or high fever.

Treatment is anti-Pitta. Anti-Pitta diet is indicated with food that promotes hair growth including milk, almonds, sesame seeds. Herbs for hair growth, as below, should be taken.

Vata (air) type hair loss involves dry skin, anxiety, insomnia, constipation, irregular digestion. It often follows fright or occurs after a severe illness.

Treatment involves anti-Vata diet and herbs. Good foods include onion, garlic, sesame, almonds, dairy, eggs, meat. Good herbs are ashwagandha, bala, amalaki and other tonics.

Warm sesame and other medicated oils should be applied to the head on a regular basis. Nasya (nasal application) of medicated oils should also be given.

Herbs for improving the hair include gotu kola, bhringaraj, amalaki, bakuchi, sandalwood, licorice. These can also be taken in medicated oils (sesame or coconut base). Formulas include Bhringaraj Oil and Brahmi Oil. Chayavan prash also nourishes the hair.

Chinese herbs include he shou wu (fo ti), rehmannia, lycium, ligustrum. Typical Chinese formulas are Shou wu pian and Rehmannia 6.

9
NERVOUS SYSTEM
DISORDERS

The ancients considered nerve impulses to be a kind of wind or air travelling through the body. Vata, the biological air humor, is the energy that moves through the brain and the nerves, controlling both voluntary and involuntary functions. Hence, Vata derangements always involve some weakness, disturbance or hypersensitivity of the nervous system.

Nervous system disorders are called 'Vatavyadhi', Vata diseases, in Sanskrit. They can also be brought on by imbalances of the other two humors. High Pitta (fire) can burn out the nervous system, causing disruption in nerve impulses. High Kapha (water) can clog it.

These disorders are due to obstruction or wrong flow of Prana or nervous energy in the subtle channels. Blockage of flow causes spasms, rigidity, numbness or paralysis. Wrong flow causes tremors and involuntary movements.

In Ayurveda, nervous system disorders are linked with mental disorders; the mind and nerves are directly connected by a system of special channels. Therefore, mental conditions should be examined carefully with any nervous disorder.

Nervous system disorders include such minor problems as insomnia, headache and tremors, major malfunctions like epilepsy or paralysis, and such degenerative nervous diseases as multiple sclerosis and Parkinson's disease, many of which are difficult to treat with Western medicine.

General Treatment

Nervous system diseases can arise either through blockage of nerve impulses or through wasting away of nerve tissue. Flow of nerve energy can be blocked by accumulation of any of the humors, as well as by Ama, the undigested food mass. Emotional or psychological blockage cause nervous diseases as well. Wasting away of nerve tissue can be caused by malnutrition, poor digestion, hyperactivity or blockage of nerve energy over a period of time. Lack of emotional nourishment or mental grounding, or excessive meditational practices are other disease-provoking factors.

For blockage conditions most nervine and antispasmodic herbs work well: they have the power to clear and open the channels. Calamus is an important herb for opening up the flow of nerve impulses and restoring nerve function. Basil, particularly holy basil (tulsi) is cleansing and clearing to the brain and nerves. Other good herbs include bayberry, camphor (in very low dosages, internally), guggul, myrrh, turmeric, bay leaves, and mint.

Gotu kola is important for clearing the nervous system and relieving inflammation. Other good herbs for overheated nerves include skullcap, bhringaraj, passion flower, hops, and betony.

For a general nervine tonic, Kapha (water) constitution individuals can take gotu kola and calamus in equal parts with honey. For Pitta (fire), gotu kola is better alone or with a slight amount of calamus (1/4 or 1/8 that of gotu kola) and taken with ghee. For Vata (air), calamus is preferable, although gotu kola in small amounts can be beneficial (up to equal amounts with calamus), taken with ghee or warm water.

For deficiency or degenerative conditions, such as MS or Parkinson's, tonic herbs and supplementation therapy are generally needed. Ashwagandha is the best herb; it can be combined with gotu kola or calamus, as above. Ashwagandha is also the main Ayurvedic herb for relieving anxiety, which comes with many nervous disorders. Other good tonic nervines are haritaki, guggul, and bala, or nervines such as calamus and gotu kola prepared in ghee or as herbal jellies (Brahma rasayan). For formulas, use the Energy tonic (no. 2) and Brain Tonic (no. 6).

A number of herbs possess special analgesic, or pain-relieving, properties and can be added to formulas to dispel nerve pain. These include the narcotic herbs, marijuana and datura, commonly used in Ayurvedic formulas, and milder herbs such as valerian, camomile, hops, corydalis, cloves, wild ginger, guggul, myrrh, and prasarini.

A good general patent formula for protecting the nervous system is the Brain Tonic (no. 6). For Vata (air) it can be taken with milk and ghee or warm water. For Pitta (fire), with milk and ghee, aloe gel or cool water. For Kapha (water), with honey.

Spiritual Therapies

As the nervous system is very subtle, the spiritual therapies of Ayurveda are also important here. Yoga therapy is an important part of treatment; it is specific to mind, nerve, and bone disorders. Sitting asanas, such as the lotus pose or siddhasana help calm internal wind, but should not be forcefully attempted. Pranayama done correctly is also essential.

Using breathing exercises, the Prana can be directed through the various channels, thereby removing blockages and restoring nutrition.

One Ayurvedic therapy is to plug one of the nostrils, as with a piece of cotton, for a period of days or weeks. This may cause some initial discomfort but it is usually quickly gotten over. Plugging the left nostril is good for conditions caused by cold and is used for nervous disorders where rigidity and lack of movement prevail, as in Parkinson's disease. Plugging the right nostril is best for conditions caused by heat or hyperactivity, as in insomnia or hallucinations. Generally, the flow of the breath will be stronger in the nostril needing to be plugged.

Mantra, meditation and visualizations are important to help guide nerve impulses back along the proper channels. The mantra, Som, is good for nourishing the nerves in wasting or long-term debilitating nervous disorders. The mantra, Sham, calms the nerves. Om itself is very effective for clearing and calming the nervous system.

Gems have strong action on the subtle level of the nervous system. A number of gems strengthen nerve function and relieve pain. Most important are those for Mercury, the planet of the nerves — emerald, jade or peridot. Those for Jupiter, ruling hormonal function, are also important — yellow sapphire, yellow topaz or citrine. Pearl, for the moon, has a calming and nurturing effect on the mind and emotions. Gold stimulates the nerves and revives function; silver calms the nerves and builds substance.

The colors of these gemstones can be used for color therapy: green (mercury) for stopping pain, gold (jupiter) for strengthening the nerves, white (the moon) for calming hypersensitivity.

General Treatment

Lowering high Vata (air) is the focus, as this is the underlying vitiated humor. Special anti-Vata herbs or an anti-Vata diet may have to be taken temporarily, even by other constitutions. Sleep, rest, relaxation or meditational retreat are often helpful.

Special emphasis is on medicated oils given externally, along with massage, as the nerves can be nourished through the skin. Simple sesame oil or almond oil can be used, or a medicated sesame oil such as Mahanarayan. For calming the nerves, oil application to the head is best; like applying an essential oil like sandalwood to the forehead. For stimulating the nerves, such essential oils as camphor, musk, myrrh, and frankincense are useful applied to the temples. Nasal application of herbs is also important; for example, take several drops of gotu kola or calamus ghee morning and night.

INSOMNIA

Insomnia is our most typical sign of nervous distress. Frequent insomnia is most commonly a Vata (air) disorder involving nervousness, anxiety, ungroundedness, hypersensitivity, and excess thought and worry. Sleep patterns include: difficulty in falling asleep, sleep easily disturbed, and difficulty in returning to sleep, once awakened. Dreams may be frightening, filled with flying, falling, nightmares, encounters with ghosts, etc.

Causes of insomnia include stress, anxiety, excessive thinking, taking of drugs or stimulants, too much travel, overwork and other Vata increasing factors.

General Treatment

Diet should be anti-Vata, emphasizing heavy or grounding foods. These include dairy, whole grains and root vegetables. Coffee, tea and other stimulants, including stimulant herbs such as ma huang or ginseng, should be avoided. Warm milk with a little nutmeg can be taken an hour before sleep. Mental activity should be avoided in the evening, including reading, listening to loud music, watching stimulating movies, etc. Sleep hours should be adjusted, so that one retires early (around 11 p.m.) and rises early (by 6 a.m.). Warm sesame oil can be applied to the feet, the top of the head or forehead, or to the whole body, followed by a warm shower.

Yoga asanas should be done, but no aerobic exercises. A calming meditation before sleep consciously releasing all the worries and tensions of the day can work wonders. Surrendering the mind to the Divine, giving complete faith to the Divine will to take care of oneself and the world is a good part of this. The bed and the sleeping room should be a place of peace, comfortable, clean, and well kept. Peace-inducing mantras such as Ram or Sham can be repeated. The mind should be concentrated on the breath or centered in the heart.

Important Ayurvedic herbs are gotu kola, nutmeg, jatamansi, valerian, and ashwagandha. Formulas include Ashwagandha compound, Saraswat powder, the Brain Tonic (no. 2) or the Herbal Sedative (no. 14), taken with ghee. A good formula can be made with 2 parts ashwagandha, 2 parts valerian, 1 part nutmeg and 1 part licorice. For chronic insomnia, take 3–6 gms. with warm milk and ghee or with water before bed.

Chinese medicine uses heavy mineral sedatives such as dragon bone and oyster shell for more severe insomnia. Heart-nourishing sedatives, zizyphus seeds and biota seeds, are for milder conditions and safer for long-term usage. Formulas include Bupleurum and Dragon Bone or Zizyphus combination.

Western herbs are valerian, skullcap, betony, hops, passion flower, and camomile. One to two teaspoons of valerian powder in a cup of warm water is usually effective in mild conditions. Skullcap and other cooling nervines are more helpful taken with the warmer ones, nutmeg or valerian, as their cold and light nature in excess can aggravate Vata.

Pitta (Fire) Type

Pitta insomnia involves turbulent emotions, irritability, anger, jealousy, resentment, and hatred. It may follow argument, or stress or be part of a febrile disease or infectious condition. Dreams may be dramatic, violent, argumentative and sleep disturbing. Sleep is agitated and broken, but one is usually able to fall back to sleep.

Causes include unresolved emotions, excessive willfulness, over-eating of hot or stimulant foods, exposure to sun and heat, etc. It may be brought on or aggravated by fever.

Diet should be anti-Pitta, avoiding all spices, stimulants, and too much sour food or salt.

Ayurvedic herbs are gotu kola, bhringaraj, jatamansi, aloe, and shatavari. Formulas include Brahmi compound or Sarasvat powder, as well as most of the formulas for Vata. Bhringaraj or Brahmi oil can be applied to the feet or the top of the head. Sandalwood is excellent.

Western herbs include skullcap, betony, hops, and passion flower. Skullcap and passion flower in equal parts is often effective. Valerian may aggravate the condition.

Kapha (Water) Type

Kapha tends towards excess sleep, so insomnia is seldom a problem unless the other humors are out of balance. It sometimes occurs as a congestive disorder. In this case calamus, nutmeg, valerian or such simple hot spices as ginger or the formula Trikatu are sufficient.

HEADACHE
MIGRAINE

Headache can be due to many causes: indigestion, constipation, colds and flus, poor posture or muscle tension. As a nerve pain condition, it is placed here, though it could go in other categories as well. Migraine, a more severe type headache, is often related to congenital factors.

Headaches often relate to hypertension and the increased pressure in the head. Many of the treatments for hypertension are helpful.

Differentiation

Headache is another more common Vata (air) disorder. Vata headache is characterized by extreme pain, anxiety, depression, constipation, and dry skin. It is aggravated by lack of sleep, irregular diet, excessive activity, and mental stimulation, worry and stress.

Pitta (fire) headache symptoms are burning sensation, red face and eyes, sensitivity to light, anger, irritability, and sometimes nose bleeds. It is often associated with liver disorders or toxic blood conditions.

Kapha (water) type is more a dull headache with feelings of heaviness and tiredness. There may be nausea, phlegm, excess salivation or vomiting. It is usually caused by congestion of phlegm in the head and may be associated with pulmonary disorders.

Treatment

For sinus and congestive headaches, those associated with common cold, cough or allergies (usually Kapha or Vata), decongestant and expectorant herbs are used: calamus, ginger, bayberry, angelica, wild ginger. Calamus powder can be snuffed or calamus ghee applied to the inner nose. The former is better for Kapha, the latter for Vata. Basil, particularly holy basil (tulsi) is excellent as a tea. Ginger paste can be applied to the lower nose and temples. Helpful essential oils for external application are camphor, wintergreen or eucalyptus.

Purgation is useful, as in all nervous disorders the colon is the main site of the problem. Vata type headaches benefit from Triphala as a purgative. Useful herbs include valerian, jatamansi, camomile, calamus and gotu kola. The formula Sarasvat powder is good. Adequate sleep is essential, so herbal sedatives are indicated.

Pitta benefits from aloe powder or rhubarb root as a purgative. The liver should also be cleansed. Gotu kola is excellent by itself or with passion flower or as Gotu kola compound. Sandalwood oil should be applied to the head. Sun and heat should be avoided; cool walks in the moonlight and flower fragrances like rose or lotus are good.

Kapha does well with formulas such as Trikatu or Clove combination. Camphorated oils can also be applied to the head. Strong exercise is often helpful.

The herbal Brain Tonic (no. 6) is useful for all these conditions, with honey for Kapha, ghee for Pitta and Vata.

Migraine headache is usually due to Pitta (fire) and Vata (air). Causes include lack of sleep, overwork, stress, poor digestion or muscular tension. It can be treated as above, but long-term tonification therapy is usually needed, with Chyavan Prash, Brahma rasayan or Ashwagandha compound.

Premenstrual headaches can be treated as under 'Dysmenorrhea'.

EPILEPSY

Epilepsy can be caused by any of the humors. In Kapha (water) types it is phlegm blocking the channels. In Pitta (fire) types it is related to nerve inflammation. For Vata (air) types it is due to hypersensitivity. Much of the treatment is as per constitution, as it is a constitutional problem.

Purgation therapy is helpful and can prevent seizures. The best purgative is castor oil, which is generally the best laxative for nervous system disorders. Triphala is also good.

Nervines such as Gotu kola compound or Brahma rasayan are excellent. Calamus, with ashwagandha, is good for Vata (with ghee) and by itself for Kapha (with honey). Chyavan prash is useful tonic between attacks. Sesame oil can be applied to the feet.

Most other tremor or seizure conditions can be treated similarly, and as per balancing the nervous system and mind.

EYE DISEASES

The eyes relate to Pitta (fire) as an organ of perception. Pitta types are often sensitive to light, prefer sunglasses and are more likely to need prescription glasses than other types. Most inflammatory diseases of the eyes, such as conjunctivitis, are Pitta disorders and treated like infectious diseases (see section).

As we age our vision and other sensory acuity tends to decrease. Increased Vata (air) causes us to gradually lose these functions. Vision can also be damaged by debilitating diseases, particularly those of the liver.

Staring at a ghee lamp is very important to improve vision. A wick of cotton or other material is placed in a small vessel with ghee. One should fix one's gaze upon it for twenty minutes daily. This is helpful for treating photophobia or photophobic headaches.

Ghee itself is the most important food for the eyes and, taken 1–2 tsps. twice a day, can improve vision. The older the ghee, the better its properties. Triphala ghee is a special medicine for the eyes. It can be used in infectious conditions but also as a general tonic.

Triphala itself can be used externally as a wash for inflamed eyes. Camomile, chrysanthemum, and rose flowers are also good eye washes for pain, irritation or inflammation. The cool infusion should be put in the eye with an eye dropper. Aloe gel or ghee can be applied to the eye lid. A paste of mung bean flour is also very soothing to the eyes. Never put essential oils or spicy herbs into the eyes. A good tonic food for the eyes is Chyavan prash, since amalaki, its main ingredient, nourishes the eyes.

Many other anti-Pitta formulas are good for improving vision. The common formulas, Sudarshan powder and Mahasudarshan powder, mean literally 'the formula for good vision' and 'the great formula for good vision'. These formulas are mainly bitter herbs as bitter taste helps cool and cleanse the eyes.

Cleansing of the eyes can also be brought about by crying. A little onion juice can be applied to the eye for this purpose. Crying also helps cleanse the nerves, the liver and the blood. Crying is a natural therapy, another route for dispelling toxins. Suppressing emotions and not crying can cause a build up of subtle toxins.

Gem therapy is an important treatment for the eyes. The right eye is the Sun and the left eye is the Moon. The gemstones for these planets help improve vision. Pearl set in silver is good for dry or inflamed eyes, photophobia, which are Vata and Pitta (fire and air) conditions. Ruby set in gold is good for lack of visual acuity, turbidity, and congestion in the eyes, and such Kapha and Vata (water and air) conditions. When these two stones are not available, moonstone and garnet can be used as substitutes. Diamond (or another Venus stone) is also good for the eyes and gives better perception of colors.

10
CONDITIONS INVOLVING THE MIND
MENTAL DISORDERS
MEDITATIONAL DISORDERS
AND ADDICTIONS

MENTAL DISORDERS
Physical and Psychological Treatment

Disease usually involves an underlying psychological or emotional imbalance. Most physical diseases result from psychological factors. We are often unable to give proper care to our bodies, because we are preoccupied with our psychological or emotional problems.

As a general rule in treatment, psychological factors tend to outweigh physical factors. A patient may have the right diet and herbs, but if the mental state is agitated or there is a negative attitude about the treatment, it will not likely be effective.

Ayurveda, as a holistic system, treats mental disorders from mild stress to severe conditions, including insanity. It has methods for enhancing mental, as well as physical, well-being. For the healing of the mind, it employs a whole series of Yogic and spiritual therapies, including meditation, pranayama, mantra, prayer, visualizations, and rituals called 'spiritual therapy' (daiva cikitsa). This is an extensive science in itself. We can only present the fundamentals of it here.

Ayurveda also employs its regular physical healing means and modalities to treat mental conditions. Physical imbalance can cause, or at least aggravate, mental imbalance. Moreover, a pattern of imbalance on the mental level, with disturbed thoughts and emotions, is usually reflected and reinforced on a physical level.

The Role of the Astral Body

According to Ayurveda and occult science, behind the gross physical is a subtle or astral body composed of the life-force, emotions and thoughts. The astral is a subtle form or underlying energy pattern of the physical, from which the physical is produced. In our waking life, we experience the astral through the physical, through our psychological states. In the dream state, the astral is free to function on its own, and we can experience it directly through conscious dreaming. There is a plane of existence, an astral universe, which we can experience through the astral body. This experience can be developed through Yoga and other occult techniques. However, it is not considered a major spiritual attainment, as all the drives of the ego still operate in the astral, sometimes inflated.

Just as there are channels in the physical body through which fluid and energy flow, so there are channels in the astral body (the emotional body) through which the life-force and emotions flow. These are the nadis, or subtle channels, which run from the different chakras, the energy centers of the astral body. Disruption of flow of these energies causes psychological disease, as disruption in the channels of the physical body causes physical disease. Our mental energy can stagnate or move in the wrong direction, resulting in various forms of misapprehension and confusion. It is important, therefore, to keep these subtle channels pure. This is one of the main purposes of Pranayama, Yogic breathing practices. Certain subtle herbs such as calamus, basil, turmeric, guggul, bayberry and camphor can help, as well as the use of incense: camphor, myrrh, frankincense and cedar.

Moreover, there are channels and energy fields connecting the physical and astral bodies, reflected in the aura. When these are disrupted, the coordination between body and mind is weakened, and mental disease can occur.

There is a shield between the astral and physical bodies protecting the physical from astral forces. When this breaks down, we can no longer discriminate between the physical and the astral, between our actual sensory perceptions and our thoughts, fantasies and emotions. When this link becomes weak, other astral influences (which may be entities from that plane or just emotional influences of the people or environment around us) can take temporary control of our physical body. We may do things we do not really wish to do, such as harming others.

According to Ayurveda, modern psychology is not yet a mature science of the psyche; it does not understand the forces of these subtle planes. It tends to treat psychological problems as personal issues. Ayurveda sees them as the imbalance of energies on an inner level. Psychological energies are woven into the whole of the collective consciousness, often with cosmic ramifications such as astrological influences. Ayurveda focuses more on providing practical tools for correcting imbalances than on analyzing the particular configuration of the imbalance in terms of personal experience.

Causes of Mental Disorders

Mental disorders are as diverse and variable as the mind itself. They are caused by emotional stress, trauma, poor upbringing, repressive religion, coming under the influence of disturbed individuals, sexual abuse or perversion, and taking of drugs. They can be brought on by excess thinking or by strain in Yogic or meditation practices. Naively opening up to the influences of the astral plane, through various occult methods, can cause mental imbalances.

As a culture, we are becoming connected with the astral plane again. As is to be expected at first, it has been mainly lower astral, the influence of the mass media, sexual liberation, and the use of mind-altering drugs. New interest in channeling, shamanism and the occult is developing. This can bring us new knowledge and is a necessary stage in the evolution of the human mind, but it can create mental disorders that are difficult to treat. Once we have opened up our minds to astral forces or entities, they have a connection with us, a power over us, which cannot be simply eradicated by the power of will or by physical methods.

The Place of Sattva (Purity of Mind)

In Ayurveda, mental disorders are caused by a vitiation of sattva; that is, by a disturbance of the inherent clear quality of the mind. This occurs through excess rajas and tamas, turbulence and darkness in the mind. Too much rajas involves excess of anger, hatred and fear, excessive nervousness, worry, and anxiety. Too much tamas involves excess sleep, dullness, apathy, inertia and the inability to perceive things as they are.

Modern society is excessively rajasic. We are constantly moving, travelling, taking on new stimulations, on the go. We are always preoccupied with one thing or another, working, playing, entertaining ourselves. We have little time for peace, silence and meditation, or for heart-to-heart communication with each other.

According to the system of Yoga, sattva, the essence of the mind, can only be truly renewed in silence. It is worn out by mental activity, including intellectual or philosophical thinking. Most of our relaxation today involves entertainment, movies, television or watching sports. These are a kind of passive mental activity that still wears out the mind. We have lost most of the sattvic mental pursuits of traditional cultures such as prayer, meditation, chanting and selfless service, which, though often turned in a dogmatic or sectarian direction, still were able to nourish the heart for those who were truly receptive. We are lacking in love, faith, openness and peace. With our agitation and distraction comes mental stress or psychological disease.

Psychological unrest is a sign of lack of connection with the soul, the source of our creative life-force and our joy. It usually occurs because we have forgotten our soul's purpose in incarnation; because we are not following a religious or spiritual path that brings us peace.

MENTAL DISORDERS AND THE BIOLOGICAL HUMORS
Vata (Air) Type

Mental, like nervous, disorders are more often due to high Vata (high air), which, as the nervous force, also governs the mind. The mind is composed of air and ether. Vata's excess of air causes instability in the mind. It involves increased rajas, a disturbed, agitated, excessively thinking nature, which causes lack of control and internal hypersensitivity. Too much exposure to the mass media, loud music, taking of drugs or stimulants, excessive exercise, overwork, excessive or unnatural sexual activity all tend to make Vata hyperactive, thus creating a predisposition for mental disturbance. Misguided meditation and excessive practice of Pranayama can also aggravate Vata.

High Vata, as excess ether, makes us ungrounded, spaced out and unrealistic. It tends to weaken our connection with the physical body, thereby disrupting our harmony with the physical world. We live too much in our thoughts; these then take the place of reality and disperse our life-force. Fear, anxiety, unrest and rapid shifts of mood begin to occur. Insanity or schizophrenia is the extreme form of this condition.

Pitta (Fire) Type

Pitta psychological disorders are also due to too much Rajas; but it is directed outwardly, against other people. There is aggression, ambition and anger. Typical Pitta is the overly critical type who cannot see any other view of things but his own. We blame other people for everything, see enemies everywhere, and are always on guard and ready for a fight. We are even often at war with ourselves and our past.

Kapha (Water) Type

Kapha psychological unrest involves excessive Tamas. There is too much sleeping, sleeping during the day, day dreaming, attachment to the past, with dullness and lethargy. The mind may be incapable of any abstract, objective or impersonal thinking. There is a lack of drive and motivation along with passivity and dependency. We want to remain a child and to be taken care of. We become preoccupied with what others think about us. We are lacking in proper self-image and tend to passively reflect our immediate environment.

Treatment of Psychological Unrest

Mild mental disorders, what we call 'neurosis', is indicated here. Such mental imbalance does not generally prevent us from functioning but makes our lives unhappy, much like a chronic disease. It is a condition that we can still treat on our own.

Treatment of psychological unrest first involves restoring Sattva, the natural clear quality of the mind. This involves a Sattvic diet (see section), being careful not to aggravate the constitutional humor in the process. Fruit harmonizes the mind, whole grains strengthen the mind, dairy products nourish the heart, ghee nourishes the nerve tissue.

Sattvic life-style should be followed (see section), again with due regard to one's constitution. Preferably, this includes arising early in the morning, 4–7 am. and practicing Yoga, asana, pranayama, mantra and meditation. Even thirty minutes of silent meditation or chanting can be very helpful if done on a regular basis.

Sattvic qualities such as faith, love, compassion, honesty and truthfulness should be cultivated. We should practise self-examination and self-inquiry. Or we can open up to the Divine in whatever form is dear to our heart, and engage in some sort of service work for the benefit of humanity, ceasing to focus on our personal unfulfillment.

Application of oils to the head is calming and nourishes the mind. Heavy fatty oils are best for sedation and to aid in sleep — sesame oil for Vata (air) and coconut oil for Pitta (fire). These can be combined with nervine herbs, gotu kola in coconut oil for Pitta (called Brahmi Oil), or ashwagandha in sesame oil for Vata.

Essential oils such as sandalwood are good to promote calm and peace. Basil, myrrh, frankincense, sage or mint will help clear the channels and promote perception.

Oils can be applied warm to the forehead (to improve perception), to the top of the head (to give greater intelligence), or to the base of the neck (to calm the unconscious).

Oils can also be applied to the nose, to directly influence the brain. Calamus ghee is best applied this way for clearing purposes (for Kapha and Vata). Gotu kola ghee is also good for calming (for Pitta and Vata).

Enemas are important for Vata conditions. Use sesame, a calming oil, or mind-nourishing herbs such as ashwagandha or haritaki.

For calming the mind and improving the psychic atmosphere, incense is important, used much like essential oils. Sandalwood is the best and most harmonizing incense. Burning of camphor or cedar cleanses the psychic environment. Myrrh and frankincense cleanse the aura and purify the air. Rose calms and nourishes the heart, as does lotus. Jasmine cleanses the emotions and increases love and compassion. Gardenia purifies the heart.

Flower remedies are helpful in this way — not only the fragrances but having the flowers around for their influence on the heart. Certain plants in the house help improve the psychic as well as the physical atmosphere. These include aloe and basil (tulsi).

Color therapy is also important. White gives peace and purity. Blue gives peace and detachment. Gold gives discrimination. Green gives harmony, balance and healing energy. Gems for the mind include pearl or moonstone to calm emotions; emerald which gives balance and equanimity; yellow sapphire or topaz to increase wisdom; and red coral which calms anger.

Ayurvedic herbs for improving Sattva (the mind) are gotu kola, calamus, holy basil (tulsi), bhringaraj, shankhapushpi, haritaki, sandalwood, ashwagandha, and guggul. They are best prepared in ghee or taken with it. Sarasvat powder is good for all types, as is the Brain Tonic (no. 6). Take these herbs with ghee for Pitta, with milk for Vata, or with honey for Kapha.

Best preparations are: Ashwagandha for Vata; gotu kola (brahmi) for Pitta; and calamus, for Kapha. These herbs work better if taken with ghee or as medicated ghees.

Chinese herbs for improving the state of the mind are mainly herbs to nourish the heart such as zizyphus, biota seeds or schizandra.

Western herbs for improving mental function include sage, bayberry, cedar, myrrh, skullcap, and camomile. Sage is good for Kapha, skullcap for Pitta, camomile for Vata. Tinctures of these herbs are preferable, as the alcohol helps draw their effects into the brain.

Herbs to nourish the heart and promote positive emotions may also be necessary. These include shatavari, saffron, rose, lotus and licorice, particularly as prepared in milk decoction. They are good for balancing negative Pitta (fiery) emotions and for calming Vata (airy) sensitivity. Formulas include Shatavari compound.

Other, more specifically nervine and sedative herbs, can be used for calming the mind. Be aware, however, that many of these have long-term Tamasic or dulling properties. Such herbs include valerian, nutmeg, passion flower, hops, and asafoetida.

INSANITY

Insanity occurs when the mental unrest is so severe that an individual is unable to function in physical reality. It is the ultimate result of neurosis or mental disturbance. Yet, some of what is called insanity may be a higher state of consciousness or a consciousness outside of social norms. According to Ayurveda and Vedanta, all of us, save the enlightened, are caught in an underlying ignorance and false perception of life. Our whole ego is an illusion. Each culture has its basic social illusion as well, so that what is sanity, and what is not, is often not as fixed as we would like to think.

Often, there are physical imbalances involved with insanity. Toxic poisoning, malnutrition, trauma and other factors may cause or aggravate it.

Differentiation

Vata (air) type insanity is characterized by excessive singing, laughing, weeping, loss of memory, incoherent talk, erratic gestures, and sometimes loss of motor function control. The individuals are usually emaciated, dry and of Vata constitution. Emotionally, they are dominated by fear, anxiety and depression. They suffer from insomnia and nightmares.

Pitta (fire) type insanity is characterized by anger and violence. There are often delusions of grandeur and power with an inflated sense of ego. Such individuals are usually very fiery, proud and contentious, wanting to impose their will on everyone. They have paranoid fantasies and feel they are oppressed by great enemies, the government or the police.

Kapha (water) type insanity is characterized by dullness, lethargy, sentimentality, attachment to the past or childhood, dependency on the parents (particularly the mother), trying too hard to please people, feeling unloved and not cared for. The individual is usually overweight and often addicted to sugar.

Treatment

Treatment is similar to mental unrest, but often stronger sedative substances have to be used. Pancha Karma is very important, as it is a stronger method.

For Vata type, nourishing and sedating herbs are required, especially ashwagandha and its various preparations. Sarpagandha, Rauwolfia serpentina, is an important Ayurvedic herb for mental disorders. From it is derived some of the chemical drugs used to treat insanity today. Other good herbs include valerian, guggul, jatamansi and calamus. Oil enemas are helpful, as above.

For Pitta type purgation, even with strong purgatives, is often helpful. The more violent the type, the more purgation is indicated. Good herbs for this include rhubarb root, senna and aloe. Gotu kola is generally the best herb; others are bhringaraj, sandalwood and passion flower. Shatavari is good for promoting sense of love and compassion and is better for weaker Pitta types.

For Kapha, spicy brain-stimulant herbs are indicated. The treatment is mainly expectorant, to clear phlegm from blocking the channels and obstructing mental functioning. Important herbs are calamus, basil, bayberry, sage, myrrh, and guggul, which have good expectorant action. Formulas include Trikatu with ghee or Calamus ghee.

POSSESSION

In most ancient cultures mental disorders were often attributed to various kinds of possession — by ghosts or evil spirits — and some sort of exorcism was prescribed. Ayurveda also shares this view but in a more sophisticated way, through the knowledge of Yoga. This view is not a naive superstition but reflects the Ayurvedic scientific knowledge of the astral plane and occult worlds. Our physical world is intimately linked up with subtler worlds, and there is a constant interplay of energies between these different dimensions. Forces from these planes can affect us in both positive and negative ways.

Ayurveda distinguishes different forms of possession, according to the entities involved.

Possession is most common in individuals who are too passive, dependent, vulnerable, open and impressionable. There is often low self-esteem, an extreme sensitivity and a capacity to take on the influences of the environment. The aura is usually weak and the sense of self is not well-defined.

Possession can also occur with groups, as in mob actions, and can affect whole countries, like Germany under the Nazis. We must respect these subtle forces, learn to recognize them, and learn to ward off their negative effects. Otherwise we are like children in the dark, and can bring upon ourselves many negative experiences that are not necessary. It is here that astrology is particularly important, giving us a picture of the astral forces at work in our lives.

General Treatment

Treatment of possession is similar to that for mental disorders and insanity but more specific exorcising methods should be used. These include chanting, incense, bells, and calling upon protective deities. Various demon-destroying deities exist in the Hindu tradition, including Durga, Rama, and the terrible form of Shiva known as Rudra. Durga is the wrathful form of the Divine Mother. Rama is the Divine Son as the protector, warrior and hero. Rudra is the terrible form of the Divine Father.

The Buddhists, particularly the Tibetans, have their demon destroyers also. But any divine power can help in clearing out negative forces in our psyche, whichever form of the Divine is closest to our heart.

Differentiation

Possession is more commonly a Vata disease, as Vata (air) types tend to be more dissociated from physical reality or the physical body. They often have low energy, so more easily come under a stronger force. Vata-type possession is most dominated by fear.

Pitta (fire) type possession usually arises from too much wrath in the nature. One is taken over by an entity that appeals to pride, ambition and power (see Asuric possession).

Kapha (water) type possession usually comes from excess sentimentality and attachment. Often souls who have died but are unwilling to leave earth, owing to excessive attachment, are able to enter us.

Poessession by Gods

The gods here are the lesser deities of the midastral world, not the truth principles of our higher pure awareness. These lesser gods enjoy a life of play, beauty, and drama in a world of vibration, color and delight. We contact their energy in the aesthetic part of the mind.

They possess human beings for the purpose of play. They do not harm their victims directly; in fact they may provide them with knowledge or inspiration. Many mediums and channels are possessed by gods and find the experience exhilarating.

According to Ayurveda and Yoga, however, any form of possession is dangerous. Possession by the gods also aggravates Vata, weakening our connection with our own soul. It can cause such Vata disorders as insomnia, arthritis or premature aging.

The gods do not like garlic and can be driven away by it. Other good herbs are nutmeg, valerian, asafoetida. They can be removed by opening up to higher Divine forces. Generally, we have to take control of our own minds and follow an appropriate life-regime.

Possession by Ghosts

Many souls are overly attached to the physical world. Death may be sudden, so it may be hard for them to pass on. Such entities can continue their stay on the earth plane by becoming connected with the living.

Calamus is a special Ayurvedic herb for clearing the effects of ghosts from the mind. Calamus ghee is good, or calamus enemas. Holy basil also cleanses our psychic environment and connects us with the immanent

Divine power (Vishnu). Clearing incense such as camphor is helpful as is the use of bells.

Remove any stagnant air in the house. Attics or basements should be cleared of old possessions and have fresh air brought in. Negative psychic entities usually require some negative air space to live in.

Consciously direct the entity away, sending it on to its next life, telling it that its fulfillment is only possible in a new birth.

Possession by Demons (Asuras)

Human life has been described as a war between the Devas and Asuras, the gods of light and the demons of darkness. The Asuras are always trying to enter into and influence human life. They run the underworld, encourage crime, and are behind most wars. Their purpose is to block human evolution, to keep us ignorant of our true spiritual nature; they serve to make us weak in our inner purpose.

This is the most dangerous form of possession. The Asuras cause the more violent forms of insanity, including psychosis. They can enter into us in a state of excess anger, hatred and fanaticism which causes us to lose self-control.

This is largely a Pitta (fire) condition and treatment is similar to Pitta mental problems. Love and forgiveness are important.

Purgation is helpful. Gotu kola with ghee is the best herb for this condition.

Mantras

'Hum' (pronounced as in our word 'whom') is the best mantra for driving off the Asuras. It is a special fire mantra and sound of Divine wrath that relates to Shiva. It can neutralize all negativity. It is also useful for warding of ghosts. But one must be pure to use it, as it will also attack any negativity that may be inside us.

'Ram' is the best mantra for giving the protection of the Divine light. It opens up our aura to the guiding intelligence of the Creator and closes it off to the lower influences of the astral plane. It is good in all mental and psychic diseases and is totally safe.

POSSIBLE SIDE-EFFECTS OF CHANNELING

Channeling is a very complex phenomena and, though it may offer us much, does have possible side-effects. Whenever we allow another entity to work through our minds, we are risking both physical and mental health.

On a physical level we have to die a little. We have to weaken the hold of our own life-force on our mind in order to let another being work through it. On a psychological level we tend to lose control of our emotional energy.

Channeling, in general, will aggravate Vata (air). Those of this constitution should be especially careful. Long-term Vata disorders including arthritis, insomnia, epilepsy or paralysis may occur. Jane Roberts, who started the whole channeling movement with her channeling of Seth, died at a relatively young age of rheumatoid arthritis, a typical Vata disorder. Ayurveda would tend to think that it was caused by her practice.

Channeling can have as many health risks as smoking and the taking of drugs. It may take a number of years for these to manifest. Those who practice channeling may notice certain disorders after a period of time.

One consideration for channelers is: unconsciousness during channeling is likely to have a damaging effect on the body and mind. If we retain our awareness, this is less likely to occur. On a physical level, it is better to be Kapha (water) types. Some weight will keep us grounded. Those who are emaciated, malnourished, with irregular appetite and lack of physical strength, face more danger.

When channeling becomes a problem, it can generally be treated under mental disorders, and specifically under possession.

Blue stones such as amethyst or blue sapphire are good for keeping any negative influences away, particularly when set in gold. Hessonite garnet is a good stone for protecting the aura.

MEDITATIONAL DISORDERS

Meditation properly practiced helps cure both physical and mental diseases. Most forms of meditation are safe; wrongly practiced, however, or done with strain, they can damage both body and mind. True meditation develops peace and the release of tension and anxiety. False meditation is indicated by restlessness, conflict and negative imaginings.

In both Ayurvedic and Tibetan medicine, cultures where a great deal of meditation is commonly practiced and often with great effort, a whole series of meditational diseases are recognized. Such disorders are not so common in the West, but with the new and sometimes naive practice of meditational techniques, we are beginning to see them here as well. Of course, Western medicine does not have a lot to offer in their treatment, as its understanding of the process of meditation is limited.

Meditation works to make the mind more subtle, which often results in the creation of more space, more ether in the mind. This mainly causes various Vata (air) disorders, and most meditational diseases are of this humor. Both symptoms and treatment are as for nervous system diseases.

Some meditation practices involve sensory deprivation. This will produce certain experiences, often colorful visions, but they may be artificial. Other practices involve sleep deprivation. These will also produce experiences, usually of a dream nature. They will tend to aggravate Vata, however. One should not confuse a Vata (high air) deranged fantasy or abnormal energy movement with spiritual awareness.

According to Yoga and Ayurveda, meditational practices should be done naturally, through our own aspiration. What we produce through harsh or forceful methods is more likely to have side effects. The mind is capable of any illusion; we should not put ourselves in positions that may artificially stimulate these.

Pranayama Disorders

Pranayama is harmonization of the breath. It often involves efforts at breath control or efforts at increasing the energy of the breath. Excessive straining at breath control can aggravate Vata (air). Exhalation or inhalation may be suppressed, thus deranging the whole flow of energy in the nervous system.

It is important, therefore, that in breathing practices one should not use force to hold the breath. The goal is not just to stop breathing; that can kill us. It is to calm the breath, and this requires peace of mind.

It is also important that in holding our breath we do not forget to breathe. For this reason, some Yoga teachers recommend retention after exhalation rather than after inhalation. Morever, we should not confuse the energy of hyperventilation, which may be brought on by rapid breathing, with spiritual awareness.

The more energetic forms of Pranayama, such breath of fire (bhastrika), are more likely to cause difficulties. Such stimulating breath control methods can agitate the mind. Pranayama should be increased gradually, a few minutes a day. If we suddenly do it for long periods of time, difficulties are more likely. Breath control can give us psychic experiences, but if our mind is not pure and our personal will is in operation, these experiences may be unwholesome.

Excessive development of Pranic energy can cause ungroundedness, anxiety, palpitations, insomnia, involuntary movements, ringing in the ears, dizziness, fainting, vertigo and other conditions of high Vata (air).

Treatment

Treatment should begin with cessation of the breathing exercises. Calming and protecting mantras such as Sham and Ram should be chanted. Anti-Vata diet should be followed, yet avoiding spices. Nothing should be taken that might overstimulate the Prana.

Herbs for strengthening the nervous system and calming the mind are indicated — ashwagandha, gotu kola, jatamansi, shankhapushpi, haritaki, and sandalwood, taken with ghee. Important formulas are Ashwagandha combination or Sarasvat powder with milk or ghee.

In severe conditions stronger sedatives — valerian, nutmeg and sarpagandha — can be taken. Avoid the nervine stimulants — coffee, tea, ephedra, and camphor.

We should apply an oil massage to the feet, head and spine using warm sesame oil or a medicated anti-Vata oil, like Mahanarayan Taila. Warm bath and sleep are prescribed. Mild exercise such as walking in the woods is all right, but strong aerobic exercise should be avoided.

Kundalini Disorders

Kundalini is the root energy of the astral body. For most of us it lays dormant at the base of the spine; a fraction or reflection of it serves to maintain our ordinary nervous activities. This power can be awakened by Pranayama, mantra, drugs or other meditational activities. It may be brought about by past karma, good or bad. Many modern recreational drugs work by artificially stimulating it but do not awaken it in full.

Most of the Ayurvedic remedies for improving Ojas, such as ghee or ashwagandha, facilitate Kundalini without artificially stimulating it. Good stimulating herbs are calamus and camphor (internally in minute amounts). Makaradhwaj, the mineral remedy, has this effect and should be taken with milk.

One method of spiritual development is to awaken this energy and follow its movement up the spine towards the awakening of cosmic consciousness. Other more direct approaches to spiritual development, may circumvent the Kundalini, and may regard it as a power of illusion to be avoided.

Kundalini is not necessarily a beneficent force. It can be aroused artificially or prematurely or be turned on too strongly. This can result in the burning out of the nervous system or various other high Vata (air) or high Pitta (fire) conditions. It may cause delusions or false imaginings to arise.

Kundalini is not a force to be toyed with; it requires the proper guidance. It is better not to use it at all than to approach without the right orientation. Before attempting to arouse it, the nature should be purified. Its awakening is more appropriately part of Rejuvenation Therapy. Soma was an ancient Vedic herbal preparation given along with Rejuvenation Therapy for this purpose. Taken by those who were impure or out of balance, it would tend to cause disease or even death.

Kundalini disorders involve pain in the lower back and often swelling pain of the genitals. There may be a burning pain along the base of the spine to the solar plexus. Sexual desire may become excessive, or other powerful emotions such as anger may become overwhelming. There will be inability to sleep, and the need for sleep will often be low. Heightened imagination will bring visions of strong colors but with lack of control. Fantasies may turn negative or destructive. Visions of heaven and hell, feelings of being a great guru, god or bodhisattva may occur. Contact with astral beings may occur, and they may encourage such fantasies.

Naturally, this is a difficult condition to recognize. The individual may mistake it for true spiritual experience. Long-term pain, anxiety and mental unrest, however, reveal its true character. Even a great Yogi may go through periods of such negative experience.

Treatment

All meditational techniques should be given up. An effortless meditation of peace and calm should be followed or simple surrender to the Divine. Rest and relaxation are important. No forceful holding of the breath or breath of fire should be done. Lunar pranayama — breathing in through the left and out through the right nostril only — can be done, or Shitali.

A combined anti-Vata, anti-Pitta diet is prescribed, avoiding spices, except for fennel and coriander. Milk and ghee can be taken but not pure forms of sugar, including honey. All drugs and alcohol should be strictly avoided. Herbal wines, generally, will not be good.

Calming and nourishing herbs like ashwagandha, shatavari, sandalwood, haritaki, amalaki, gotu kola and aloe gel are to be taken. Stimulant herbs, calamus, camphor, bayberry and sage, should not be used.

Good formulas are Ashwagandha compound, Ashwagandha ghee, Brahmi ghee or Brahma rasayan, or Shatavari compound.

Oil massage should be done with warm sesame oil to the pelvic region, genitals and base of the spine. Brahmi oil to the head is particularly good.

Essential oils such as sandalwood, rose and lotus should be applied to the top the head, the third eye and navel chakras.

Helpful gems for balancing and regulating Kundalini energy are yellow sapphire, yellow topaz, emerald, jade, pearl, moonstone. Ruby, garnet and cat's eye should not be used. The latter is particularly good for stimulating Kundalini.

Best mantras for calming Kundalini are 'sham' and 'ram'. Om in excess can arouse it. The mantra 'hum' is strongest to arouse it and should be done with care.

ADDICTIONS

Addictions are another form of mental disorder. They occur from too much tamas or inertia in the mind. This is often caused by excess rajas, or mental disturbance, which is compensated for by providing an artificial calm.

All addictions tend to increase Vata (air) by creating nervous dependency. The individual becomes mentally destabilized and is not able to look at the condition objectively.

Kapha (water) individuals, with the strongest physiques, can stand more bad habits such as smoking, drinking, taking of stimulants or drugs. They will also have the greatest difficulty in giving up addictions.

Vata (air) types will be damaged by them very easily. They can give them up short term but tend to return to them, or to shift from one habit to another.

Pitta (fire) types, with their stronger self-righteousness, will have more difficulty in giving them up unless they are convinced it is their own best choice in the matter. The typical drinker turned fundamentalist religious fanatic is usually of Pitta constitution.

Treatment

Ayurvedic treatment of different addictions is similar. The humoral imbalance behind the problem must be addressed. Specific herbs to help reduce the emotional need for addicting substances are nervines such as calamus, gotu kola, skullcap or camomile. Other herbs are necessary for the tissue damage done by the addictive substance: lung tonics for smoking, liver tonics for drinking, brain or nerve tonics for drugs.

Addictions indicate wrong life-style, so our whole life-regime needs to be examined. All addictions are part of a psychological pattern of dependency. This must be addressed. Efforts should be made to contact the true Self that is independent and transcends environmental influences. For this the Yoga of knowledge is indicated.

SMOKING

Addiction to smoking can occur in any of the three humors. Vata (air) types like to smoke as a nervous habit to calm anxiety and give distraction from worry. Pitta (fire) types like the addition of more fire into their systems and the increased feeling of power. Kapha (water) types like the clearing and stimulating effect of tobacco, which activates them and removes lethargy. Smoking of mainly spicy herbs is often recommended for Kapha problems.

The herb calamus helps counter the nervous habit behind addictions. It can be added in small amounts to cigarettes or taken as a powder or ghee; in the latter form it is particularly good to apply several drops to the nose two or three times a day.

Gotu kola is excellent for addictions in Pitta and Kapha types. Ashwagandha is good for Vata types. Camomile can be used for calming the nerves in most addictions. Kapha types often benefit from herbal cigarettes and can take these as a substitute.

Treatment

Kapha (water) types often experience congestion after giving up smoking. They will do best with more spices and expectorants — calamus or cloves with honey — or formulas such as Clove compound or Trikatu. Milk decoctions of long pepper (pippali) can be used to rebuild the lungs. Elecampane can be taken in this way.

Smoking often causes lung weakness, dry cough and constipation in Vata (air) types. Tonic foods for the lungs, milk, almonds, pine nuts and sesame are good. Tonic herbs for the lungs — ashwagandha, shatavari, bala, ginseng, comfrey root, and marshmallow — are beneficial. These are better taken in milk decoctions with raw sugar and ghee, 1–2 tsps. of herbs per cup. Formulas include Ashwagandha compound.

Smoking in Pitta (fire) types causes infectious diseases of the lungs, liver and blood. Detoxification is more strongly required. Good herbs include aloe gel, bayberry, shatavari, and burdock. Formulas such as Sudarshan churna are good.

ALCOHOLISM

Taking of alcohol is the addition of fire to the body. It tends to damage the liver and the blood, and creates various Pitta (fire) disorders.

Alcohol is also a sugar. Addiction to it may be part of or a substitution for sugar addiction. This occurs more in Kapha (water) and Vata (air) types.

Herbal wines can be given as substitutes for alcohol and will help reduce dependency.

Aloe is the best herb for balancing liver function. The gel or herbal wine is preferable. Gotu kola is the best herb for clearing out toxins from the brain tissue and reducing disturbed emotions in the liver. Bitters, such as katuka or gentian, are helpful for cleansing the liver and blood. Turmeric and barberry together help clear congested emotions from the liver. Good formulas include Brahma rasayan and Saraswat powder.

Skullcap is a good Western herb for calming addiction and also helps cleanse the liver. Passion flower, betony, hops and other cooling nervine herbs are helpful in both Pitta and Kapha types. Bitters, in general, are very good.

For detoxifying the liver in most addictions, equal parts turmeric, barberry and gotu kola can be used. To these, Vata types can add licorice, Pitta types can add burdock and Kapha types can add dry ginger.

The Chinese herb bupleurum has been found to be good for cleansing the liver, as well as reducing emotional factors behind drinking and other addictions.

DRUG DISORDERS

We live in a culture of drug abuse, both recreational and medicinal. Long-term taking of drugs severely aggravates Vata, the biological air humor. Hence, most drug disorders are also mainly Vata disorders. Many drugs are diuretic and have a drying affect, causing constipation and weakening the kidneys. They tend to deplete Ojas.

Stimulant drugs, particularly in their short-term use, aggravate Pitta (fire) and can burn out the nervous system and damage the eyes.

Drugs tend to damage Sattva, the basic clear nature of the mind. Artificially driving the mind and nerves, they create tamas, dullness, inertia, darkness and loss of perception, even though their temporary action may be opposite this.

Hallucinogenic drugs function mainly by increasing Tejas, the mental fire. This results in the experience of color and heightened perception, which may give us a sense of the deeper powers of our consciousness. But these drugs function by burning up Ojas, our subtle vital reserve, causing long-term depletion of our primary vitality. Once Ojas is brought below a certain threshold, it is very difficult for it to reconstitute itself. The result is drug burnout, a vegetative state of mind. Hence, the number of times we can take such drugs in a positive way is very limited.

Sleep-inducing medicines, in the long run, tend to cause insomnia, just as laxatives cause constipation.

Amphetamines and other stimulants also overly increase Vata and Pitta. Downers usually increase Kapha (Tamas).

Marijuana, particularly when smoked, is much like tobacco addiction and can be treated in a similar way. Also, like tobacco, it causes lung and liver cancer.

Treatment

Diet should be according to humor, usually anti-Vata, anti-Pitta. Ghee should be taken, 1–2 tsps. 2–3 times a day, to nourish the nerve tissue. Spices should be avoided for Pitta except coriander, fennel and saffron. Garlic, asafoetida, nutmeg and other grounding spices are good for Vata.

Gotu kola is the best herb to help cleanse hallucinogenic drugs from the liver and brain. Gotu kola ghee or Brahmi rasayan is good for cooling and calming high fire in the mind (too much Tejas).

Ashwagandha is the best herb for helping to rebuild the nervous system depleted by drug use. Shatavari helps restore emotional sensitivity and balance.

Calamus is most important for restoring mental faculties, including perceptual acuity and power of self-expression. It is especially good for the dullness and depression or the vegetative state that follows excessive use of drugs.

Valerian is good to counteract the effects of stimulants and is an effective sedative in drug disorders; 3 tsps. per cup of warm water.

All of these herbs are best taken with ghee.

Guggul or myrrh is also important for cleansing and fortifying the deeper tissues. Yogaraj guggul and Mahayogaraj guggul are best. Triphala guggul has better cleansing, but weaker tonifying action.

The Chinese herb, zizyphus seed, is particularly good for nourishing and tonifying brain tissue damaged through excess use of drugs.

PART III

REMEDIAL MEASURES

Section I of this book examines the basic principles and therapies of Ayurveda. Section II, the treatment of common diseases, introduces a number of formulas. In Section III more information is given on these formulas, as well as additional Ayurvedic healing modalities of oils, incense, gems, mantras and spiritual measures.

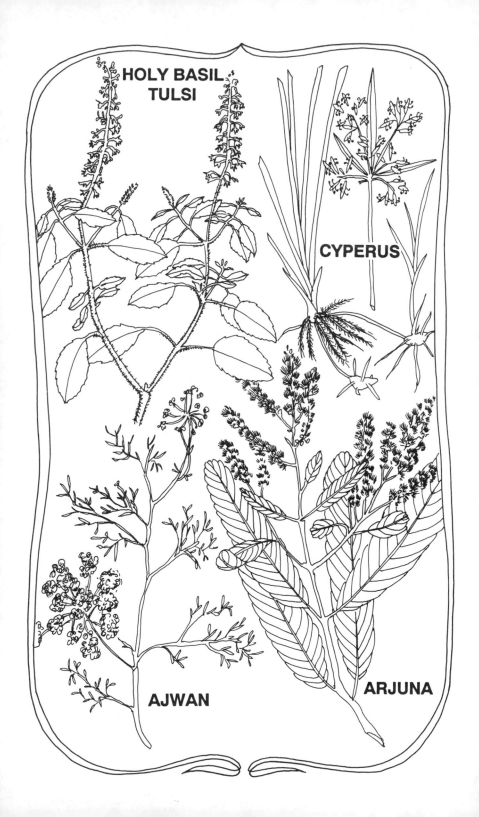

HYMN TO THE PLANTS — *RIG VEDA X. 97.*

*Plants, which as receptacles of light were
born three ages before the Gods, I honor
your myriad colors and your seven hundred
natures.*

*A hundred, oh Mothers, are your natures
and a thousand are your growths. May you
of a hundred powers make whole what has
been hurt.*

*Plants, as Mothers, as Goddesses, I address
you. May I gain the energy, the light, the
sustenance, your soul, you who are the
human being.*

*Where the herbs are gathered together like
kings in an assembly, there the doctor is
called a sage, who destroys evil, and averts
disease.*

*As they fell from Heaven, the plants said,
"The living soul we pervade, that man will
suffer no harm."*

*The herbs which are in the kingdom of the
Moon, manifold with a hundred eyes, I take
you as the best of them, for the fulfillment of
wishes, as peace to the heart.*

*The plants which are queens of the Soma,
spread over all the Earth, generated by the
Lord of Prayer, may your energy combine
within this herb.*

1
CLASSICAL AYURVEDIC
FORMULAS

A representative selection of classical Ayurvedic formulas is mentioned in this book. The formulas are chosen to reflect both common usage in Ayurveda and familiarity or accessibility of main ingredients in the West. There are many other formulas, of equal quality. The formulas are limited primarily to purely herbal products. Ayurvedic mineral preparations or compounds of minerals and herbs are very common and often have better potency but are not yet available here.

The same herb or formula may be offered in several forms; powder, tablet, herbal jelly, herbal wine, etc. Ayurveda offers the largest variety of herbal preparations of any herbal tradition. The form does not always matter; taste, manner of taking, or duration of potency more often determines use. Generally, different preparations of the same herb or formula can be used in the same way.

Powders have the shortest shelf life, up to one year; tablets are good up to two years if well coated; herbal oils, wines and jellies up to three years. Medicated ghees may last only six months.

Powders, tablets, pills and gugguls are taken with appropriate vehicles (anupanas): warm or cool water, milk, buttermilk, ghee, honey, butter, yogurt, or teas of other single herbs. Appropriate vehicles are listed after each formula.

It should be noted that formulas are not always specific for lowering one of the biological humors. The humor a formula treats can be modified by the vehicle used with it or the formulas with which it is combined. Many formulas are good for lowering two.

Dosages and times of taking vary according to conditions. This information is general, to be adapted per principles (as in *The Yoga of Herbs,* pgs. 88 and 92).

Properties of formulas are usually determined by that of the primary herb they are named after. When the formula is not available, a decoction of the main herb or chief ingredients is generally sufficient.

Most of these classical formulas come from various ancient Ayurvedic source books. However, ingredients and their proportions vary according to different formulations, modern adjustments, or the standards of the company which manufactures them. Usages generally remain the same. Some of the formulas are given new names by their manufacturers for modern appeal. I have translated their Ayurvedic names when this can be done easily.

POWDERS
TABLETS

Many herbal powders are used in Ayurveda. Herbs are seldom used in the raw form, partly because raw herbs deteriorate quickly in India's tropical climate. Powders are prepared by reducing the herbs to a fine powder and mixing together. As they tend to deteriorate more quickly, many powders are now made into tablets, particularly for export to the West, and are given special protective coatings.

Tablets, however, are not made only of powders. Many use herbal pastes and herbal extracts, which give them a superior quality over simple tableted powders.

Asafoetida 8 Compound
Hingashtak Churna

Ingredients	Asafoetida, trikatu, rock salt, cumin, black cumin, ajwan.
Properties	Carminative, stimulant, antispasmodic. Decreases Vata and Kapha, for Vata indigestion, increases Pitta.
Uses	Abdominal distention, gas, colic, indigestion.
Dose	1–4 gms. or 2–8 tablets, 2–3 times a day.
Vehicle	Warm water.

Ashwagandha Compound Powder
Ashwagandhadi Churna

Ingredients	Ashwagandha, vidari kanda.
Properties	Tonic, aphrodisiac, antirheumatic, astringent, analgesic. Lowers high Vata, mildly increases Kapha and Pitta.
Uses	Arthritis, debility, wasting diseases, impotence, nocturnal emissions, leucorrhea, anxiety, insomnia, general. tonic for elderly, convalescence or high Vata.
Dose	1–6 gms. or 2–12 tablets, 2–3 times a day.
Vehicle	Milk or ghee.

Avipattikar Churna

Ingredients	Trikatu, triphala, cyperus, vidanga, cardamom, cinnamon leaf, cloves, trivrit, raw sugar.
Properties	Laxative, carminative, cholagogue.
Uses	Hyperacidity, heartburn, biliousness, vomiting, indigestion, dropsy, rheumatism. Good for Pitta type digestive disorders.
Dose	1–4 gms. or 2–8 tablets, 2–3 times a day, after meals.
Vehicle	Warm water.

Bilva Compound Powder
Bilvadi Churna

Ingredients	Bilva, ginger, fennel, cardamom, bombax, woodfordia, and others.
Properties	Astringent, alterative.
Uses	Diarrhea, dysentery, malabsorption.
Dose	1–3 gms. or 2–6 tablets, 2–3 times a day.
Vehicle	Buttermilk, water.

Cardamom Compound
Eladi Churna

Ingredients	Cardamom, cloves, keshara, kolamajja, laja, priyangu, cyperus, sandalwood, long pepper.
Properties	Carminative, antiemetic, stomachic.
Uses	Vomiting, cough, asthma, indigestion, anorexia.
Dose	1–4 gms. or 2–8 tablets, 2–3 times a day.
Vehicle	Honey or raw sugar (some formulations of it already contain raisins or other forms of sugar).

Chitrak Compound Tablets
Chitrakadi Bati

Ingredients	Chitrak, 5 salts, trikatu, ajwan, chavya, asafoetida.
Properties	Stomachic, antacid, carminative.
Uses	Indigestion, gas, hyperacidity, colic.
Dose	2–4 tablets twice a day after meals.
Vehicle	Warm water.

Cloves Compound
Lavangadi Churna

Ingredients	Cloves, camphor, cardamom, cinnamon, nagakeshar, nutmeg, vetivert, ginger, cumin, valerian, bamboo manna, jatamansi, long pepper, sandalwood, cubeb, raw sugar.
Properties	Diaphoretic, expectorant, antitussive, antispasmodic. Very good for Kapha conditions, also reduces Vata, increases Agni and Pitta.
Uses	Colds, cough, whooping cough, intestinal gas, colic, diarrhea, nausea, vomiting, lack of appetite, lumbago.
Dose	1–4 gms. or 2–8 tablets, 2–3 times a day.
Vehicle	Honey.

Dhatupaushtic Churna
(Tissue-Strengthening Powder)

Ingredients	Shatavari, gokshura, cannabis seed, vamsha rochana, sarsaparilla, cubeb, mucuna, black musali, white musali, trikatu, dioscorea, ashwagandha, nishotha.
Properties	Tonic, rejuvenative, aphrodisiac.
Uses	Debility, convalescence, senility.
Dose	2–5 gms. or 4–10 tablets, 2–3 times a day.
Vehicle	Milk.

Garlic Compound Tablet
Lashunadi Bati

Ingredients	Garlic, cumin, rock salt, sulphur, trikatu, asafoetida, lemon juice.
Properties	Stimulant, carminative, laxative.
Uses	Loss of appetite, distention, gas, borborygmus, constipation, parasites.
Dose	2–4 pills (1–2 gms.), 2–3 times a day.
Vehicle	Warm water.

Gotu Kola Compound Tablet
Brahmi Bati

Ingredients	Gotu kola, shankhapushpi, calamus, black pepper, often with various minerals.

Properties	Sedative, antispasmodic, nervine tonic.
Uses	Mental weakness, poor memory, neurasthenia, epilepsy, coma, paralysis.
Dose	2 pills (1 gm.) twice a day.
Vehicle	Honey.

Guduchi Sattva
Tinospora Extract

Ingredients	Water soluble extract (starch) of guduchi.
Properties	Bitter tonic, diuretic, alterative.
Uses	Liver disorders, fever, malaria, headache, urinary disorders, convalescence.
Dose	1–2 gms. twice a day.
Vehicle	Ghee or water.

Kutajghan Bati

Ingredients	Kutaj, ghan, atish.
Properties	Alterative, astringent, amoebicide.
Uses	Diarrhea, dysentery, hemorrhoids, hematuria. Specific antibacterial and amoebicidal for dysentery.
Dose	2–4 pills (1–2 gms.), three times a day.
Vehicle	Warm water, buttermilk or yogurt.

Lavanbhaskar Churna
Five Salts Compound Powder

Ingredients	5 salts, fennel, long pepper, long pepper root, black cumin, cinnamon leaf, nagakeshar, talisha, rhubarb root, pomegranate seeds, cinnamon, cardamom.
Properties	Stimulant, carminative, laxative. Decreases Vata, increases Agni and Pitta.
Uses	Loss of appetite, malabsorption, constipation, abdominal pain, tumors.
Dose	1–4 gms. or 2–8 tablets, 2–3 times a day.
Vehicle	Warm water, buttermilk.

Licorice Powder
Yashtimadhu Churna

Ingredients	Licorice.
Properties	Demulcent, tonic, expectorant, laxative.
Uses	Cough, sore throat, chronic constipation, debility.
Dose	2–4 gms. or 4–8 tablets, 2–3 times a day.
Vehicle	Honey (as laxative or expectorant), milk (as nutritive tonic).

Mahasudarshan Powder

Ingredients	Bitters (such as chiretta, guduchi, barberry), trikatu, triphala, cannabis.
Properties	Antipyretic, diaphoretic, diuretic.
Uses	Fever, intermittent fever, debility after fevers, nausea, enlargement of liver and spleen. Mainly anti-Pitta.
Dose	1–4 gms. or 2–8 tablets, 2–3 times a day.
Vehicle	Water.

Nutmeg Compound
Jatiphaladi Churna

Ingredients	Nutmeg, cloves, cardamom, cinnamon leaf, cinnamon, nagakeshar, camphor, bamboo manna, valerian, amalaki, haritaki, trikatu, chitrak, cumin, vidanga, cannabis, raw sugar.
Properties	Sedative, astringent, antispasmodic, hemostatic.
Uses	Diarrhea, dysentery, malabsorption, lack of appetite, cough, asthma, migraine headache, dysmenorrhea, menorrhagia.
Dose	1–3 gms. or 2–6 tablets, 2–3 times a day.
Vehicle	With honey.

Rasayana Churna
Rejuvenation Powder

Ingredients	Guduchi, gokshura, amalaki.
Properties	Bitter tonic, demulcent, alterative, diuretic, antacid.

Uses	General debility, sexual debility, venereal diseases, skin rashes, allergies, chronic fevers or infections. Good rejuvenative tonic for Pitta, in particular after febrile diseases.
Dose	1–4 gms. or 2–8 tablets, 2–3 times a day.
Vehicle	Raw sugar and ghee, in milk.

Sarasvat Powder

Ingredients	Ashwagandha, calamus, shankhapushpi, ajwan, cumin, trikatu, rock salt, and others.
Properties	Nervine tonic and stimulant.
Uses	Mental weakness, nervous strain, mania, epilepsy, hemiplegia, weakness of voice. Mainly for Vata disorders.
Dose	1–4 gms. or 2–8 tablets, 2–3 times a day.
Vehicle	Honey and ghee, in milk.

Sitopaladi Churna
(Rock Candy Compound Powder)

Ingredients	Rock candy, bamboo manna, long pepper, cardamom, cinnamon.
Properties	Expectorant, antitussive.
Uses	Colds, cough, lack of appetite, fever, debility, burning sensation in extremities. Major anti-Kapha formula, also reduces Vata.
Dose	1–4 gms. or 2–8 tablets, 2–4 times a day.
Vehicle	Honcy, ghee.

Sandalwood Compound Powder
Chandrnadi Churna

Ingredients	Sandalwood, fennel, long pepper, long pepper root, black pepper, cloves.
Properties	Diuretic, alterative, febrifuge, urinary antiseptic.
Uses	Urinary tract infections, cough, asthma, fever, venereal diseases.
Dose	1–4 gms. or 2–8 tablets, 2–3 times a day.
Vehicle	Water, milk.

Sarsaparilla Compound Powder
Chopchinyadi Churna

Ingredients	Sarsaparilla, fennel, pippali, pippali root, black pepper, cloves, ginger, cinnamon, and others.
Properties	Alterative, sedative, antirheumatic.
Uses	Venereal diseases, sexual debility, gout, arthritis, epilepsy.
Dose	1–4 gms. or 2–8 tablets, 2–3 times a day.
Vehicle	Milk.

Shatavari Compound
Shatavaryadi Churna

Ingredients	Shatavari, gokshura, atibala, and others.
Properties	Tonic, nutritive, demulcent, diuretic, aphrodisiac.
Uses	Debility, convalescence, impotence, infertility. Good tonic for Pitta and Vata.
Dose	1–6 gms. or 2–12 tablets, 2–3 times a day.
Vehicle	Milk, ghee.

Sudarshan Churna

Ingredients	Chiretta and various mainly bitter or pungent herbs.
Properties	Anti-pyretic, alterative, antiperiodic.
Uses	Fever (old), intermittent fever, debility, weak digestion, liver disorders, enlargement of liver and spleen. Mainly anti-Pitta.
Dose	1–4 gms. or 2–8 tablets, 2–3 times a day.
Vehicle	Warm water.

Talisadi Churna

Ingredients	Talisha, trikatu, bamboo manna, cardamom, cinnamon, raw sugar.
Properties	Expectorant, antitussive, stimulant.
Uses	Colds, flus, bronchitis, loss of appetite, indigestion, chronic fever. Mainly anti-Kapha.
Dose	1–4 gms. or 2–8 tablets, 2 times a day.
Vehicle	Honey.

Trikatu Powder

Ingredients	Black pepper, long pepper, dry ginger.
Properties	Stimulant, expectorant.
Uses	Lack of appetite, indigestion, cough, congestion. Specific for low Agni and high Ama, weak digestive fire and accumulation of toxins; reduces Kapha and Vata, increases Pitta.
Dose	1–3 gms. or 2–6 tablets, 2–3 times a day.
Vehicle	Honey, warm water.

Triphala Churna

Ingredients	Haritaki, amalaki, bibhitaki.
Properties	Laxative, tonic, rejuvenative, astringent.
Uses	Chronic constipation, abdominal gas and distention, diabetes, eye diseases, chronic diarrhea. Good for all three humors, best and safest laxative.
Dose	2–10 gms. or 4–10 tablets, before sleep.
Vehicle	Ghee, honey, warm water.

Trisugandhi Churna
(Three Aromatics Powder)

Ingredients	Cinnamon, cinnamon leaf, cardamom.
Properties	Stimulant, carminative, diaphoretic.
Uses	Indigestion, lack of appetite, vomiting, gas, distention. Good like Trikatu for improving the digestion of food and herbs; bay leaf can be used in place of cinnamon leaf.
Dose	1–3 gms. or 2–6 tablets, 2–3 times a day.
Vehicle	Honey or warm water.

ADDITIONAL TRADITIONAL COMPOUNDS

The following are famous formulas usually made as powders. Their formulation today often varies, with many substitutions for the original plants or plant parts. Hence, we will treat them in a more general way.

Dashamula
Ten Roots

This formula is very good for Vata conditions as a tonic and sedative. It is often used in enema therapy and in medicated oils.

Tikta
Bitter
A compound of bitter herbs, good for all the general indications of bitter taste and often used like Sudarshan churna.

GUGGULS
Gugguls are special pills made with the resin of guggul, Commiphora mukul, a relative of myrrh. They are mainly for treating arthritis, nervous system disorders, skin diseases and obesity, many of the same conditions Western herbalists treat with myrrh. Their advantage over myrrh is that they are purified so that the resin cannot damage kidney function. Guggul is purified by boiling it in various herbal decoctions, like Triphala, and straining out the purified resin. Western herbalists may find this way of preparing guggul to be useful in preparing myrrh. Herbal powders or extracts are added to the purified guggul resin, often with ghee.

Gokshuradi Guggul
Tribulis Compound Guggul

Ingredients	Guggul, gokshura, trikatu, triphala, cyperus.
Properties	Diuretic, alterative, demulcent.
Uses	Difficult urination, urinary tract stones, diabetes, leucorrhea, gonorrhea, arthritis.
Dose	2–5 pills, 2–3 times a day.
Vehicle	Cyperus tea, pashanabheda tea, vetivert tea.

Mahayogaraj Guggul

Ingredients	Guggul, triphala and the ashes of lead, silver, tin, iron, mica, iron sulphate and mercuric sulfide, along with many different, primarily pungent herbs.
Properties	Antirheumatic, alterative, sedative, astringent.
Uses	Arthritis, gout, diabetes, nervous disorders, epilepsy, asthma, tumors. This is the main Ayurvedic formula for severe and degenerative arthritis and for difficult nervous disorders like paralysis, MS, Parkinson's disease.
Dose	1–3 pills, 2–3 times a day.
Vehicle	Galangal tea, triphala tea or honey.

Triphala Guggul

Ingredients	Guggul, triphala and long pepper.
Properties	Alterative, anti-inflammatory, antibiotic, antiseptic.
Uses	Oils, carbuncles, abscesses, ulcers, hemorrhoids, nasal polyps, edema, arthritis. Very cleansing and detoxifying for Vata, particularly in Sama conditions or when Vata has entered the lymph or blood.
Dose	2–5 pills, 2–3 times a day.
Vehicle	Warm water.

Yogaraj Guggul

Ingredients	Guggul, triphala, ginger, black pepper, chavya, asafoetida, ajwan, galangal, vidanga, atish, calamus, chitrak, and others.
Uses	Arthritis, gout, nervous diseases, hemorrhoids, epilepsy, anemia.
Dose	2–5 pills, 2–3 times a day.
Vehicle	Galangal tea, garlic juice, honey.

HERBAL WINES

Herbal wines are self-generated herbal fermentations. They are prepared similar to grape wine, in big wooden vats. They are quite different than tinctures, though tinctures can substitute for them to some extent. There are two types, asavas and arishtas. Asavas are made without boiling the herbs used in them; usually fresh herbal juices are used. Arishtas are made with decoctions. Fermentation is brought about by the addition of dhataki flowers.

These medicinal wines not only last longer than powders and pills, but they also make the herbs more digestible. Many contain additional spices for improving their assimilation. Their sour taste makes them particularly good for Vata.

Draksha is already being made in this country. Herbal wines are a new field of herb preparation for us. At some point, we will learn to produce many varieties of our own.

Aloe Herbal Wine
Kumaryasava

Ingredients	Aloe gel, jaggery and honey, with trikatu, triphala and other predominately spicy herbs.

Properties	Alterative, tonic, hematinic.
Uses	Anemia, poor endocrine function, cough, asthma, constipation, liver disorders, chronic hepatitis.
Dose	2–4 ounces with meals.

Arjunarishta
Arjuna Herbal Wine

Ingredients	Arjuna, raisins, madhuka flower, dhataki and jaggery.
Properties	Heart tonic, cardiac stimulant.
Uses	All cardiac and pulmonary disorders, heart weakness.
Dose	2–4 ounces with meals.

Ashokarishta
Ashoka Herbal Wine

Ingredients	Ashoka, dhataki, jaggery, cumin, triphala, ginger, sandalwood, and others.
Properties	Alterative, astringent, hemostatic.
Uses	Menorrhagia, leucorrhea, dysmenorrhea, hematuria.
Dose	2–4 ounces with meals.

Ashwagandharishta
Ashwagandha Herbal Wine

Ingredients	Ashwagandha, white musali, madder, licorice, turmeric, trikatu, sandalwood, calamus, dhataki and jaggery.
Properties	Nervine tonic, sedative.
Uses	Nervous debility, loss of memory, epilepsy, insanity. Another good way to take ashwagandha, particularly for its nervine properties.
Dose	2–4 ounces with meals.

Balarishta
Bala Herbal Wine

Ingredients	Bala, ashwagandha, lily, cardamom, galangal, cloves, vetivert, gokshura, castor root, dhataki, jaggery.
Properties	Tonic, nutritive, antirheumatic, diuretic.
Uses	Arthritis, paralysis, debility, high Vata.
Dose	2–4 ounces with meals.

Draksha
Grape Herbal Wine

Ingredients	Mainly raisins and various spices; some varieties made with nuts have better tonification properties.
Properties	Stimulant, carminative, diuretic.
Uses	Loss of appetite, indigestion, general debility, insomnia, cough, pulmonary diseases. Particularly good for Vata type weak digestion.
Dose	2–4 ounces with meals.

Kutajarishta
Kutaj Herbal Wine

Ingredients	Kutaja, raisins, madhuka, gmetina, dhataki, jaggery.
Properties	Astringent, hemostatic, antiperiodic.
Uses	Diarrhea, dysentery, malabsorption, parasites.
Dose	2–4 ounces with meals.

Saraswztarishta
Saraswat Herbal Wine

Ingredients	Gotu kola, shatavari, vidari kanda, haritaki, vetivert, fresh ginger, fennel, honey, raw sugar, dhataki and other herbs and spices.
Properties	Nervine tonic, sedative.
Uses	Nervous debility, convulsions, stammering, memory loss, sexual debility.
Dose	2–4 ounces with meals.

HERBAL JELLIES

Herbal jellies are prepared with raw sugar such as jaggery or honey. They are herbal confections. The sugar acts as a preservative, improves the taste of the herbs and enhances their tonic properties. Herbal jellies serve as herbal foods and are good for tonification therapy. Not all of them, however, taste good.

Brahma Rasayan
Gotukola Herbal Jelly

Ingredients	Haritaki, amalaki, gotu kola, shankha pushpi, vidang, sandalwood, agaru, calamus, dashamula, raw sugar, and others.
Properties	Alterative, tonic, nervine, rejuvenative.
Uses	Mental weakness, loss of memory, general debilit, senility, neurasthenia, cough. Good brain and meditation food.
Dose	1–2 tsps., 2–3 times a day.
Vehicle	Milk.

Chyavan Prash

Ingredients	Amalaki, long pepper, bamboo manna, cloves, cinnamon, cardamom, cubebs, ghee, raw sugar, and others (many varieties are available, some with silver or gold foil).
Properties	Nutritive tonic, rejuvenative.
Uses	General debility, old age debility, anemia, sexual debility, cough, tuberculosis. This is the most famous and widely useful of the herbal jellies, good for almost any weakness condition or as an energy supplement. Many kinds are available, some with gold, silver or other minerals. It is considered a good tonic for all three humors. Most Indian markets and restaurants in this country carry it. The same formula can be found as a pill or powder. The best quality is made with fresh Amalaki. This is not done by companies today because the fresh fruit is only available seasonally.
Dose	1–2 tsps., 2–3 times a day.
Vehicle	Milk.

Musli Pak

Ingredients	White musali, ghee, sugar, trikatu, cinnamon, cardamom, chitrak, ashwagandha, cloves, nutmeg and special minerals.
Properties	Nutritive tonic, aphrodisiac.
Uses	Sexual debility, infertility, emaciation, lack of strength.
Dose	1–2 tsps. 2–3 times a day.
Vehicle	Milk.

Vasavaleha
Vasa Herbal Jelly

Ingredients	Vasa, haritaki, bamboo manna, long pepper, caturjat.
Properties	Antispasmodic, expectorant, laxative, alterative.
Uses	Asthma, bronchitis, cough, bleeding from the lungs.
Dose	1–2 tsps., 2–3 times a day.
Vehicle	Milk.

MEDICATED OILS

Medicated oils (tailas) are prepared mainly with sesame oil. They are mainly for external use. Dose is largely as needed for massage; Ayurveda uses larger amounts of oil for massage, requiring a shower afterwards to remove excess oil.

These medicated oils are an Ayurvedic specialty. No other herbal system uses so many different herbs in a heavy oil base. Most others are essential oils in a light alcohol base, or else heavier ointments. Ayurveda uses many tonic herbs prepared in oil for external nourishment, as well as more special analgesic herbs (see also chapter on 'Oils and Incense').

Medicated oils are not just supplements; they are a primary treatment and can be a treatment in themselves. They are very important in oleation (snehana) therapy.

Some modern companies are preparing these oils with more pleasant fragrances and better absorbability.

Simple oils can be made by adding herbs to sesame oil and water, boiling the water away and straining the herbs.

Bhringaraj Taila
Eclipta Oil

Ingredients	Bhringaraj juice and sesame oil.
Properties	Antiseptic, hair tonic, nervine.
Uses	Premature graying or balding, alopecia, pruritus of the scalp. Can use as a good hair and scalp conditioner, also for calming the mind.

Brahmi Taila
Gotu Kola Oil

Ingredients	Gotu kola and other nervine herbs in coconut oil base.
Properties	Nervine, sedative, antipyretic.

Uses   Insomnia, mental agitation, headache, eye-ache, premature
                    greying or balding. Generally as brain tonic; some varieties
                    commonly sold in this country.

Chandanadi Tailas
Sandalwood Compound Oil

Ingredients   Sandalwood, licorice, saussurea, etc. and sesame oil.

Properties   Antipyretic, hemostatic, sedative.

Uses   Fever, headache, neuralgia, burning sensation, nose bleed,
                    hemoptysis.

Chandan Bala Lakshadi Taila

Ingredients   Sandalwood, bala, sumac, deodar, saussurea, manjishta,
                    ashwagandha, etc. and sesame oil.

Properties   Antipyretic, antispasmodic, antiseptic, analgesic.

Uses   Fever, cough, asthma, headache, skin diseases, arthritis.

Mahamasha Taila

Ingredients   Masha, dashamula, castor root, and sesame oil.

Properties   Demulcent, emollient, analgesic.

Uses   All kinds of pain, paralysis, earache.

Mahanarayan Taila

Ingredients   Shatavari, castor root, brihati, bala, and sesame oil.

Properties   Demulcent, emollient, analgesic.

Uses   Arthritis, rheumatism, gout, paralysis. Most commonly
                    used oil for arthritis.

Narayan Taila

Ingredients   Shatavari, ashwagandha, bilva root, brihati, neem,
                    dashamula, milk, sesame oil.

Properties   Demulcent, emollient, analgesic.

Uses   Rheumatic pain, paralysis, fever.

Pinda Taila

Ingredients   Manjishta, sariva, sarjarasa, licorice, wax, castor oil.

Properties   Anti-inflammatory, analgesic.

Uses   Rheumatism, gout.

Vishagarbha Taila

Ingredients	Vatsanabha, vitex juice, bhringaraj juice, and sesame oil.
Properties	Analgesic, sedative.
Uses	Good for any kind of muscle ache, neuralgia, gout, rheumatism, earache, sciatica.

MEDICATED GHEE

Medicated ghees are good as nervine tonics, as ghee nourishes the brain and nerves. Ghee also combines well with bitter herbs, enhancing their properties by its Pitta reducing action. Most nervines, or bitters, gain in strength when prepared in ghee or taken with ghee.

Ghees do not require vehicles (anupanas) to take them with, but they are usually followed with milk.

Simple ghees can be prepared like medicated oils. Ghee, itself, is prepared by cooking raw unsalted butter over a low flame until all the milk fats settle to the bottom, then straining off the clear liquid.

Ashwagandha Compound Ghee
Ashwagandha Ghrita

Ingredients	Ashwagandha and ghee.
Properties	Tonic, nervine, aphrodisiac.
Uses	General debility, nervous debility, insomnia, lack of sexual vitality.
Dose	1–2 tsps. twice a day.
Vehicle	Milk.

Gotu kola Compound Ghee
Brahmi Ghrita

Ingredients	Gotu kola, calamus, saussurea, shankhapushpi, ghee.
Properties	Sedative, nervine tonic.
Uses	Insanity, epilepsy, weakness of voice, as brain tonic.
Dose	1–2 tsps., twice a day.
Vehicle	Milk.

Note: a simpler version of this formula can be made with gotu kola 3 parts and calamus or bayberry 1 part. Cook two ounces of the herbs in one pint of water; simmer slowly down to one cup. Add to one cup of ghee and slowly cook until the water evaporates.

Mahatikta Ghrita

Ingredients	Katuka, vasa, mainly bitter tonics and ghee.
Properties	Bitter tonic, alterative.
Uses	In diseases, boils, carbuncles.
Dose	1–2 tsps. twice a day.
Vehicle	Milk.

Phala Ghrita

Ingredients	Triphala, saussurea, katuka, calamus, sariva, galangal, bamboo manna, ghee.
Properties	Tonic, endocrine stimulant.
Uses	Sexual debility and infertility in women.
Dose	1–2 tsps. twice a day.
Vehicle	Milk.

Purana Ghrita
Old Ghee

Ingredients	Ghee at least 1 year old, the older the better, (very old ghee, ten years or more, is said to be able to cure all diseases).
Properties	Tonic, expectorant, emollient, antiseptic.
Uses	Pulmonary disorders, general debility, externally for sores, boils, carbuncles etc.

Shatodhara Ghrita

Ingredients	Ghee that has been triturated with water in a copper vessel.
Properties	Demulcent, emollient, antiinflammatory, antiseptic.
Uses	Externally (only) for skin rashes, itch, skin sores, burns.

Triphala Ghrita
Triphala Ghee

Ingredients	Triphala, vasa, bhringaraj, ghee.
Properties	Tonic and alterative for the eyes.
Uses	Conjunctivitis, weakening of vision.

Dose	1–2 tsps. twice a day.
Vehicle	Milk.

MINERAL AND ANIMAL PREPARATIONS
These are all specially prepared and are safe for human usage. Hundreds like them exist in Ayurveda.

Godanti Bhasma
Gypsum Ash

Ingredients	Gypsum, aloe juice.
Properties	Alterative, antacid, febrifuge.
Uses	Fever, cough, flu, headache, malaria.
Dose	250–500 mg., 2–3 times a day.
Vehicle	Honey.

Navayas Loha Guti
Iron Tablets

Ingredients	Iron ash, trikatu, triphala, cloves, nutmeg, cardamom.
Properties	Blood tonic and alterative. One of the main Ayurvedic iron supplements.
Uses	Anemia, amenorrhea, dropsy.
Dose	1–3 gms., 2–3 times a day.
Vehicle	Water or punarnava tea.

Shankha Bhasma
Conch Shell Ash

Ingredients	Mainly conch shell.
Properties	Carminative, antacid, analgesic.
Uses	Hyperacidity, indigestion, gas and distention.
Dose	250 mg. to 1 gm., 2–3 times a day.
Vehicle	Water.

Shilajit Compound

Ingredients	Shilajit, gurmar, neem, various minerals.
Properties	Tonic, diuretic, alterative, aphrodisiac.

Uses	Urinary tract disorders, kidney stones, edema, sexual debility, diabetes, venereal diseases.
Dose	1–2 pills (500 mg. to 1 gm.) twice a day.
Vehicle	Honey.

Shilajit by itself is also effective for such conditions.

Shringa Bhasma
Deer Horn Ash

Ingredients	Deer horn and aloe juice.
Properties	Expectorant, diaphoretic.
Uses	Lung diseases, cough, pneumonia, chest pain.
Dose	125–500 mg.
Vehicle	Honey.

RASA PREPARATIONS

These are special very powerful Ayurvedic herbal preparations using minerals, primarily purified sulfur and mercury. While important to Ayurvedic practice, they are part of an old spiritual, alchemical tradition now lost in the West (and for the most part, in China). Though we cannot import them, owing to F.D.A. restrictions, we can get them in India. We want to introduce them to acquaint the public with their power.

The toxic metals are purified by various procedures. These include soaking and boiling in various herbal preparations and repeated incinerations (up to one thousand times). The result is a usually a white powder, an oxide of the metal or gem, which is 'humanized' or rendered safe for human consumption. Clinical tests in India prove these products, in the normal dosage, do not leave any toxic residues in the tissues.

MAKARADHVAJ

This is the most famous Ayurvedic rasa preparation, consisting of purified sulfur and mercury, to which herbs like camphor, nutmeg, cloves and black pepper, and other minerals like gold may be added depending upon the formulation. It is stimulant, alterative, aphrodisiac and heart tonic. It is unexcelled for reviving energy in low vitality or chronic diseases. It is a great energy tonic for the nervous system. Dosage is 500 mg. to 1 gm. daily for periods up to one month, usually in the winter.

2
MODERN
AYURVEDIC FORMULAS

Ayurvedic practitioners not only use classical formulas, they devise their own formulas. These are usually based on classical models, modified according to experience. Ayurvedic companies have their special proprietary medicines. We, ourselves, can make Ayurvedic formulas using Ayurvedic principles with herbs we are familiar with. The following are such modern formulas. They are largely balanced (Tridosha) medicines; but the vehicle we use to take them with, like honey or ghee, can serve to direct their effects to the different humors.

Additional modern Ayurvedic medicines may be made of only a single herb, like bhumyamalaki (phyllanthus), arjuna, ashwagandha, guggul or shilajit. They may be potentized by preparation along with the fresh juice or decoction of the herb. They may be as effective as more complex formulas but sometimes require higher dosages.

While premade and over the counter formulas can be good, usually what we make for ourselves with raw herbs is stronger and has the additional power of bringing us in more direct contact with the herbs and the healing process. Many of the following formulas are simple enough for us to do on our own or to use as models for such formulas we make for ourselves.

1. Digestive Stimulant
Trikatu Plus

Ingredients	Dry ginger, black pepper, long pepper, coriander, nutmeg, ajwan (when ajwan is not available cloves can be used); all equal parts.
Properties	Stimulant, expectorant, carminative.
Uses	Lack of appetite, indigestion, nausea, vomiting, colic, intestinal gas, malabsorption, candida, metabolic disorders (overweight or underweight), cough, cold, congestion, poor circulation. Can be used wherever Trikatu is indicated and is safer and more balanced for long term usage. Decreases Kapha and Vata, increases Pitta, burns up Ama.

Dose	1–4 gms. three times a day, before meals to increase appetite, after to promote digestion.
Vehicle	Honey for Kapha, warm water for Pitta and Vata. Pitta can take more safely with aloe gel.

2. Energy Tonic
Ashwagandha Compound

Ingredients	Ashwagandha 4, shatavari 2, pueraria (kudzu) 2, long pepper (pippali) 1.
Properties	Tonic, rejuvenative, aphrodisiac, expectorant, antirheumatic, analgesic.
Uses	Lack of energy, low vitality, sexual debility, infertility, nervous debility, insomnia, nerve degeneration, emaciation, arthritis, diabetes, weak immune function, chronic bronchitis. Can be used wherever Ashwagandha or its preparations are indicated. More balanced and safer for long term usage or usage as a general tonic for all three humors than Ashwagandha by itself. Decreases Vata, increases Kapha and Pitta.
Dose	2–5 gms. three times a day with meals.
Vehicle	Warm milk or warm water. Milk is preferable as a vehicle for its nutritive properties.

3. Lung Tonic

Ingredients	Bala or solomon's seal 2, holy basil (tulsi) 2, elecampane 1, vasa or mullein 1, cinnamon 1.
Properties	Expectorant, stimulant, diaphoretic, decongestant.
Uses	Cough, colds, flu, congestion, asthma, bronchitis, weak lungs, shortness of breath, indigestion. Decreases Kapha and Vata, increases Pitta.
Dose	2–4 gms. every two hours for acute conditions; 1–4 gms. twice a day as a lung tonic.
Vehicle	Warm water or honey for its dispersing and expectorant action, as a tonic with milk.

4. Woman's Tonic
Shatavari Compound

Ingredients	Shatavari 3, comfrey root 2, cyperus 1, red raspberry 1, saffron 1/4.

Properties	Emmenagogue, tonic, alterative, laxative. Can be used whenever Shatavari is indicated in treating female reproductive, blood or liver disorders. Decreases Vata and Pitta, does not overly increase Kapha.
Uses	Menstrual disorders (PMS, amenorrhea, dysmenorrhea), menopause, female debility, infertility, anemia, swollen breasts, breast or uterine tumors, chronic hepatitis, cirrhosis.
Dose	1–4 gms. three times a day before meals.
Vehicle	Milk (with ghee) as a tonic, warm water or fresh ginger tea to promote menstruation, aloe gel for Pitta.

5. Colon Tonic
Triphala Plus

Ingredients	Haritaki 2, amalaki 1, bibhitaki 1, ginger 1.
Properties	Laxative, astringent, tonic, rejuvenative.
Uses	Chronic constipation, colitis, diverticulitis, hemorrhoids, arthritis, nervous debility. Can be used whenever Triphala is indicated. Stronger in action and requires lower dosage (Triphala by itself traditionally requires 3–15 gms. for a normal dosage). Good for all three humors.
Dose	1–4 gms. three times a day, before meals or on an empty stomach; 3–10 gms. before sleep as a purgative.
Vehicle	Water generally, for Kapha with honey.

6. Brain Tonic
Gotu Kola Compound

Ingredients	Gotu kola 4, ashwagandha 2, calamus 1, sandalwood 1, licorice 1.
Properties	Nervine, antispasmodic, diuretic.
Uses	Insomnia, headaches, nervousness, irritability, anxiety, mental weakness, poor memory, poor concentration, hypertension, drug detoxification, to counter addictions. Can be used whenever Gotu Kola is indicated. Balanced for all three humors and a good tonic for the mind.
Dose	1–4 gms. three times a day after meals; an additional dosage can be taken before sleep.
Vehicle	With cool water to cool the mind, with ghee (clarified butter) or warm milk as a tonic.

7. Herbal Febrifuge
Blood Purifier

Ingredients	Sandalwood 2, vetivert 2, lemon grass 1, katuka (or barberry) 2, dry ginger 1.
Properties	Antipyretic, alterative, refrigerant.
Uses	Fever, swollen glands, sore throat, boils, skin rashes, acne, sunstroke, burns, flu, bronchitis, headaches. Decreases Pitta and Kapha, increases Vata.
Dose	1–4 gms. three times a day for general blood cleansing, every 2–3 hours for fever.
Vehicle	Ghee or cool water for old fevers, warm water for new.

8. Liver Tonic

Ingredients	Bhumyamalaki (phyllanthus) 2, katuka 2, turmeric 1, barberry 1, gotu kola 1, coriander 1.
Properties	Hepatic, alterative, bitter tonic.
Uses	Hepatitis, jaundice, gall stones, cirrhosis, genital herpes, venereal diseases. An excellent anti-Pitta formula, cuts to the root of many Pitta disorders by decongesting the bile. Helpful for many Kapha conditions also; may increase Vata.
Dose	1–4 gms. three times a day (double dosage during fever).
Vehicle	Generally with cool water or ghee.

9. Herbal Absorption Compound

Ingredients	Nutmeg, cardamom, cyperus, long pepper (pippali), camomile, licorice; all equal parts.
Properties	Stimulant, carminative, astringent.
Uses	Lack of appetite, indigestion, gas and abdominal distention, colic, nervous indigestion, candida, chronic diarrhea or loose stool, malabsorption. Decreases Vata and Kapha, increases Pitta.
Dose	1–4 gms. three times a day before meals.
Vehicle	Water, buttermilk, draksha. Buttermilk is the main vehicle for all humors.

10. Kidney Tonic

Ingredients	Gokshura 2, pashana bheda (or gravel root) 2, corn silk 1, lemon grass 1, coriander 1, fennel 1.

Properties	Diuretic, lithotriptic, tonic.
Uses	Difficult, painful or burning urination, urinary tract infections, sciatica, lower back pain, kidney stones. Decreases Kapha and Pitta, does not overly increase Vata.
Dose	1–4 gms. three times a day.
Vehicle	For Kapha with honey, for Pitta or infectious conditions with cool water or aloe gel, for Vata and as a tonic with milk.

11. Heart Tonic
Arjuna Compound

Ingredients	Arjuna 4, ashwagandha 2, guggul 2, sandalwood 1.
Properties	Circulatory stimulant, tonic, alterative, hemostatic.
Uses	Heart weakness, palpitations, arteriosclerosis, hypertension, coronary heart diseases, angina, after heart attacks, postsurgery, cardiac edema. Can be used wherever arjuna is indicated, balanced for all three humors.
Dose	1–4 three times a day.
Vehicle	Warm water, milk for tonic action.

NOTE: Another effective heart tonic can be made with arjuna 2, guggul 1, gotu kola 1 and elecampane 1.

12. Antacid Formula

Ingredients	Amalaki 1, shatavari 1, licorice 1, dry ginger 1/2, gentian 1/2.
Properties	Antacid, demulcent, analgesic.
Uses	Indigestion, hyperacidity, heartburn, ulcers, gastritis Decreases Pitta and Vata, mildly increases Kapha.
Dose	1–4 gms. three times a day, after meals.
Vehicle	With warm water or milk generally.

13. Antirheumatic Formula
Guggul compound

Ingredients	Guggul 4, shallaki (or myrrh) 2, cyperus 1, galangal 1.
Properties	Antirheumatic, alterative, analgesic.

Uses	Arthritis, gout, rheumatoid arthritis, bone or ligament in-juries, useful in sports medicine. Good wherever guggul is indicated. Decreases Vata and Kapha, does not overly in-crease Pitta.
Dose	1–4 gms. morning and evening.
Vehicle	Warm water generally; with honey for Kapha.

14. Herbal Sedative

Ingredients	Gotu kola 2, jatamansi (or valerian) 2, shankha pushpi 1, nutmeg 1.
Properties	Sedative, nervine, antispasmodic.
Uses	Insomnia, anxiety, hypertension, nervousness, tremors, pal-pitations. Generally balancing but specific for lowering Vata. Dose 2–6 gms. in the evening or as needed.
Vehicle	Warm milk or ghee for increasing calming action on all three humors.

15. Weight Reduction Formula

Ingredients	Haritaki 2, amalaki 2, bibhitaki 2, katuka (or gentian) 2, dry ginger 1, gotu kola 1.
Properties	Laxative, alterative.
Use	Obesity, overeating, hypertension, chronic constipation, sugar addictions. Specific for Kapha but balances all three humors.
Dose	1–4 gms. before meals.
Vehicle	Best taken with honey or warm water by all types.
Precautions	Emaciation, chronic low weight or sudden weight loss.

16. Chyavan Combination

Chyavan prash is the most famous Ayurvedic herbal tonic food. The jelly, however, is not always convenient to take. This formula is one of the oldest versions; it can be taken whenever Chyavan prash is indicated: its properties and use are the same.

Ingredients	Amalaki, gokshura, bhumyamalaki, guduchi, ash-wagandha, shatavari, kapikacchu, cyperus, cinnamon leaf and nagakeshar.
Dose	1–3 gms. or two to three tablets twice a day morning and evening.
Vehicle	Warm milk.

17. Sexual Vitality Formula

Ingredients	Gokshura, Asteracantha longifolia, kapikacchu, ashwagandha, shatavari; all equal parts.
Properties	Tonic, stimulant, aphrodisiac, rejuvenative.
Uses	Sexual debility, impotence, swollen prostate, low vitality, poor immune function, lower back pain. Decreases Vata and increases Kapha, does not overly increase Pitta.
Dose	1–4 gms. morning and evening.
Vehicle	Warm milk (and ghee) — these are also considered aphrodisiacs.

3
OIL THERAPY,
AROMAS AND INCENSE

Various oils are commonly used in herbal systems throughout the world, but they have their greatest diversity and importance in Ayurveda.

Oil is specific for Vata (air or wind) disorders. As these constitute the majority of diseases, oil therapy is essential for most forms of treatment. It is indicated in diseases of the nervous system, bones and the deeper tissues. It is useful for the other humors as well. Ayurvedic oils are mainly for external use, but some can be taken internally. Simple oils can be homemade, or special preparations can be purchased.

External usage in Ayurveda includes application of oils to the nasal passage, the ears, mouth and other orifices and in medicated enemas, as well as massage. Essential oils can be placed on various sites on the skin, like the points of the seven chakras (especially the third eye).

Oils are usually of two types, which can be combined. First, there are heavy or fatty oils. These are vegetable oils like sesame and animal oils like ghee (clarified butter) or animal fat. With their nutritive properties they combine well with tonic herbs like licorice or ashwagandha.

The second are essential oils: subtle aromatic oils from fragrant or pungent plants like mint or jasmine. They are active in small amounts and, when combined with heavier oils, help activate them and give them greater powers of penetration. They work well in alcohol. They should never be taken internally in their pure form, nor applied directly to any mucus membranes, as their action can be highly irritant with many side effects.

OIL THERAPY AND THE DIFFERENT HUMORS

VATA (AIR)
For Vata the best general oil is sesame. It is warm, heavy, lubricating, nourishing to the skin, bones and nerves and calms the mind. It is said to be the only oil that has the power to penetrate all seven layers of the skin and to nourish all the organs and tissues. Almond or olive oil are also good but cannot substitute for sesame in severe diseases.

Many tonic herbs are good prepared in sesame oil, such as ashwagandha, shatavari, and bala. The nutritive, softening, demulcent action of the oils and tonic herbs works synergistically. This combination is necessary for lowering high Vata.

Special Ayurvedic oils for Vata include Mahanarayan and Narayan. Most Ayurvedic oils are good for Vata.

Essential Oils

Best for Vata are warm, stimulating essential oils like camphor, wintergreen, cinnamon, musk, galangal or cyperus, combined with calming, nutritive and grounding oils like sandalwood, rose or jasmine. Both do better added to the heavy oils and tonics mentioned above. In an alcohol base they may be too light to really alleviate Vata, which may be irritated by fragrances that are too strong or perfumy.

PITTA (FIRE)

For Pitta the best general oil for external usage is coconut oil. It is cooling and calming and relieves thirst and burning sensations. Sunflower oil is also helpful and can be used for inflammatory skin conditions. Sometimes sesame oil is used as a base for anti-Pitta oils with the addition of cooling herbs that neutralize its slightly warming energy. Some Pitta types who cannot tolerate sesame oil (it causes itching) do well with olive oil.

Ghee (clarified butter) is usually the best oil for Pitta, but mainly for internal usage. However, it can be used externally and was in Vedic times, particularly if aged in a copper or silver vessel.

Cooling and calming tonic herbs should be added to these oil bases, including shatavari, gotu kola, bhringaraj. Formulas include Brahmi oil and Bhringaraj oil.

Essential Oils

Pitta types enjoy fragrant flowers as most flowers have cooling and calming properties. Good flowery oils for Pitta include gardenia, jasmine, rose, honeysuckle, violet, iris, and lotus. The best essential oil for Pitta is sandalwood, especially when applied regularly to the third eye. Other good cooling oils that can be applied to the head are lemon grass, lavender, mint, henna and vetivert.

KAPHA (WATER)

For Kapha the best general oil is mustard oil. It is warm, light and stimulating and dispels phlegm. Another good drying oil for Kapha is flaxseed (linseed) oil. When Kapha is very high, however, all oils may have to be avoided.

Essential Oils

Kapha does best with essential oils that are warm, light, stimulating and expectorant. Good oils include sage, cedar, pine, myrrh, camphor, musk, patchouli, and cinnamon. Kapha can tolerate and should use strong, sharp and stimulating fragrances, though may prefer those that are sweet. Plasters of these herbs or the oils in rubbing alcohol can be applied when Kapha cannot tolerate any heavy oils.

INCENSE

Incense has been used in the Orient not only for religious purposes but for healing, particularly for the treatment of mental disorders. It is a good preventative to ward off disease and promote longevity. It should be used on a daily basis.

Incense is important for calming the mind. All incenses generally balance the mind, equalize the humors and increase sattva, mental clarity. Incense purifies the air and the physical environment, the aura and astral environment, increasing prana. It helps counter negative emotions, negative attitudes and confused thoughts, and drives out negative influences and negative entities. Drawing down the energies of the gods (beneficent cosmic powers), it increases faith, devotion, peace and perception.

The properties and application of incense are similar to those of essential oils.

VATA (AIR)

Vata types benefit from incense to calm the mind and strengthen the nerves, to relieve restlessness, anxiety and fear, and to counter hypersensitivity.

For Vata, good incenses are those that are warming and energizing yet grounding, stabilizing and give peace and strength — sandalwood, myrrh, frankincense, almond, musk, basil and camphor.

PITTA (FIRE)

Pitta benefits from incense to calm the emotions and cool the mind, to relieve agitation, aggression and anger.

The best incense for Pitta is sandalwood. Also good are rose, saffron, jasmine, gardenia, geranium, plumeria, and most flower fragrances.

KAPHA (WATER)

Kapha benefits from incense to stimulate the mind, promote perception and counter dullness. Essential oils of flowers, which increase Kapha and promote Kapha emotions like love, faith and compassion, are better for Pitta and Vata. Incense from tree resins like pine or myrrh are good for Kapha, as they have expectorant and cleansing properties.

Good incenses for Kapha are myrrh, frankincense, cedar, sage, basil, camphor, and musk.

4
HERB
USAGE

DOSAGE

The sections on various diseases in the book list individual herbs that are good for different conditions. These can be taken as single remedies, usually one ounce of the herb per pint of boiling water, taken daily in two or three portions. If the herbs are very pungent or very bitter, like cayenne or golden seal, lower dosages can be used, one-quarter to one-half. The same herbs can be taken as powders, 1–4 gms. (four grams is one teaspoon or a little more for most powdered herbs), two or three times daily. Again, the lower dosage is for the stronger tasting herbs. The appropriate vehicles, like honey for Kapha (water), ghee for Pitta (fire) or warm milk for Vata (air), should be used. The same dosages and manner of taking can be used for those who wish to prepare for themselves the formulas listed in the text. For premade medicines, dosages are listed under them in the formula section.

FORMULA DEVELOPMENT

To devise our own formulas based on Ayurvedic principles, we must first comprehend the main principles of formula development. We can build on classical Ayurvedic formulas or combinations (Trikatu, for instance), or use similar ideas to make our own base formulas. We can use Western or Chinese herbs and combinations once we understand their energetics. Devising our own formulas and using raw herbs, rather than premade pills and tablets, we can make stronger preparations and have greater variability in our treatment approach. It also allows us to make a remedy when the appropriate Ayurvedic herbs or premade formulas are not available. However, it is less convenient and requires a certain skill and familiarity with herbs that can take some time to acquire.

There is no great mystery about formula development. There are a few major principles with adaptations according to conditions. Yet certain combinations, theoretically no better than others, are found to work especially well.

A good starting principle is to use two to four herbs, usually three, that most typify the action one wishes to achieve. We have the famous three pungent herbs, the Trikatu formula of Ayurveda, just mentioned. Imagine that we want a formula with primarily bitter taste, which can treat a large variety of Pitta and Kapha conditions. We can make a simple formula with three common bitters as gentian, barberry and golden seal.

To such a base formula we add various supplementary herbs to adjust or modify it in various directions. We might add herbs to strengthen its action along related lines or balancing agents to prevent its action from being too extreme.

Diuretics would aid in its cleansing properties; uva ursi or pipsissewa, also mainly bitter, would strengthen its antibiotic properties against bladder infections.

We could add alteratives — dandelion or isatis — to aid in its blood-cleansing action for dealing with boils or severe infections.

Purgatives to aid in its bile cleansing action could be rhubarb root and aloe powder, also bitter.

To increase its weight-reducing action and to prevent these bitter herbs from weakening the digestive fire, we could add spices like dry ginger. This would be especially good for Kapha types.

As it is a fairly reducing formula, we might want to add some tonifying herbs. Licorice, marshmallow or shatavari, would do this, giving it some nourishing properties but retaining its anti-Pitta action. Moreover, their demulcent property, combined with the bitter, makes a good combination for ulcers and hyperacidity, adding soothing action on the mucus membranes.

As all disease tends to involve stress, tension and disturbed mental or emotional states, we might want to add a nervine or antispasmodic herb. Gotu kola or bhringaraj would be good; they aid in the basic liver-cleansing action of the three bitters. Such a combination would also be good for dealing with alcohol and other substances that make the liver toxic.

Disease is commonly based on a stagnation of energy or blockage of the channels. We might want to add some turmeric for opening up the liver and pancreas and relieving any blockage in their systems.

Putting these principles together for a liver-cleansing formula for a strong Kapha type who has eaten too much meat, sugar and fats, we might use gentian, golden seal and barberry, along with dry ginger, turmeric and gotu kola, taken with honey.

For a weak Pitta type suffering from chronic hepatitis, we might use the three bitters with shatavari, licorice, turmeric and gotu kola, taken with ghee. We might even take out one of the bitters, like golden seal, to prevent the formula from being too reducing.

With the appropriate strategy, avoiding any excessive or one-sided action, we have much latitude in combining herbs to treat conditions. Yet, whatever the condition, we must take care to treat the underlying humor and not just proceed symptomatically. We must then adjust the formula based upon the experience of the patient. In this process we can learn to make our combinations more effective. Herbs, whether classically formed and commercially made or formulas made by ourselves, do not always have the expected result, even if all factors appear correct. Experience must always be our final teacher. Using these Ayurvedic herbs and formulas, we may find that their effectiveness varies according to time, place and culture, requiring some adaptation and adjustment.

POTENTIZATION OF HERBS

Not only must we have the right diagnosis and right prescription to adequately treat a condition, the herbs must also have the right potency. Many old or commercially-prepared herbs may lack this.

Potentization of herbs is not just a physical or chemical matter. It requires strengthening the life-force in the herbs, which in turn requires an act of consciousness. It cannot be done by mechanical methods alone. A physically-oriented medicine must fail, as it cannot serve as a vehicle for the life-force. So too, a physical or descriptive herbalism is inherently limited.

Many of these methods of potentization overlap. Some are discussed in more detail in other parts of the book.

HOW TO PREPARE HERBS WITH POWER

In some respects it is misleading to speak of the general properties of an herb. These vary, particularly by degree, according to how the herb is grown, prepared and combined. They are general guidelines, not rigid rules. Miraculous powers can be found in very ordinary herbs when they are specially grown and prepared. All herbs are vehicles of the life-force or cosmic healing power. As such, they all possess a certain neutrality and can be made into vehicles for that power on different levels.

Specially Powerful Herbs

Some herbs, like ginseng or ashwagandha, are endowed with special power. They tend to retain this power even when other supporting factors are lacking. Generally, roots hold their power longer than other plant parts, then barks and fruit; leaves and flowers deteriorate first.

Specially Grown Herbs

Fresh herbs maintain a special power, have more Prana or chi, more life-force, than dry ones. Their juice is particularly strong. Growing methods, in terms of soil, sunlight, etc., are important. Fresh herbs, even singly or in small dosages, can affect the body and mind more directly, and have better healing power, than large amounts of old herbs. Homegrown herbs, grown with love and attention, possess more gentle, yet consistent, healing power.

How an herb is grown is as important a factor in healing as what the herb is. A few well grown or prepared herbs can cure diseases that many herbs otherwise cannot touch. Some herbalists, therefore, choose to use a few herbs, perhaps very common ones, grown and prepared with care. This is not a lack of sophistication but sophistication of a different nature.

Wild Herbs

Wild herbs possess the strongest life-force. Handpick your own with care, love and respect. They transmit the force of Nature herself. Wildcrafted herbs also tend to be stronger than those cultivated.

Special Combinations of Herbs

The right combination of herbs allows the individual herbs to function synergistically, with geometrically increased powers. Each herbal tradition has such combinations. We can discover others ourselves.

Special Extraction

The active ingredients of herbs are best extracted by the appropriate medium. These include water, alcohol, vinegar, milk, honey and oils. These may be used as vehicles for taking the herbs also.

Addition of Potentizing Herbs

Some herbs are able to potentize others in different directions and can be added as an activating principle. These include stimulants such as cayenne, ginger, camphor, and mint, which often serve as guiding herbs. Vehicles (anupanas) or special media such as honey or ghee also help to direct the effects of herbs.

Herbal Preparations

Herbal wines, oils and jellies not only extend the life of herbs but also can heighten their powers.

Trituration

This process involves stirring an herb in a mortar and pestle. Usually a powder or a liquid paste is used. Juices or decoctions of the herb or other herbs can be added. This allows a more uniform energy to the herbal preparation as well as greater strength. The properties of the substance the mortar and pestle are made of is important. Stone, copper, silver or gold add their special qualities to the herbs triturated in them.

Alchemical Preparations

Spagyric tinctures are very powerful.

The combination of herbs with specially incinerated minerals is commonly used in Ayurveda.

Gems and Minerals

Gems can be used to energize plants, as gem waters, gem tinctures or used to focus energy on an herbal preparation. See chapter on 'Spiritual Remedial Measures'.

Gold, silver, copper and iron can also help energize herbs. Prepared or cooked in vessels of these metals, herbs gain their mineral power. Tinctures of these metals transmit their properties to the herbs without causing any toxicity.

Gold aids in reducing Vata and Kapha (air and water). Silver reduces Pitta and Vata (fire and air). Copper reduces Kapha (water). Iron reduces Vata (air). Bronze reduces Pitta (fire).

Attunement Methods

Attunement is the growing, preparing or prescribing of herbs according to the right time. Astrology is the main attunement method. Proper power and aspect of the Moon is important, as it rules plants generally. Mercury, which rules healing, Jupiter, which gives vitality; are also considered.

Mental Methods

Methods of mental empowerment are mantra, meditation and prayer. They may involve the energization of a particular wish or intention. Some use an energy pattern in the mind on a subtle level to empower that in the herb on a gross level. Others concentrate on a certain deity or divine power to work through the herb.

Some may be part of or involve physical actions or rituals. All preparation of herbs is a ritual; that is, a sacred action, in harmony with the rhythm of the cosmos, to facilitate the cosmic healing force.

Such methods are essential to any form of holistic healing. Otherwise, on a subtle or astral level the herbs, with their sensitivity and neutrality, may pick up negative energies.

Mantras for Potentizing Herbs

Many different mantras can be used for potentizing herbs. Deities may be called on as part of this process, as each mantra is a Divine Name. 'Om', used generally, affirms and empowers whatever we direct it towards. It also empowers other mantras (see 'Spiritual Remedial Measures'). The mantra 'Som' increases the energy of plants.

Other Factors

Herbs have better effect when applied close to the site of the problem; for instance, the use of enemas for Vata.

Also, herbs have to be integrated into an appropriate life-regime in harmony with an individual's nature. They can only work through the tree of our own soul.

5
SPIRITUAL REMEDIAL MEASURES:
AYURVEDA, ASTROLOGY,
GEM THERAPY AND MANTRA

Ayurveda and Astrology

Ayurveda and astrology were originally part of a single spiritual science. While Ayurveda primarily diagnoses and treats the physical body, astrology primarily diagnoses and treats the subtle body or mind. Using both together, we can achieve a more integral treatment. Ayurveda gives us a more specific view on present physical imbalances; astrology shows us the long-term trends of the life and vitality.

Spiritual Therapies of Ayurveda

Ayurveda uses various spiritual therapies to treat subtle disorders. These are more specifically aligned with astrology but can be applied on their own as well. Hence, in this section we also present gems, mantra and color therapy.

Astrology and Gem Therapy

In the Vedic system of astrology used in India certain gems are correlated to the planets and used to balance out their influences. In this way gems have been used astrologically to treat physical, mental and spiritual disorders. Gem therapy is the main astrological treatment and is prescribed according to astrological indications.

Gems prescribed to be worn according to Vedic astrology can be taken internally for similar effects in Ayurveda. However, for internal usage they are specially treated by complex processes to render them safe and non-toxic to the body. These gem preparations are still used in Ayurvedic medicines today. They are not available in the United States, but we can use gems externally or use gem tinctures that do not actually involve taking the mineral itself.

Gems are worn externally as rings or as pendants hanging down to the throat or heart chakras. According to the Vedic system the fingers of the hand and the elements correspond: the little finger is earth, the ring finger water, the middle finger air, the index finger ether, and the thumb fire (the being the size of the thumb in the Vedas is Agni). The planets ruling these fingers are Mercury (earth), Sun or Moon (water), Saturn (air) and Jupiter (ether). No specific planet rules the thumb. By wearing the gems relating to these respective elements or planets on the appropriate fingers, we can strengthen their influences. It is always best if the gems are set so as to actually touch the skin.

Gem tinctures, like herb tinctures, are prepared by soaking the gem for a period of time in a 50–100% alcohol solution. Hard gems like diamond or sapphire can be soaked for one month (from full moon to full moon). Soft, usually opaque gems, like pearl and coral, are soaked for shorter periods of time, or in weaker solutions. Chanting of the planetary mantras aids in giving power to the tincture.

Gem therapy, though mainly forgotten for centuries, has gained a new popularity in the Western world today. There is a strong new interest in the healing properties of crystals, gems and minerals. There is, however, much difference of opinion as to what each gem does or to what it corresponds.

The Vedic use of gems, on the other hand, is grounded in a many thousand year old medical and astrological system. It is integrated, as well, with the use of colors and mantras as part of the system of Yoga originated by enlightened sages. Ayurvedic doctors have carefully noted the internal effects of gem oxides. Hence, the Vedic system presents the oldest, most continually used and most validated system of gem therapy. Its insights should be carefully considered in any new gem therapy today.

The following are some introductory ideas. Medical astrology is a subject in itself. I have dealt with it in detail in my Vedic Astrology correspondence course and in my forthcoming book on the subject, *The Astrology of the Seers.*

GEMS AND THE PLANETS

The classical Vedic correspondence between the major precious gems and the planets is as follows.

The Sun	Ruby.
The Moon	Pearl.
Mars	Red Coral.
Mercury	Emerald.
Jupiter	Yellow Sapphire.
Venus	Diamond.
Saturn	Blue Sapphire.

The Vedic system also used the lunar nodes. For the north node or dragon's head, a hessonite (golden grossularite) garnet, was prescribed. For the south node or dragon's tail, it was a cat's eye (chrysoberyl).

Uranus, Neptune and Pluto were not known to the ancients. Pluto appears to relate to dark stones such as black coral or onyx. Neptune may have much in common with opals, particularly the iridescent type. Uranus is associated with the dark blue Saturn stones, or amethyst.

Since most of these gem stones are very expensive, the following are recommended as substitutes. Red coral is not expensive so substitution for it is not necessary.

For ruby	Garnet or sunstone.
For pearl	Moonstone.
For emerald	Peridot or jade.
For yellow sapphire	Yellow topaz or citrine.
For diamond	Clear zircon.
For blue sapphire	Amethyst.

TRADITIONAL USAGE OF GEMS IN ASTROLOGY AND AYURVEDA

While gems do have influence on the physical body, their main action is on the level of the life-force. Not all are strongly related to one of the biological humors. Many, as subtle or mental remedies, can help balance all three humors. We can direct or balance their humoral action according to the metal we set them in (which serves as the vehicle).

The more expensive gem stones, worn as rings, should be two or more carats. The less expensive or substitutes are better in four or more. Even larger stones can be used, particularly for pendants or necklaces (in which case a good substitute stone would be better than a small size primary stone). Gem stones have stronger effects if they touch the skin. Hence rings made according to the Vedic system are open below, set to come into direct contact with the skin.

Below I list the main properties of the primary gem stones. Their substitutes have similar but weaker qualities.

Ruby

Ruby is used in astrology for strengthening the heart, improving digestion, promoting circulation, reviving fire and increasing energy. It increases Pitta and decreases Kapha and Vata. It is hot in energy and composed of the elements of fire, air and ether. Ruby strengthens the will, promotes independence, gives insight and enhances power; it was the gem of kings. It is usually set in gold and worn on the ring finger of the right hand.

Ruby ash (Manikya bhasma) is regarded as a stimulant, nervine and heart tonic for weakness of the heart and nerves, and for general debility.

Pearl

Pearl is good for promoting body fluids and the blood, nourishing the body tissues and the nerves. It increases Kapha and decreases Pitta and Vata. It is slightly cold in energy and composed of water, earth and ether. Pearl strengthens the female reproductive system, improves fertility, and calms the emotions. It is usually set in silver and worn on the ring finger of the left hand.

Pearl ash (Moti bhasma) is said to be tonic, alterative, sedative, nervine and antacid. It is used for hyperacidity, ulcers, epistaxis, hemoptysis, liver and kidney ailments, nervous excitability, hysteria and as a good general tonic for women and infants.

Red Coral

Red coral strengthens the blood and reproductive system, improves energy and calms emotion. It harmonizes Pitta, decreases Vata but in excess can increase Kapha. It is slightly warm in energy and composed of earth, water and fire. Red coral is an aphrodisiac, particularly for the male, builds flesh and muscle, gives courage and improves work capacity. It is usually set in silver and worn on the ring or index finger.

Red coral ash (Praval bhasma) is alterative, antacid, tonic. It is used for cough, asthma, swollen glands, hyperacidity, impotence, bleeding from the lungs, anemia, and sexual debility.

Emerald

Emerald calms mental agitation, regulates the nervous system, helps stop nerve pain and improves speech and intelligence. It harmonizes Vata, decreases Pitta but can slightly increase Kapha. It is cool in energy and composed of ether, water and air. Emerald promotes healing, energizes the breath, strengthens the lungs and increases flexibility and adaptability of mind. It is a harmonizing stone, good for cancer and other degenerative diseases. For Vata and Kapha it is set in gold, for Pitta silver. It is worn on the middle or little finger.

Emerald ash (Panna bhasma) is nervine, alterative and tonic. It is used for nervous debility, neurasthenia, general debility and as a heart tonic. It is good for asthma, ulcers, skin diseases, fevers and infections and as a tonic for children.

Yellow Sapphire

Yellow sapphire gives energy and vitality and is the best general stone for promoting health. It regulates the hormonal system and increases Ojas. It is slightly warm in energy. It generally balances all the humors but is particularly good for lowering high Vata. In excess or not balanced properly it can aggravate Pitta. Yellow sapphire is good for diabetes and all wasting diseases, and for convalescence. It is composed of ether, fire and water. It is usually set in gold and worn on the index finger.

Yellow sapphire ash is tonic, alterative and nervine. It improves digestion, strengthens the heart and brings about increase of intelligence.

Diamond

Diamond is neutral in energy and composed of all five elements. It decreases Vata and Pitta but mildly increases Kapha. It strengthens the kidneys and reproductive system and enhances Ojas. Diamond gives beauty, power and charm and enhances our creative abilities. It protects our life in extreme diseases. It is usually set in white gold and worn on the middle or little finger.

Diamond ash (Hira bhasma) is tonic, nutritive and aphrodisiac. It gives strength and firmness to the body, protects the life, increases sexual power and Ojas.

Zircon ash (Vaikrant bhasma) can be used as a substitute.

Blue Sapphire

Blue sapphire is cold in energy and is composed of the elements of ether and air. It clears infections and wards off all negative energies. It is antitumor and antifat and good for reducing therapy. Blue sapphire strengthens the bones, increases longevity and helps calm the nerves and emotions. It promotes calm, peace and detachment. For Vata and Kapha it is set in gold, for Pitta, silver. It is worn on the middle finger.

Blue sapphire ash is used as an alterative, nervine and antiseptic. It is good for arthritis, rheumatism, fevers, infections, nerve pain, and paralysis.

Hessonite Garnet

Hessonite garnet is neutral in energy and composed of the elements of fire, water and ether. Like the yellow sapphire, golden hessonite is a good balancing stone. It calms the nerves, quiets the mind, relieves depression. This stone is recommended for almost everyone, as it counters the negative influence of Maya (illusion). The north lunar node is thought to indicate the influence of Maya, which is predominant in the dark age in which we live. Hessonite garnet is usually set in gold and worn on the middle finger. No ash of it is commonly made.

Cat's Eye

Cat's eye is hot in energy and composed of the elements of fire, air and ether. It increases Pitta and decreases Kapha and Vata. It stimulates Tejas, mental fire, and is good for promoting psychic and spiritual perception. Cat's eye is a good nervine stimulant and is helpful for mental disorders. It is the gem stone of seers and astrologers. It also is not usually found as an ash.

Quartz Crystal

The commonly used quartz crystal is also used in the Vedic system. Clear quartz is considered a Venus stone, cloudy or milky is a Moon stone. Clear quartz has an action similar to diamond but much weaker. It is regarded as a very impressionable stone that magnifies whatever influence, good or bad, is around it. Hence, it should be purified and energized properly through mantra and meditation.

Rock crystal ash (Sphatika bhasma) is alterative, hemostatic and tonic and used to treat bleeding disorders, anemia, chronic fever, jaundice, asthma, constipation and general debility.

HERBS AND ASTROLOGY

Herbs were traditionally used along with astrology in both early Eastern and Western herbalism. Famous European herbalists, such as Culpepper were typical of this approach. Herbs were associated with certain signs and planets and were prescribed according to special planetary configurations. Today herbal and naturalistic healing systems are again being correlated with astrology in the Western world, as they have been continuously in the East.

HERBS AND THE PLANETS

The following herbs increase the energy of the planets to which they correspond. They decrease the energy of planets of opposite qualities. Many herbs have energies relating to two or more planets.

The Sun	Hot, spicy or pungent herbs: cayenne, black pepper, ginger, long pepper, cinnamon, cloves, calamus, bayberry, cardamom, galangal.
	These are largely stimulants and increase digestion, promote circulation, improve perception and promote functional activity. In Chinese medicine they are usually yang, warming herbs.

The Moon	Cool, sweet or salty herbs: sandalwood, shatavari, slippery elm, comfrey root, marshmallow, Irish moss, Iceland moss, chickweed. These are largely demulcent and emollient herbs. They may be lung tonics. In Chinese medicine they are usually yin tonics.
Mars	Warm, pungent, stimulant herbs: garlic, asafoetida, mustard, damiana, aconite, coffee, tobacco, wine, marijuana. These are largely stimulants, like the herbs for the Sun, but possess grosser properties. In large amounts some serve as depressants. Many aphrodisiacs, particularly for the male, come under Mars also.
Mercury	Mild, harmonizing and nervine herbs: gotu kola, skullcap, betony, mint, fennel, bhringaraj, jatamansi. Most of the herbs that work on the nerves and mind and help balance all three humors are here.
Jupiter	Sweet, tonic herbs and substances: licorice, ashwagandha, bala, ginseng, ghee, sesame oil, olive oil. Jupiter rules over oils and fats. Most of the energy tonics of Oriental medicine are under this category.
Venus	Sweet, cooling herbs, often fragrant flowers: lotus, rose, hibiscus, red raspberry, saffron, safflower, gardenia, aloe. These work largely on the heart, kidneys and the reproductive system (particularly female).
Saturn	Cold, bitter, astringent, detoxifying herbs: golden seal, gentian, barberry, coptis, isatis, uva ursi, violet, dandelion, selfheal. These are the natural antibiotics, antitumor and anti-fever herbs.

GEMS AND HERBS

The properties of hot, spicy herbs can be increased by taking them with a ruby tincture or by wearing a ruby or its substitutes.

The properties of tonic and rejuvenative herbs can be increased by taking them with a tincture of yellow sapphire or yellow topaz or by wearing these stones or their substitutes.

The properties of herbs to clear heat, cleanse the blood, detoxify the liver and reduce tumors can be increased by taking them with a blue sapphire tincture or by wearing the stone or its substitutes.

The properties of nervine and harmonizing herbs can be increased by taking with an emerald tincture or by wearing an emerald or its substitutes.

The properties of stimulant and aphrodisiac herbs can be increased by taking with a red coral tincture or by wearing red coral.

The properties of emmenagogue herbs or tonics to the reproductive system can be increased by taking with a diamond tincture or by wearing diamond or its substitute.

The properties of demulcent and nutritive tonic herbs can be increased by taking with pearl tincture or by wearing pearl and its substitute.

COLOR THERAPY

Herbs work largely through the green ray of the planet Mercury, which possesses the greatest force of healing and harmonization.

Color therapy can be used in the same way as gems of a specific planet. The body can be bathed in light of the particular color, or exposed to more of that color through clothes, environment, etc. All colors used should be sattvic or harmonious in nature, not excessively bright, loud, flashy or artificial. Please see section on 'Life Regimes' for more information on color therapy and the humors.

Planetary Colors

Sun	Red.
Moon	White.
Mars	Dark red.
Mercury	Green.
Jupiter	Yellow, gold.
Venus	Transparent, variegated.
Saturn	Dark blue, black.
Rahu	Ultraviolet.
Ketu	Infrared.

MANTRA

Mantras and the Planets

Herbs can be energized by the mantra which corresponds to the planet which rules them. These mantras, along with Om, can also be used by themselves for spiritual treatment of the diseases caused by their respective planets.

The Sun	Sum (pronounced 'soom').
The Moon	Som (pronounced like Om).
Mars	Am (pronounced 'um').
Mercury	Bum (the u pronounced as in put).
Jupiter	Gum (same u sound as above).
Venus	Shum (same u sound as above).
Saturn	Sham (pronounced 'shum').

North Node   Ram (the a pronounced as in father).
South Node   Kem (the e pronounced as a long 'a' as in came).

Other Important Healing Sounds

OM: Om is the most important mantra. It serves to energize or empower all things and all processes. Therefore, all mantras begin and end with Om. It clears the mind, opens the channels and increases Ojas. In ancient books it is the sound of the Sun.

SHRIM: ('shreem'). This is the best mantra for promoting general health, beauty, creativity and prosperity. It has lunar and venusian properties and can strengthen the feminine nature.

RAM: (the same as for the North Node of the Moon). This is the best mantra for drawing down the protective light and grace of the Divine. It gives strength, calm, rest and peace and is particularly good for high Vata (air) and mental disorders.

HUM: (the 'u' sound as in put). This is the best mantra for warding off negative influences attacking us, whether disease-causing pathogens, negative emotions or even black magic. It is also the best mantra for awakening Agni and promoting the digestive fire.

AIM: ('aym'). This is the best mantra for the mind, for improving concentration, thinking, for rational powers and for improving speech. It is helpful in mental and nervous disorders. It has a Mercury energy and corresponds to the Goddess of Wisdom, Saraswati.

KRIM: ('cream'). This mantra gives the capacity for work and action and gives power and efficacy to what we do. It is good for chanting while making preparations, as it allows them to work better.

KLIM: ('kleem') gives strength, sexual vitality and control of the emotional nature.

SHAM: the mantra for Saturn can be used generally for promoting peace, calm, detachment and contentment. It is good for mental and nervous disorders.

HRIM: ('hreem') is a mantra of cleansing and purification. It gives energy, joy and ecstasy but only after atonement. It aids any detoxification process.

Mantras for the Elements

The five elements can be strengthened by their respective mantras. These are Lam for Earth, Vam for Water, Ram for Fire, Yam for Air and Ham for Ether. In each case the 'a' sound is short, like the vowel sound in 'the'.

6
VEDIC AND YOGIC
SCIENCE

Those who marvel at the beauty and profundity of Ayurveda should realize that these qualities are shared by all aspects of Vedic Science, of which Ayurveda is a part.

Throughout a long history, the sages and people of India have looked back to a great enlightened Golden Age called the 'Vedic Age'. At that time, the country was ruled by kings who followed the will of the sages. Spirituality permeated the whole of life, which was centered around various internal and external offerings to every form of the Divine. All life was Yoga.

The Vedic Age was well over by the time of Krishna, some centuries before the Buddha, who marks the beginning of what from the Vedic perspective can be called modern Indian historic times. The old integral Vedic teaching broke into several lines and different, often conflicting, systems of spiritual teachings arose. Much of the Vedic spirit was incorporated in Yoga and Vedanta and continued as the guiding light of the culture. We can also call Vedic Science, 'Yogic Science'. The term Yoga first occurs in the Vedic mantras as controlling the mind for spiritual illumination (*Rig Veda, V.80. 1.*).

Of all the branches of Vedic knowledge, Ayurveda has perhaps best preserved the original Vedic terminology (like Agni and Soma), though much of the spiritual implication of these terms was forgotten.

The original Vedic texts themselves, were not seriously studied in India after the time of Krishna, over three thousand years ago. European curiosity revived native interest in them over a century ago. Several great modern Vedic and Vedantic interpreters arose, the most important of which were Swami Vivekananda, Swami Rama Tirtha, Sri Aurobindo, Gangadhar Tilak and Swami Dayananda Saraswati, who were all well known and respected in India.

Based on the model of Vedic Science and incorporating the principles of Yoga and Ayurveda, the essence of the system is shown below. From my own work with the Vedas and my writings on them, I have tried to present an integral approach.

PRINCIPLES OF AN INTEGRAL HEALING SCIENCE
ACCORDING TO THE MODEL OF VEDIC SCIENCE

In this system we can recognize four levels of knowledge, each of which has its own methods of integration or healing. These levels follow the three bodies and our true Self, the embodied being. The physical body is composed of matter; the astral body of thoughts and emotions; the causal body, the reincarnating entity of ideals and archetypes.

1. SELF-KNOWLEDGE — transcendent healing science: Self-inquiry; predominately the higher aspect of the Yoga of knowledge, though surrender to the Divine, the essence of the Yoga of devotion leads one here also.

2. YOGA — causal healing science: Yoga and meditation; includes all the main systems of Yoga in their higher forms, knowledge, devotion, work and techniques, including tantra in its higher aspect.

3. ASTROLOGY — astral healing science: mantra, gems, color therapy and rituals; the systems of Yoga in their lower or occult forms are also useful here.

4. AYURVEDA — physical healing science, diet, herbs, and bodywork.

Five Sheaths and Healing Modalities

According to this system, the individual is composed of three bodies and five sheaths. Of these, the vital sheath connects the physical and astral; the intelligence sheath connects the astral and causal.

Physical sheath	Diet and herbs and asana.
Vital sheath	Herbs, gems and pranayama.
Mental sheath	Mantra (pratyahara).
Intelligence sheath	Meditation (dharana, dhyana).
Bliss sheath	Union, absorption (samadhi).

YOGA AND AYURVEDA

These healing modalities of the five sheaths reflect the eight limbs of the classical Yoga system. The first two, yama and niyama, are the factors of internal and external cleanliness, including right attitude and spiritual values in life, right life-style and life regime for all five sheaths. These two are the foundation of Yoga, without which Yogic practices may have unwholesome results.

The yamas are non-violence, truthfulness, control of sexual energy, non-stealing and non-clinging. The niyamas are self-study, purity, contentment, self-discipline and surrender to the Divine. A traditional Ayurvedic physician was expected to live up to such a standard of ethical behavior.

The next three make up the outer process of Yoga and harmonize the outer nature, allowing us to open up to our true being.

Asana is posture, which is the right alignment of the energies of the physical body along the spine. This gives physical peace.

Pranayama is harmonization and expansion of the life force. This gives emotional peace and calms the vital nature. Pratyahara is withdrawal from distraction, drawing attention inward. This gives peace to the mind.

The last three constitute the inner process of Yoga, the essence of the system. They can be done with form, on a particular object, or without form, on our own Self or on pure consciousness itself. The latter is the true or higher form of meditation; the former is still involved with the outer process of Yoga.

Dharana is attention; the consciousness is concentrated fully on what we direct it towards.

Dhyana is meditation; the consciousness merges into the object of our attention. These two allow intelligence to function.

Samadhi is absorption or unification of the consciousness into the object of our meditation. It is the direct perception of truth in which the observer is the observed.

For these modalities to work, one must have viveka and vairagya. Viveka is discernment, whereby one can discriminate between reality and unreality, truth and falsehood, the eternal and the transient, true joy and passing pleasure. Vairagya is absence of egoistic emotional reactions, which cloud our perception. From these comes abhyasa, our continual practice, the practice of who we are in daily life and action. What we implement in abhyasa determines the success of our Yoga.

It is the purpose of Ayurveda to give us the means of health and healing on a physical and psychological level so that we can pursue the path of Yoga. Ayurveda is most aligned with the outer process of Yoga as asana and pranayama — postures and breath control — which are emphasized in Hatha Yoga (the Yoga of the physical body). Ayurvedic life regimes should be based upon the foundation of Yoga as yama and niyama, inner and outer purity.

This Yoga/Ayurveda system is the natural evolution of life towards reintegration with its Divine source, not a particular religious dogma we should follow. It can be used with all religions or apart from all of them, for the true religion is being itself.

PART IV

APPENDICES

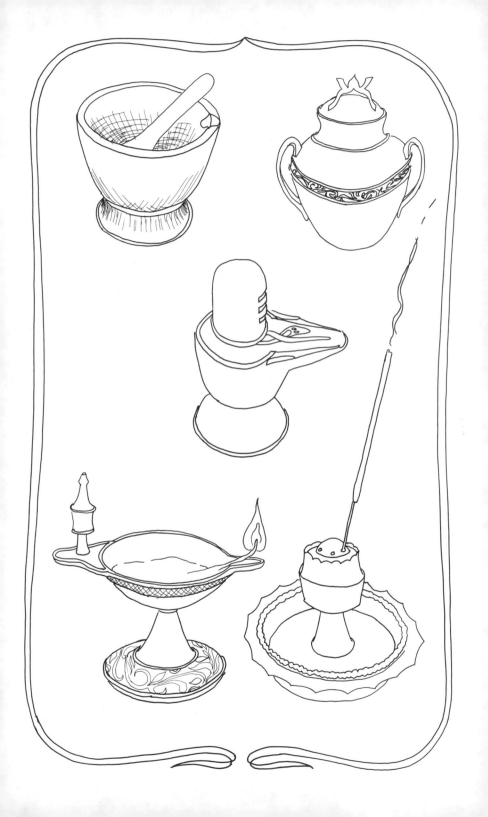

1

ENGLISH

GLOSSARY

Alopecia	natural or abnormal baldness; loss of hair
Alterative	tending to restore normal health; cleanses and purifies the blood; alters existing nutritive and excretory processes gradually restoring normal body functions
Amenorrhea	absence or suppession of menstruation
Anabolic	constructive phase of metabolism; building up (repair and growth) of body substance Analgesic relieves pain
Anthelmintic	helps destroy and dispel parasites (includes vermides and vermifuges; in Ayurveda parasites include worms, bacteria, fungus and yeast)
Antibiotic	inhibits growth of or destroys microorganisms
Antipyretic	dispels heat, fire and fever
Antispasmodic	relieves spasms of voluntary and involuntary muscles
Aperient	a mild laxative
Aphrodisiac	reinvigorates the body by reinvigorating the sexual organs
Aromatic	herbs which contain volatile, essential oils which aid digestion and relieve gas
Astringent	firms tissues and organs; reduces discharges and secretions
Bitter tonic	bitter herbs which in small amounts stimulate digestion and otherwise help regulate fire in the body
Carminative	relieves intestinal gas, pain and distention; promotes peristalsis

Catabolic	destructive phase of metabolism
Cathartic	strong laxative which causes rapid evacuation
Demulcent	soothes, protects and nurtures internal membranes
Diaphoretic	causes perspiration and increased elimination through the skin
Diuretic	promotes activity of kidney and bladder and increases urination
Dysmenorrhea	painful or difficult menstruation
Dyspnea	difficulty in breathing
Emetic	induces vomiting
Emmenagogue	helps promote and regulate menstruation
Emollient	soothes, softens and protects the skin
Enteritis	inflammation of the small intestine
Epistaxis	nosebleed
Expectorant	promotes discharge of phlegm and mucus from lungs and throat
Febrilfuge	reduces fever
Gastritis	inflammation of the stomach
Hematemesis	vomiting of blood
Hemoptysis	spitting up of blood from the lungs or bronchial tubes
Hemostatic	stops the flow of blood; type of astringent that stops internal bleeding or hemorrhaging
Laxative	promotes bowel movements
Lithotriptic	substance that dissolves and discharges gall bladder and urinary stones and gravel
Malabsorption	inadequate absorption of nutrients from the intestinal tract
Menorrhagia	excessive bleeding during menstruation
Nephritis	inflammation of the kidney
Nervine	strenghtens functional activity of nervous system; may be stimulants and sedatives
Neurasthenia	severe nerve weakness, nervous exhaustion

Nutritive tonic	Increases weight and density and nourishes the body
Paroxymal fever	periodic, recurring fevers
Refrigerant	reduces body temperature and relieves thirst
Rejuvenative	prevents decay, postpones aging, revitalizes the organs
Sedative	calms or tranquilizes by lowering functional activity of organ or body part
Stimulant	increases internal heat, dispels internal chill and strengthens metabolism and circulation
Stomachic	strengthens stomach function
Suppuration	pus formation and discharge
Vasodilator	causes relaxation of the blood vessels
Vermicidal	kills parasites in the intestines
Vulnerary	assists in healing of wounds by protecting against infection and stimulating cell growth

2
SANSKRIT
TERMS

Alochak Pitta	form of fire governing vision
Ama	toxins, the undigested food mass
Ambhuvahasrotas	channels carrying water
Annavahasrotas	channels carrying food
Apana	downward moving air
Arishta	herbal wine made with decoctions
Artavavahasrotas	channels carrying menstrual fluid
Asanas	yoga postures
Asava	herbal wine made with juice of herbs
Asthi	bone
Atma	true Self
avalambak Kapha	form of water giving support
Avaleha	herbal jelly
Ayurveda	Vedic science of life or longevity
Bhakti	devotion
Bhasma	specially incinerated mineral preparation
Bhrajak Pitta	form of fire governing complexion
Bodhak Kapha	form of water governing taste
Brahma	reality; the absolute
Brahmacharya	control of sexuality; celibacy
Brimhana	tonification or building therapy
Buddha	the enlightened one; an incarnation of Vishnu
Chikitsa	Ayurvedic treatment

Churna	herbal powder
Dhanvantari	traditional deity of Ayurveda
Dharana	attention
Dhyana	meditation
Ghee	clarified butter
Ghrita	clarified butter
Guggul	pills made with guggul (Commiphora mukul)
Guna	prime quality of nature (Prakriti)
Jnana	knowledge
Jyotish	Vedic or Hindu astrology
Kapha	biological water-humor
Karma	action
Kledak Kapha	form of water governing digestion
Kratu	inner will
Kundalini	energy of the subtle body
Langhana	reduction or lightening therapy
Majja	marrow and nerve tissue
Majjavahasrotas	channels supplying marrow and nerve tissue
Mamsa	muscle
Mamsavahasrotas	channels supplying muscle
Manas	mind
Manovahasrotas	channels carrying thought
Mantra	healing sounds, sacred words
Medas	fat tissue
Medovahasrotas	channels supplying fat tissue
Mutra	urine
Mutravahasrotas	channels carrying urine
Nasya	nasal application of herbs and oils
Nirama	conditions without Ama

Niyama	yogic observances
Ojas	prime energy of the body
Pachak Pitta	form of fire governing digestion
Pancha Karma	the five purification practices of Ayurveda
Pariksha	examination, diagnosis
Pitta	biological fire-humor
Prana	life-force; inward-moving air
Pranavahasrotas	channels carrying the life-force
Pranayama	breath control, yogic breathing practices
Prakriti	primal Nature; biological constitution
Prash	herbal jelly
Pratyahara	yogic control of the senses
Puja	devotional worship or flower offering
Purisha	feces
Purishavahasrotas	channels carrying feces
Purusha	pure Spirit
Ranjak Pitta	form of fire coloring the blood
Rajas	quality of energy, turbulence and distraction
Rakta	blood
Rakta Moksha	blood purification
Raktavahasrotas	channels carrying the blood
Rasa	plasma; special Ayurvedic mineral reparations
Rasayana	rejuvenative
Rasavahasrotas	channels carrying plasma
Rig Veda	most ancient scripture of India
Sadhak Pitta	form of fire governing intelligence
Sama Kapha	Ama condition of Kapha
Sama Pitta	Ama condition of Pitta
Sama Vata	Ama condition of Vata

Samadhi	yogic absorption
Samana	equalizing air, governs digestion
Sattva	quality of clarity and harmony, the mind in its natural state
Shamana	palliation therapy
Shodhana	purification therapy
Shukra	reproductive tissue
Shukravahasrotas	channels supplying the reproductive tissue
Sleshak Kapha	form of water lubricating the joints
Snehana	oil application
Srotas	channel systems of the body
Stanyavahasrotas	channels carrying the breast milk
Sveda	sweat
Svedana	therapeutic sweating, steam therapy
Svedavahasrotas	channels carrying sweat
Taila	medicated oil, mainly with sesame oil
Tapas	asceticism; spiritual work
Tarpak Kapha	form of water governing emotion
Udana	upward moving air
Upanishads	ancient spiritual teachings of India
Vamana	emesis; therapeutic vomiting
Vata	biological air-humor
Vedas	ancient scriptures of India
Vedanta	final or summary portion of the Vedas
Vikriti	disease nature
Virechana	purgation
Vyana	diffusive or outward moving air
Yama	yogic attitudes
Yoga	practise of spiritual reintegration

3
GLOSSARY
OF HERBS

WESTERN HERBS
AND COMMONLY KNOWN AYURVEDIC HERBS

English	Latin	Sanskrit or Hindi
Agrimony	Agrimonia eupatori	
Alfalfa	Medicago sativa	Lasunghas
Almond	Amygdalus communis	Vatatma
Aloe	Aloe spp.	Kumari
Alum root	Heuchera americana	
American ginseng	Panax quinquifolium	
Angelica	Angelica spp.	Choraka
Apricot seeds	Prunus armenica	Jardalu
Arnica	Arnica montana	
Barberry	Berberis spp.	Daruharidra
Basil	Ocimum spp.	Tulsi
Bay leaves	Laurus nobilis	
Bayberry	Myrica spp.	Katiphala
Betony	Stachys betonica	
Black cohosh	Cimicifuga racemosa	
Black pepper	Piper nigrum	Marich
Burdock	Arctium lappa	
Calamus	Acorus calamus	Vacha
Calendula	Calendula officinalis	Zergul
Camomile	Anthemum nobilis	Babuna
Camphor	Cinnamomum camphora	Karpura
Cardamom	Eletarria cardamomum	Ela

English	Latin	Sanskrit or Hindi
Cascara sagrada	Rhamnus purshianus	
Castor oil	Ricinis communis	Eranda
Catechu	Acacia catechu	Khadir
Catnip	Nepeta cataria	Zufa
Cattail	Typha spp.	Eraka
Cayenne pepper	Capsicum frutescens	Katuvira
Cedar	Cedrus spp.	Devadaru
Chaparral	Larrea divaracata	
Chickweed	Stellaria media	
Chicory	Cichorium intybus	Kasani
Chrysanthemum	Chrysanthemum indicum	Sevanti
Cilantro	Coriandrum sativum (leaf)	Dhanyaka
Cinnamon	Cinnamomum zeylonica	Tvak
Cleavers	Galium spp.	
Cloves	Syzgium aromaticum	Lavanga
Cocklebur	Xanthium strumarium	Arista
Coltsfoot	Tussilago farfara	Fanjuim
Comfrey	Symphytum officinale	
Coptis	Coptis spp.	Mishamitita
Coriander	Coriandrum sativum (seed)	Dhanyaka
Corn silk	Zea mays	Yavanala
Cubebs	Piper cubeba	Kankola
Cumin	Cumin cyminum	Jiraka
Damiana	Turnera aphrodisiaca	
Dandelion	Taraxacum vulgare	Dughdapheni
Dates	Phoenix dactylifera	Kharjur
Datura	Datura alba	Kanaka-dattura
Dill	Anthemum vulgaris	Mishreya
Echinacea	Echinacea angustifolia	
Elecampane	Inula spp.	Pushkaramula
Elder flowers	Sambucus glauca	

English	Latin	Sanskrit or Hindi
Ephedra	Ephedra spp.	Somalata
Evening Primrose	Oenethra biennis	
Eucalyptus	Eucalyptus globulis	Tailaparni
Fennel	Foeniculum vulgare	Shatapushpa
Fenugreek	Trigonella foenum-graecum	Methi
Flaxseed	Linum usitatissimum	Uma
Fo ti	Polygonum multiflorum	
Frankincense	Boswellia carteri	Dhup
Galangal	Alpinia officinarum	Rasna
Gardenia	Gardenia floribunda	Nadihingu
Garlic	Allium sativum	Lashuna
Gentian	Gentiana spp.	Trayamana
Ginger	Zingiberis officinalis	Ardra (fresh) Shunthi (dry)
Ginseng	Panax ginseng	Lakshmana
Golden seal	Hydrastis canadensis	
Gotu kola	Centella asiatica	Brahmi
Gravel root	Eupatorium purpuerum	
Grindelia	Grindelia robusta	
Hawthorn berries	Crataegus oxycantha	Ban-sangli
Henna	Lawsonia spp.	Mendhi
Hibiscus	Hibiscus rosa-sinensis	Japa
Horehound	Marrubium vulgare	Farasiyun
Horsetail	Equisetum spp.	
Hyssop	Hyssopus officinalis	Zupha
Iris	Iris spp.	Padma-pushkara
Irish moss	Chondrus crispus	
Jasmine	Jasminum grandiflorum	Jati
Juniper berries	Juniperus spp.	Hapusha
Kelp	Fucus visiculosis	
Lavender	Lavendula spp.	Dharu

English	Latin	Sanskrit or Hindi
Lemon	Citrus limonum	Limpaka
Lemon balm	Melissa officinalis	
Lemon grass	Cymbopogon citratus	Rohisha
Licorice	Glycyzrrhiza spp.	Yashtimadhu
Lime	Citrus acida	Nimbuka
Liquidamber	Liquidamber spp.	
Lobelia	Lobelia inflata	Dhavala
Lotus	Nelumbo nucifera	Padma
Male fern	Dryopteris felix-mas	
Marigold	Tagetes erecta	Jhandu
Marshmallow	Althea officinalis	Gulkairo
Mint	Mentha arvensis	Phudina
Motherwort	Leonurus cardiaca	Guma
Mugwort	Artemesia vulgaris	Nagadamani
Mustard	Brassica alba	Svetasarisha
Myrrh	Commiphora myrrha	Bola
Nettle	Urtica urens	Bichu
Nutmeg	Myristica fragrans	Jatiphala
Oak bark	Quercus spp.	Majuphul
Orange peel	Citrus aurantium	Svadu-narin-ga
Oregano	Origanum vulgare	Sathra
Osha	Ligusticum porteri	
Parsley	Petroselium spp.	
Passion flower	Passiflora incarnata	Mukkopira
Pau d'arco	Tabebuia avellenada	
Peach seeds	Prunus persica	Pichu
Pennyroyal	Mentha pulegium	
Peppermint	Mentha piperata	Gamathi phudina
Pine	Pinus spp.	Shriveshtaka
Pink root	Spigelia marilandica	
Pipsissewa	Chimaphilla umbellata	

English	Latin	Sanskrit or Hindi
Plantain	Plantago spp.	Lahuriya
Plumeria	Plumeria alba	
Potentilla	Potentilla spp.	Spangjha
Prickly ash	Zanthoxylum spp.	Tumburu
Pomegranate	Punica granatum	Dadima
Pumpkin seeds	Curcubito pepo	Kurlaru
Purslane	Portulaca oleracea	Loni
Psyllium	Plantago psyllium	Snigdha-jira
Red clover	Trifolium pratense	Trepatra
Red raspberry	Rubus spp.	Gauriphal
Rhubarb root	Rheum spp.	Amlavetasa
Rose	Rosa spp.	Shatapatra
Rosemary	Rosemarinus officinalis	Rusmari
Rue	Ruta graveolens	Sadapaha
Safflower	Carthamus tinctorius	Kusumba
Saffron	Crocus sativa	Kumkum
Sage	Salvia spp.	Shati
Sandalwood	Santalum alba	Chandana
Santonica	Artemesia santonica	Gadadhar
Sarsaparilla	Smilax spp.	Chopchini
Sassafras	Sassafras officinale	
Saw palmetto	Serenoa repens	
Self-heal	Prunella vulgaris	
Senna	Cassia acutifolia	Nripadruma
Sesame	Sesamum indicum	Til
Siberian ginseng	Eleuthrococcus senticosus	
Skullcap	Scutellaria spp.	
Slippery elm	Ulmus fulva	
Spearmint	Mentha spictata	Pahadi phudina
Spikenard	Aralia racemosus	
Squaw vine	Mitchella repens	

English	Latin	Sanskrit or Hindi
Solomon's seal	Polygonatum officinalis	Mahameda
Southernwood	Artemesia abrotanum	
Strawberry leaf	Fragaria spp.	
Sumac	Rhus glabra	Karkata shringi
Tansy	Tanacatum vulgare	
Thyme	Thymus vulgarus	Ipar
Turmeric	Curcuma longa	Haridra
Usnea	Usnea barbata	
Uva ursi	Arctostaphylos uva-ursi	
Valerian	Valeriana spp.	Tagara
Vetivert	Andropogon muricatus	Ushira
Violet	Viola spp.	Banafshah
Wild cherry bark	Prunus virginiana	
Wild ginger	Asarum spp.	Upana
Wintergreen	Gaultheria procumbens	Gandapura
Witch hazel	Hamamelis virgiana	
Wormseed	Chenopodium abthelminiticum	Chandanbatva
Wormwood	Artemesia absinthium	Indhana
Yarrow	Achillea millefolium	Rojmari
Yellow dock	Rumex crispus	Amlavetasa
Yerba santa	Eriodityon glutinosum	
Yohimbe	Caryanthe yohimbe	
Yucca	Yucca spp.	

Additional Special Ayurvedic Herbs

First is the common name and then the Latin and Sanskrit. When the Sanskrit is the common name it is not repeated.

Common	Latin	Sanskrit
Aconite	Aconitum napellus	Visa
Ajwan	Apium graveolens	Ajamoda
Amalaki	Emblica officinalis	

Common	Latin	Sanskrit
Arjuna	Terminalia arjuna	
Asafoetida	Ferula asafoetida	Hingu
Ashok	Saraca indica	
Ashwagandha	Withania somnifera	
Atmagupta	Mucuna pruriens	Kapikacchu
Bakuchi	Psoralea corylifolia	
Bala	Sida cordifolia	
Betel nuts	Areca catechu	Kramuka
Bhallataka	Semecarpus anacardium	
Bhringaraj	Eclipta alba	
Bhumyamalaki	Phyllanthus niruri	
Bibhitaki	Terminalia belerica	
Black musali	Curculigo orchiodes	Kala musali
Chiretta	Swertia chiratata	Kirata tikta
Chitrak	Plumbago zeylonica	
Cuscuta	Cuscuta reflexa	Amaravalli
Cyperus	Cyperus rotundus	Musta
Dhataki	Woodfordia floribunda	
Gokshura	Tribulis terrestris	
Guduchi	Tinospora cordifolia	Amrit
Guggul	Commiphora mukul	
Gurmar	Gymena sylvestre	Meshashringi
Haritaki	Terminalia chebula	
Holy Basil	Ocimum sanctum	Tulsi
Indian sarasaparilla	Hemedesmis indica	Anantamul
Isatis	Isatis spp.	Nila
Jatamansi	Nardostachys jatamansi	
Kapikacchu	Mucuna pruriens	
Katuka	Picrorrhiza kurroa	
Kutaj	Holarrhena antidysenterica	
Lodhra	Symplocus racemosus	

Common	Latin	Sanskrit
Long Pepper	Piper longum	Pippali
Manjishta (Indian madder)	Rubia cordifolium	
Neem	Azadiracta indica	Nimbu
Nirgundi	Vitex negundo	
Nishot	Ipomoea turpethum	
Pashana bheda	Bergenia spp.	
Prasarini	Paedaria foetida	
Punarnava	Boerrhavia diffusa	
Sarpagandha	Rawolfia serpentina	
Saussurea	Saussurea lappa	Kushta
Shankhapushpi	Crotalaria verrucosa	
Shatavari	Asparagus racemosus	
Shilajit	Asphaltum	
Vamsha rochana	Bambusa arundinacea	
Vidanga	Embelia ribes	
White musali	Asparagus adscendens	Shveta musali
Zedoaria	Curcuma zedoaria	Kachura

Special Chinese Herbs

First is the common name, then the Latin and Chinese. When the common name is the Chinese, it is not repeated.

Common	Latin	Chinese
Astragalus	Astragalus mongolicus	Huang qi
Biota seeds	Biota orientalis	Bai zi ren
Bupleurum	Bupleurum falcatum	Chai hu
Cimicifuga	Cimicifuga racemosa	Sheng ma
Citrus peel	Citrus reticulata	Chen pi
Corydalis	Corydalis	Yuan hu suo
Dang shen	Codonopsis pilosula	
Desmodian	Desmodian styracifolium	Jin qian cao

Common	Latin	Chinese
Dioscorea	Dioscorea opposita	Shan yao
Du huo	Angelica dahurica	
Eucommia	Eucommia ulmoidis	Du Zhong
Forsythia	Forsythia suspensa	Lian qiao
Fritillary	Fritillaria cirrhosa	Chuan bei mu
Gentiana macrophylla		Qin jiao
He shou wu (fo ti)	Polygonum multiflorum	
Hoelen	Poria cocos	Fu ling
Honeysuckle	Lonicera	Jin yin hua
Ligusticum	Ligusticum wallichi	Chuan xion
Ligustrum	Ligustrum lucidum	Nu zhen zi
Loranthus	Loranthus parasiticus	Sang ji sheng
Lycium	Lycium chinense	Go ji zi
Lygodium	Lygodium japonicum	Hai jin sha
Magnolia bark	Magnolia officinalis	Hou pu
Magnolia flower	Magnolia liliflora	Xin yi hua
Ma Huang	Ephedra sinica	
Oldenlandia	Oldenlandia diffusa	Bai hua she she ao
Ophiopogon	Ophiopogon japonicus	Mai men dong
Phellodendron	Phellodendron amurense	Huang bai
Perilla leaf	Perilla frutescens	Zi su ye
Pinellia	Pinellia ternata	Ban xia
Pseudoginseng	Panax pseudoginseng	San qi
Pueraria (kudzu)	Pueraria lobata	Ge gen
Qiang huo	Notopterygium incisum	
Red Peony	Paeonia obovata	Chi shao yao
Rehmannia	Rehmannia glutinosa	Di huang
Salvia	Salvia miltorrhiza	Dan shen
Schizandra	Schizandra chinensis	Wu wei zi
Scute	Scutellaria baicalensis	Huang qin
Spargania	Sparganium simplex	San leng

Common	Latin	Chinese
Tang kuei	Angelica sinensis	Dang gui
Trichosanthes root	Trichosanthes kirlowii	Tian hua fe
White atractylodes	Atractylodes alba	Bai zhu
White peony	Paeonia lactiflora	Bai shao yao
Zizyphus	Zizyphus spinosa	Suan cao ren

CHINESE HERBAL FORMULAS

Common	Chinese
Anemarrhena, Phellodendron and Rehmannia	Zhi bai di huang wan
Bupleurum and Tang kuei	Xiao yao san
Cannabis seed comb.	Ma zi ren wan
Capillaris comb.	Yin chen hao tang
Cinnamon branch decoction	Gui zhi tang
Citrus and Craetagus	Bao he wan
Coptis and Rhubarb	San huang xie xin tang
Coptis & Scute	Huang lien jie du tang
Dianthus comb.	Ba zheng san
Four Gentlemen	Si jun zi tang
Four Materials	Si wu tang
Gentian comb.	Long dan xie gan tang
Gypsum comb.	Bai hu tang
Honeysuckle and Forsythia	Yin qiao san
Magnolia and Ginger	Ping wei san
Ma huang decoction	Ma huang tang
Minor Bupleurum	Xiao chai hu tang
Minor Pinellia and Hoelen	Xiao ban xia jia fu ling tang
Minor Rhubarb	Xiao cheng qi tang
Major Blue Dragon	Da qing long tang
Major Bupleurum	Da chai hu tang
Major Rhubarb	Da cheng qi tang

Common	Chinese
Ophiopogon comb.	Mai men dong tang
Persica and Rhubarb	Tao he cheng qi tang
Polyporus combination	Zhu ling tang
Pueraria, Coptis and Scute	Ge gen huang qin huang lian tang
Rehmannia 6	Liu wei di huang wan
Rehmannia 8	Jing gui shen qi wan
Shou wu pian	
Tang kuei and Gelatin	Jiao ai tang
Tang kuei and Peony	Dang gui shao yao san
Ten Major Tonification formula	Shi quan da bu tang
Woman's Precious Pill	Ba zhen tang

4
BIBLIOGRAPHY

Books

Agarwal, R.S. *Secrets of Indian Medicine.* Pondicherry, India: Sri Aurobindo Ashram, 1983.

Bensky, Dan, Andrew Gamble. *Chinese Herbal Medicine Materia Medica.* Seattle WA: Eastland Press, 1986.

Christopher, John R. *School of Natural Healing.* Provo, Utah: BiWorld, 1976.

Dash, Bhagwan. *Alchemy and Metallic Medicines in Ayurveda.* New Delhi, India: Concept Publishing Company, 1986.

Dash, Bhagwan, Manfred Junius. *A Hand Book of Ayurveda.* New Delhi, India: Concept Publishing Company, 1983.

Dash, Bhagwan, Lalitesh Kashyap. *Materia Medica of Ayurveda.* New Delhi, India: Concept Publishing Company, 1980.

Ficino, Marsilio. *The Book of Life.* Irving, Texas: Spring Publications, Inc., 1980.

Frawley, David, Vasant Lad. *The Yoga of Herbs.* Santa Fe, New Mexico, Lotus Press, 1986.

Gupta, Sen. *The Ayurvedic System of Medicine,* Volumes I and II. New Delhi, India: Logos Press, 1984 (reprint).

Hsu, Hong-Yen, Chau-Shin Hsu. *Commonly Used Chinese Herb Formulas with Illustration.* Los Angeles, CA: Oriental Healing Arts Institute, 1980.

Lad, Vasant. *Ayurveda: The Science of Self-Healing.* Santa Fe, New Mexico, Lotus Press, 1984.

Lust, John. *The Herb Book.* New York, NY: Bantam Books, 1974.

Nadkarni, K.M. *Indian Materia Medica.* Bombay, India: Popular Prakashan, 1976.

Pathak, Dr. R.R. *Therapeutic Guide to Ayurvedic Medicine.* Patna, India: Baidyanath Ayurved Bhawan, 1980.

Rapgay, Lobsang. *Tibetan Medicine.* Dharmsala, India: Lobsang Rapgay, 1985.

Srikantamurthy, K.R. *Clinical Methods in Ayurveda.* Varanasi, India: Chaukhambha Orientalia, 1983.

Strehlow, Dr. Wighard and Gottfried Hertzka. *Hildegard of Bingen's Medicine.* Santa Fe, NM: Bear and Co., 1988.

Tierra, Michael. *Planetary Herbology.* Santa Fe, Lotus Press: 1988.

The Way of Herbs. New York, NY: Washington Square Press, 1983.

Verma, Ganpati Singh. *Miracles of Indian Herbs.* New Delhi, India: Rasayan Pharmacy, 1982.

Yeung, Him-che, *Hankbook of Chinese Herbs and Formulas* (two volumes). Los Angeles, CA: Institute of Chinese Medicine, 1985.

SANSKRIT TEXTS USED

Charaka. *Charaka Samhita*

Krishna. *Bhagavad Gita*

Krishna Ishwara. *Sanhkhya Karika*

Patanjali. *Yoga Sutras*

Rig Veda Samhita

Sushruta. *Sushruta Samhita*

Upanishads

Vagbhatta. *Ashtanga Hridaya*

MARATHI

Gogate, Vishnu Mahadeva. *Dravyagunavijnana.* Pune, India: Continental Publishers, 1982.

AYURVEDIC CORRESPONDENCE COURSE

We offer a comprehensive correspondence course in Ayurveda based upon and the complementary to *Ayurvedic Healing.* It covers all the main aspects of Ayurvedic Medicine and explains Ayurveda as part of the science of Yoga.

Part I is Introduction, Historical and Spiritual Background, and a comprehensive examination of Ayurvedic Anatomy and Physiology (Doshas, Dhatus, Malas, Srotas, Kalas, and Organs).

Part II is Constitutional Analysis, Mental Nature, the Disease Process, Examination of Disease, Diagnosis (pulse, tongue, and abdomen) and Patient Examination, Yoga and Ayurvedic Psychology.

Part III is Dietary Therapy, Herbal Therapy, Ayurvedic Therapeutic Approaches (including Pancha Karma), Subtle Healing Modalities of Ayurveda and Practical Application of Yoga Psychology.

The course has been approved by well-known Ayurvedic doctors in India. Additional study tapes are available, as well as options for advanced study.

VEDIC ASTROLOGY CORRESPONDENCE COURSE

Vedic astrology, also called Hindu astrology or Jyotish, is the traditional astrology of India, often used along with Ayurveda and Yoga.

This course teaches the fundamentals of Vedic astrology through an explanation of the planets, signs, houses, aspects, harmonic charts, planetary periods and principles of chart interpretation. In addition, it sets forth the astrology of healing based upon the combined use of Ayurveda and Vedic astrology, explaining remedial measures of diet, herbs, gems, colors, mantras, yantras and deities. Spiritual and karmic aspects of astrology are stressed, astrology as a means of self-knowledge and attunement to the cosmic mind.

The course, perhaps the only one of its kind in this regard, presents the system in clear, practical and modern terms and is adapted toward western culture. Options for advanced study are also available.

For Courses send a S.A.S.E. to:

AMERICAN INSTITUTE OF VEDIC STUDIES
P.O. BOX 8357, SANTA FE, NM 87504-8357

BIODATA

Dr. David Frawley is a modern teacher of the comprehensive system of Vedic and Yogic Science, much like the Vedic seers of old. He is the coauthor (along with Dr. Vasant Lad) of *The Yoga of Herbs* and Editor of Michael Tierra's *Planetary Herbology*. He has a doctor's degree (O.M.D.) in Chinese medicine and is on the International Advisory Committee of the Interdisciplinary School of Ayurvedic Medicine at University of Poona, India. He is also recognized in India as a Vedacharya or teacher of the ancient wisdom. In addition he practices Vedic (Hindu) Astrology and is a Sanskrit scholar. He has written many books and articles on different aspects of the spiritual and healing traditions of India, particularly the ancient Vedic texts on which he is a recognized modern authority. He is the director of the American Institute of Vedic Studies.

His Indian books include *Hymns From the Golden Age* (1986), *Beyond the Mind* (1984) and *The Creative Vision of the Early Upanishads* (1982). His American titles include *The Yoga of Herbs* (1986), *From the River of Heaven* (1990), *The Astrology of the Seers* (1990) and *Gods, Sages and Kings* (1991). He also has a doctor's degree (O.M.D.) in Chinese medicine and is a published *I Ching* scholar both in the United States and China.

Dr. Frawley is the director of the American Institute of Vedic Studies, which aims to provide educational material for a modern restoration of

Vedic knowledge, including Ayurveda, Vedic astrology, Vedic studies and Yoga. His forthcoming books through Passage Press are: *Wisdom of the Ancient Seers, Secrets of the Rig Veda; The Upanishadic Vision;* and *Beyond the Mind.*

The following are reviews of his various books on Vedic knowledge published in India:

"Frawley is superb when he discusses in what sense the world is a creation of the word. His note on the Mantra is as chiselled as the Vedic Mantra itself." — M. P. Pandit, *The Mountain Path*

"With such spiritual translation and interpretation of the Vedic mantras, he deserves a place amongst the great spiritual commentators of the Veda like Swami Atmananda, Swami Dayananda, Sri Aurobindo and V.S. Agrawal." — Prof. K. D. Shastri; *Haryana Sahitya Academy Journal of Indological Studies*

"The work is an exceptionally admirable attempt to understand the Vedic vision. After Sri Aurobindo, it is perhaps the most original hermeneutical exercise in Vedic studies." — Dr. S. P. Duby; *Prabuddha Bharata*

"The author discloses an acute sensitivity for the sound and spiritual meaning of the Vedic mantras." — P. Nagaraja Rao; *The Madras Hindu*

VEDIC ASTROLOGY COMPUTER PROGRAM

PC-JYOTISH, a Vedic (Hindu) astrology computer program, is now available. Its features include: South & North India chart styles; Rasi (sign) and Bhava (house) charts; Navamsa and other Varga (divisional) charts; Summary Tables — relationships & locations; Sign/house qualities & relationships; Nakshatras — lords/sublords & pada lords; Vimshopak; Planetary Significators; Ashtaka Varga — complete; Vimshottari dashas, bhuktis & sub-bhuktis; (365¼ or 360 days year); Pop-up Transit window with Ashtaka Varga & Nakshatra divisions; Aspects Table; and a range of Ayanamshas. It is an easy to use, user driven program which includes: mouse support; changing input data immediately alters on-screen tables & charts; Pull-down menus; print to file or any ASCII printer; complete on-screen functions; as many charts & tables on-screen as user desires; user arranges windows on-screen; chart storage limited only by disk space; manual with Glossary by David Frawley; program range: 1500 BC to 2200 AD; color/mono, hi-res mode — no graphics card required, and more. DEMO program available.

For more information call or write:
Passage Press
P.O. Box 21713
Salt Lake City, UT 84121-0713
(801) 942-1440

General Index

A

abdominal distention, 270, 292
abdominal pain, 273
abortion, habitual, 210
abscesses, 279
acne, 292
addictions, 261, 291; treatment, 261
Agni, 4, 117, 145; low, 277
AIDS, 39, 197; treatment, 197
alchemical tradition, 13
alcoholism, 262
allergic rhinitis, 169; treatment, 170
allergies, 275
allergies, food, 145, 148 –149;
    general treatment, 149
alochaka pitta, 8; site, 9
aloe gel, 99–100
alopacia, 283
ama, 88–89, 100, 214; conditions,
    96; high, 277; treatment of, 120
amenorrhea, 203, 287, 291; treat-
    ment, 203
amphetamines, 57
anemia, 158, 179, 279–280, 282,
    287, 291; differentiation, 180;
    general treatment, 180; specific
    treatment, 181
angina, 171, 293
anorexia, 159, 271; treatment, 159–
    160
anti-amadiet; animal products, 101;
    beans, 101; beverages, 102; dairy,
    101; dietetics, 102; fruit, 100;
    grains, 100; nuts and seeds, 101;
    oils, 101; spices, 101; sweeterners,
    101; vegetables, 100
anti-Kapha, 276
anti-Kapha formula, 275
anti-Pitta, 276
anxiety, 38, 270, 291, 294

apana vata, 7; derangements of, 8;
    site, 8
Apollonius of Tyanna, 12
appendicitis, 126
appetite; lack of, 272, 274, 275–277,
    289, 292; loss of, 273, 281
arteriosclerosis, 171, 176, 293
arthritis, 40, 91, 154, 223, 270, 276,
    278–280, 284, 290–291, 294; dif-
    ferentiation, 225; general treat-
    ment, 223; medicated sesame oils,
    224; specific treatment, 225
asthma, 40, 161, 167, 271, 274–275,
    278, 280, 283–284, 290; differen-
    tiation, 168; differentiation and
    treatment, 169; general treatment,
    168
astrology, 49, 254, 305; and the aura,
    112; and yurveda, 307; gem
    therapy, 307; and mental nature,
    28; Vedic, xi
Atman, site, 171
aura, the, 112; strengthening, 112;
    weakened by, 112–113
avalambaka kapha, 9; site, 9
Ayurveda, xv
Ayurveda and Modern Medicine, xii
Ayurveda Revisited, xii
Ayurvedic mineral preparations, 269

B

back pain, lower, 293, 295
baldness, premature, 238
bhrajaka pitta, 8; site, 8
bile, 5
biliousness, 271
bleeding, 177; differentiation, 178;
    general treatment, 178; Kapha
    (water) type, 179; Pitta (fire) type,
    179; Vata (air) type, 179
bleeding gums, 230
bleeding therapy, 94
blue sapphire, 311
bodhaka kapha, 9; site, 9
boils, 286, 292

HERBAL INDEX

A